Refinements in Facial and Body Contouring

Refinements in Facial and Body Contouring

Luiz S. Toledo, M.D.
São Paulo, Brazil

Illustrations by
Arthur Baldissara

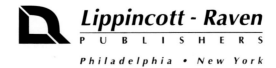

Lippincott - Raven
PUBLISHERS

Philadelphia • New York

Acquisitions Editor: Danette Knopp
Developmental Editor: Keith Donnellan
Manufacturing Manager: Dennis Teston
Production Manager: Cassie Moore
Production Editor: Rosemary Palumbo
Cover Designer: Kevin Kall
Indexer: Susan Thomas
Compositor: Maryland Composition Company, Inc.

Printed and bound in Singapore

9 8 7 6 5 4 3 2 1

Library of Congress Cataloging-in-Publication Data

Toledo, Luiz Sergio.
    Refinements in facial and body contouring / Luiz S. Toledo ;
illustrations by Arthur Baldissara.
       p.   cm.
    Includes bibliographical references and index.
    ISBN 0-397-51600-2
    1. Lipposculpture. 2. Face—Surgery. I. Title.
    [DNLM: 1. Surgery, Plastic—methods. 2. Lipectomy—methods.
3. Lipectomy—instrumentation. 4. Face—surgery.   WO 600 T649r
1999]
RD119.5.L55T64 1999
617.9′5—dc21
DNLM/DLC
for Library of Congress   98-17731
                                        CIP

To my parents, Pedro and Yvonne,
my three children, Juliano, Isabella, and Valentina,
and my wife Kate, who is always there for me.
Gibraltar may tumble. . .

Contents

Section III: Facial Contouring

Foreword

It is with great pleasure that I write this foreword to Luiz Toledo's work. Luiz Toledo has been a colleague and a friend for many years. He is a prolific writer who has published over 30 papers and has been editor of numerous annals and abstract books. Dr. Toledo is a prominent and popular figure in Brazilian and international plastic surgery, and is dedicated to all aspects of aesthetic plastic surgery.

Several papers on syringe liposuction, video endoscopic face-lifting, and other new procedures have proven Dr. Toledo's dedication to the advancement of aesthetic surgery into new territories. Over the years, his contribution of new techniques and surgical details has been of great help to many. *Refinements in Facial and Body Contouring* evaluates recent advances in the field of plastic surgery and will certainly be a useful addition to any aesthetic surgeon's library.

Dr. Toledo has coauthored two previous books. *Circumareolar Techniques for Breast Surgery*, which he wrote with Drs. Wilkinson and Aiache, shows great precision in historical details. *Superficial Liposculpture*, coauthored with Drs. Lewis and Gasparotti, explained the philosophy, technique, and advantages of liposuction concisely, and has proven to be a model manual in the field. His three Annals of Recent Advances in Plastic Surgery (RAPS) International Symposiums gave many the opportunity to benefit from recent advances in the early nineties.

Dr. Toledo's new publication meets the high standards to which we have become accustomed. His position at the forefront of facial and body contouring has been proven through surgery and lecturing in many countries.

Dr. Toledo has been a member of the International Society of Aesthetic Plastic Surgery (ISAPS) for many years, and is currently the ISAPS Instructional Course Director. Since he gave his first ISAPS postgraduate course in Sydney in 1994, many have benefitted from his vast experience. With Dr. Toledo's fine organizational talents, backed by the ISAPS Educational Foundation Chairman, Yann Levet, we will no doubt see a new era in the ISAPS educational field, in addition to the achievements realized so far.

I wish Dr. Toledo every success with this publication, which he justly deserves. But no one is solely responsible for success, not even a plastic surgeon! The cliche, ''Behind every great man is a great woman,'' is very true in his case, and his wife Kate should share in this achievement too.

Ulrich T. Hinderer, M.D., Ph.D.

Preface

When I was putting my ideas together for this book, I was invited to coauthor the book *Superficial Liposculpture*, published in 1993. At that time, I had been using the superficial liposculpture technique for a few years. The possibility of treating the superficial layer of fat was a new tactic, not a new technique, and became an overnight sensation within the specialty. It seemed that there was no space for other ideas. Suddenly everything was ''superficial.''

My coauthors and I sensed a need for correct information in the form of a manual of technique. Although the approach itself proved prudent, in the course of helping many surgeons to understand the possibilities and the limits of this particular technique, some misunderstandings came about. The worst misunderstanding was the notion that every patient should be treated with the superficial technique. I will try to correct this misconception in this book.

The book is presented in three sections. The first deals with basic principles: the concept of beauty, the importance of good photography, instruments, anesthesia, positioning of the patient, incision points, the principles of fat aspiration and injection, and postoperative care. The second section demonstrates the treatments of particular areas of the body. In the third section I present my approach to facial contouring, which is based on simple procedures with short recovery periods.

My approach to this book was influenced by one of the landmarks in plastic surgery literature, Tord Skoog's *Atlas of Plastic Surgery* (1973), a book that left its mark on a whole generation of young plastic surgeons. Skoog knew that plastic surgery as a whole would be too vast a subject to be approached satisfactorily in one book. Like Skoog, I limit myself to selected subjects, particularly techniques that I have developed or perfected. Each technique is illustrated by typical cases. Drawings complement the points that would not be clear with photographs alone.

The concept of beauty varies from country to country. Brazilians have different preferences in the shape of their bodies than do Europeans and North Americans.

I discuss a variety of options and indications of procedures, and explain why I choose one rather than another. This is a very personal approach to problems that are often treated in a more traditional manner.

The trend in modern plastic surgery over the past decade has been towards minimally-invasive surgical techniques, minimal scarring, and short recovery periods. The use of the syringe rather than the aspirator and the improvement of local anesthesia formulas has allowed treatment of patients who might not have undergone surgery because of their fear of long scars, general anesthesia, or prolonged recovery periods. Due to the precision of the syringe method, the indications for surgery have changed, and within a short period, my results improved. In this book, I explain the techniques that have changed my practice for the better; I hope you find it valuable.

Luiz S. Toledo

Acknowledgments

I would like to thank the following people:

Dr. William Callia, my professor, who ignited the spark that made me want to be a plastic surgeon and who taught me surgical simplicity.

Dr. Tord Skoog, whose book opened my mind and whom I wish I had met.

Drs. Yves Gerard Illouz and Pierre Fournier, the two French pioneers, who I am glad I have met.

Dr. Carson Lewis, a friend.

Dr. Marco Gasparotti, for inspiration.

Dr. Ivo Pitanguy, who got there first, and stayed there.

Drs. Tolbert Wilkinson, Garry Brody, Jaime and Jordi Planas, Baker, Gordon, Stuzin, and Baker, to my colleagues at the International Society of Aesthetic Plastic Surgery (ISAPS), the American Society for Aesthetic Plastic Surgery (ASAPS), the American Society of Plastic and Reconstructive Surgery (ASPRS), and the Lipoplasty Society of North America (LSNA), who give me a chance to teach what I learn, and to learn what I teach.

My assistant Gilberto de Almeida and my anesthesiologist Manoel Mosquera.

The women in the clinic.

Baldissara, my illustrator.

Sebastião Gonçalves de Oliveira, from Ph Color photo laboratory, São Paulo, who has processed my photos for 20 years. He is responsible for the color reproductions for this book and for all of my photographic lab work. A professional.

The blue smoke of a good robusto.

Introduction

BREAKING THE RULES

The first revolution in body contouring, and to this day the most important one, was the advent of liposuction in the late 1970s. For the first time, we could alter body shape through minimal incisions. The second revolution was the development of syringe liposculpture, in the mid-1980s. The aspirator could be substituted by disposable syringes, and it was possible to measure precisely how much fat was aspirated, but its best advantage was the possibility of reinjecting fat. In 1987, tumescent anesthesia made all body contour procedures safer outpatient procedures. In 1989, superficial syringe liposculpture allowed us to remove more fat and to improve the body contour of patients with a more flaccid skin tone.

LIPOSCULPTURE

Liposculpture is the technique that uses disposable syringes to aspirate localized fat deposits and, if necessary, reinject it where needed (1,2). When fat is not reinjected, the procedure is called reduction liposculpture.

I prefer to use the term *reduction liposculpture* rather than *liposuction* to differentiate this gentler syringe technique from the traditional liposuction method performed with the aspirator. This is not just a matter of semantics; the techniques are different, although the principle (fat suction) and the objective (improving body contour) are the same.

The advantages of the syringe method are many: It is light, cheap, disposable, precise, safe, and silent. Those who work with an aspirator every day can really appreciate how cumbersome it is in comparison to working with a light syringe. While the aspirator costs a few thousand dollars, the syringe costs only a few cents. If the aspirator breaks down during a procedure and there is not a second unit available, or if there is a power cut, you will not be able to finish the surgery.

So it is good to have a syringe system, if only for backup. If the syringe breaks, just reach for another one.

The precision of the syringe is especially apparent when treating small adiposities or pair adiposities, where the same amount should be aspirated from each side. With a syringe, the exact amount of anesthesia injected is known (this is difficult to know precisely when one uses an infiltrator), and the amount of fat aspirated and reinjected is also measurable.

When using the aspirator, a maximum of 2 liters of fat can be safely removed, due to bleeding. We can remove more with the syringe, because there is much less blood loss. In cases in which aspirated fat is reinjected, the syringe method is obviously superior; fat has no contact with air (hence no oxidation), and no vaporization. There are no risks of dangerous fat or blood aerosols. Cells can be washed in a closed technique, and sterilized, or can be immediately reinjected. Fat removed with a syringe is pure, and is usually reinjected immediately. If there is any trace of blood, we use Ringer's lactate to gently wash the fat cells, and decant the washing solutions and blood before injection.

It is possible to treat the whole body with the syringe. Some surgeons still think of the syringe as only useful for "touch ups" or small localized fat deposits (LFDs), but I use it to treat much larger areas. The surgery takes the same time as it would with a machine, but the work is more precise and the results are better. Once the cannula is inserted into the area to be treated, the plunger is locked to form a vacuum in the syringe. If the cannula gauge is the same in both methods, suction takes the same amount of time, because the vacuum is the same. A smaller-gauge cannula or a smaller orifice at the tip of the syringe slows the suction time. Suction performed with a 10-mm gauge cannula is a good deal faster than with a 4-mm gauge, but finer cannulas give much more precision, and decrease the chance of producing irregularities. Body liposculpture involves refinement and art to produce a good result. Time is seondary, because the objective is not just to remove the bulk of the fat.

Beginners often waste time when changing syringes. I avoid this by having my assistant hand me an empty syringe with the same cannula as soon as the first syringe is full. I work with an assistant and a scrub nurse for liposculpture. An assistant is mandatory in Brazil. For this type of surgery, there must be at least 2 surgeons in the field. A nurse is optional, but I find her presence essential, not only to handle instruments, but to treat the aspirated fat for possible reinjection. The nurse decants the syringes and records the amount of total aspirated fluid and pure fat removed with each syringe, for each area treated. We complete the surgery with a map that outlines the exact amounts of aspirated and infiltrated fat.

One of the main differences between using the syringe and using the aspirator is that in order to maintain the vacuum, the incision point should be at least 3 or 4 cm away from the area to be treated. When the cannula is removed from the body and the vacuum is lost we cover the cannula tip with a swab to eliminate air from the syringe before restarting suctioning. This will avoid splashing fat when pulling the plunger back to position.

When suctioning smaller areas, however, I will lock the plunger with my thumb instead of the lock. If pressure is lost, I just pull back the plunger a little more and continue suctioning until the syringe is full.

FUTURE POSSIBILITIES

In the early 1990s, ultrasonic liposuction appeared, with the promise of removing even more fat and retracting skin even better. In 1997, external ultrasound (lipotripsy) promised the removal of small fat deposits through a noninvasive method. Endermology, the French noninvasive suction massage method, promises correction of cellulite and superficial irregularities.

REFERENCES

1. Fournier P. *Liposculpture—ma technique.* Paris: Arnette, 1989.
2. Toledo LS. Total liposculpture. In: Gasparotti M, Lewis CM, Toledo LS. *Superficial liposculpture.* New York: Springer-Verlag, 1993:44.

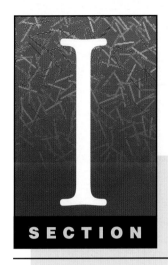

SECTION I

Introduction to Basic Principles

1

Beauty

WHAT IS BEAUTY?

The devotion to beauty and to the creation of beautiful things, is the test of all great civilizations.

Oscar Wilde

Philosophers have always raised questions about values: What is beauty? How can the beautiful be distinguished from the ugly? It is easy to identify physical beauty when we see it. Sculptures such as the Venus de Milo and Michelangelo's David, and modern movie stars, athletes, and especially top models show the importance we give to the appreciation of physical attributes.

Beautiful faces and bodies can go in and out of fashion. Yet in every era certain people are considered truly "beautiful." What, then, are the standards of beauty, and how are people chosen as representatives of an ideal (1)?

Scientific investigation is of little help in determining answers to questions that deal with matters of opinion rather than fact. But beauty can be found in balanced proportions, which can be precisely measured. The perfect balance is something that has always been sought by artists and philosophers from the Ancient Greeks through the Renaissance to the modern age. Plato discussed proportion as the source of beauty; Polyclitus, one of the foremost Greek sculptors of the 5th century B.C., was noted for his statues of athletes, which embodied his theories of human proportion (2). In the 15th century, Renaissance artists made efforts to discover the correct laws of proportion for architecture and for the representation of the human body. Leonardo da Vinci's perfectly proportioned drawing of a Vitruvian man (1485–1490) exemplified the ideals of the Renaissance.

BEAUTY TODAY

Without emotion there is no beauty.

Diana Vreeland

Today, plastic surgeons do not have to refer to old sculptures or paintings. It is not difficult to find beauty daily in newspapers and magazines. Perfection can be found represented in everyday life by the top models. Their existence dictates not ''a'' pattern of beauty, but ''the'' pattern of beauty (3). The beauty of the top model does not come from an artist's imagination. It comes from a correct genetic combination, plus the long-term ingestion of the right amount of proteins, a certain lifestyle, and a bit of luck with the law of probability.

BEAUTY AND MONEY

Economists have shown that men and women considered ''ugly'' generally make 10% to 20% less money than those considered ''beautiful'' (4). Obese people also make less money than slim people, even if they do not have any health problems related to obesity. Hamermesh and Biddle (4) question this preference for beauty, which may be akin to the reason racists avoid people of different color; or perhaps attractive people do better in job interviews because they have more self-confidence and a sense of leadership.

BEAUTY AND WEIGHT

I've never met a person I couldn't call a beauty. Every person has beauty in some point in their lifetime. Usually in different degrees. Sometimes they have the looks when they're a baby and they don't have it when they're grown up, but then they could get it back again when they're older. Or they might be fat but have a beautiful face. Or have bow-legs but a beautiful body. Or be the number one female beauty and have no tits. Or be the number one male beauty and have a small you-know-what.

Andy Warhol

The fear of being overweight and thoughts about dieting start in female adolescence and reflect the greater aesthetic value that contemporary society places on thinness for women (5). An excessive preoccupation with weight and dieting in either male or female adolescents suggests psychological problems.

The social pressure to diet occurs across all weight categories. The strong emphasis placed on appearance and on being slim has provoked intense body preoccupation in many people, patients will try almost any strategy to loose weight. It has been shown that a ''strong correlation between attractiveness and perceived fitness, a good body image, and feelings of self-worth'' (6) exists. Most studies find that children acquire values of beauty before adolescence, and that thinness is desirable to girls well before puberty (7). Although very young children may seem to have an established body type, only after the onset of puberty does the waist-hip ratio seem to be an indicator of body fat distribution (8).

The effects of sex, age, and body shape were estimated by the Self-Rating Body Image (SRBI) test in 687 adolescents in Japan (9). The study suggests that female adolescents want to be thinner and that the body image shows critical changes during the early and middle periods of adolescence, ultimately leading to unsatisfactory body images. The same test was also used in patients with eating disorders such as anorexia nervosa and bulimia, and revealed that both the anorexic and bulimic patients showed a distortion of body image (9), but the anorexic patients had distorted images of more parts of the body than the bulimic patients.

SOMATOTYPES

The types of bodies we operate on can be classified into three categories:

- ''A'' shaped body or gynoid, who accumulate more fat below the waist.

- "V" shaped body or android, who accumulate more fat above the waist.
- "O" shaped body, a combination of A and V shaped bodies.

We can also follow the method established by sports medicine for analyzing physical types. Anthropometric determinations include height, body mass, lean body mass, percentage of fat, and somatotype. The Health-Carter somatotype classification defines the morphology of each individual. The following measurements are used: to find the Health-Carter anthropometric somatotype weight, height, skin folds (triceps, subscapular, suprailiac, and mid-calf), circumference of arm and leg, and diameters of humeral bi-epicondyle and femoral bi-epicondyle. Although it is good to know that we can precisely classify every type of body we treat, I find this method too complicated for everyday use. A body contouring procedure will not alter patients somatotypes; it will only remove excess localized fat. Complementing the surgical treatment with diet and exercise can provide individuals with the best body shape possible within their genetic constitution.

BEAUTY AND GEOGRAPHY

I hate that aesthetic game of the eye and the mind, played by these connoisseurs, these mandarins who "appreciate" beauty. What is beauty, anyway? There's no such thing. I never "appreciate," any more than I "like." I love or I hate.

Pablo Picasso

The concept of beauty varies according to geography, culture, age, and race. African and European students rated 24 drawings of male and female figures ranging from obese to anorexic. Ugandans, as opposed to the British, rated the more obese female and the more anorexic male figures as more attractive (10). These results show cross-cultural differences in body image, attractiveness, and eating disorders. A comparative study of facial proportions showed that the appreciation of vertical proportions in the African-American face and the white face were similar (11). Appreciation of horizontal dimensions, however, varied significantly between racial groups. The individual with the "right" form, proportion, and features is immediately presumed intelligent, strong, charming, good, or any of a number of other socially esteemed characteristics. In a highly competitive society, it is no wonder we strive for the edge that beauty bestows (12).

BEAUTY AND PLASTIC SURGERY

Even beauties can be unattractive. If you catch a beauty in the wrong light at the right time, forget it. I believe in low lights and trick mirrors. I believe in plastic surgery.

Andy Warhol

Does plastic surgery improve self-image? Studies have shown that patients rated their appearance as noticeably improved after surgery, their self-esteem rose significantly, and they reported more social adeptness and acceptance at home and at school (13). Even if other people observe only subtle changes, quality of life apparently improves for patients due to increased self-esteem and confidence, which free them to overcome social barriers (14).

Surgeons believe that most plastic surgery patients seek normality and through that, acceptance by their peers, but some patients seek beauty or the improvement of an existing beautiful feature. The presence of prominent zygomas, a subtle cheek hollow, flat nasolabial folds, and a well-defined jawline are considered beautiful. An average face shape can be attractive, but may not be beautiful. Aesthetic judgments of face shape are similar across different cultural backgrounds. It has been shown that highly attractive faces are not average (15). Attractive faces can be made more attractive by exaggerating some features.

The benefits of cosmetic surgery were found by Harris (16) to be psychotherapeutic. "The distress symptoms caused by self-consciousness of abnormal appearance are cured by an operation that normalizes the abnormality as the patient sees it" (12). But surgery should not be the only treatment to achieve the desired figure. We have to keep in mind that the best results are achieved when we combine the best surgical technique with diet and exercise. Juneau et al. (16) found that "Moderate-intensity, home-based, self-monitored exercise training significantly increases functional capacity in healthy, middle-aged men and women."

REFERENCES

1. Romm S. The changing face of beauty. *Aesthetic Plast Surg* 1989;13:91–98.
2. Dinsmoor A. In: Richter GMA, *Sculpture and sculptors of the Greeks,* 4th ed., Robertson CM. *A History of Greek Art,* 1975.
3. Ascher N. Top models and zero degree of beauty. *Folha de São Paulo* April 2, 1995:3–5.
4. Hamermesh D, Biddle J. Estudo indica que homem feio ganha menos que bonito. *O Estado de São Paulo,* January 28, 1994.
5. Casper RC, Offer D. Weight and dieting concerns in adolescents, fashion or symptom? *Pediatrics* 1990;86:384–390.
6. Rodin J. Cultural and psychosocial determinants of weight concerns. *Ann Intern Med* 1993;119:643–645.
7. Feldman W, Feldman E, Goodman JT. Culture versus biology: children's attitudes toward thinness and fatness. *Pediatrics* 1988;81:190–194.
8. Kalker U, Hovels O, Kolbe-Saborowski H. [Obese children and adolescents. Waist-hip ratio and cardiovascular risk]. *Monatsschr Kinderheilkd* [German] 1993;141:36–41.
9. Tadai T, Kanai H, Nakamura M, Nakejima T. Body image changes in adolescents. I. The development of self-rating body image (SRBI) test and effects of sex, age and body shape. *Jpn J Psychiatry Neurol* 1994;48:533–539.
10. Furnham A, Baguma P. Cross-cultural differences in the evaluation of male and female body shapes. *Int J Eat Disord* 1994;15:81–89.
11. Jeffries JM III, Di Bernardo B, Rauscher GE. Computer analysis of the African-American face. *Ann Plast Surg* 1995;34:318–321.
12. Arndt EM, Travis F, Lefebvre A, Niec A, Munro IR. Beauty and the eye of the beholder: social consequences and personal adjustments for facial patients. *Br J Plast Surg* (Scotland), 1986;39:81–84.
13. Truppman ES, Schwartz BM. Aesthetic breast surgery. *J Fla Med Assoc* 1989;76:609–612.
14. Harris D. The benefits and hazards of cosmetic surgery. *Br J Hosp Med* 1989;41:540–545.
15. Perrett DI, May KA, Yoshikawa S. Facial shape and judgments of female attractiveness. *Nature (England)* 1994;368:239–242.
16. Juneau M, Rogers F, De Santos V, et al. Effectiveness of self-monitored, home-based, moderate-intensity exercise training in middle-aged men and women. *Am J Cardiol* 1987;60:66–70.

2

Photography

The secret to taking good, comparable pre- and postoperative pictures is to always use the same camera, lens, film, light, focal distance, and angle of shot, with the patient in the same position against the same background. Good photographic equipment is one of the best investments plastic surgeons can make when opening their first office. The camera does not have to be new, but it does have to produce top-quality pictures. Part of the start-up office budget should be allocated to instruction in proper camera use. The purchase, processing, and correct storage of film should represent part of the annual operating budget. A system of cataloguing pre- and postoperative pictures and slides must be established. Lighting should be present with little need for arrangement, pose positions should be standardized, and the quality of each roll of film developed should be checked. The goal is to obtain consistent and reproducible pre- and postoperative photographs (1). It is important to begin the standardization of positions and illumination early in one's career in order to have comparable recordings for patient information, lecture material, and the publishing of new ideas and techniques. Today we can appreciate results obtained by surgeons more than 120 years ago because they kept good photographic records of their work (2,3).

Some surgeons prefer to send their patients to professional photographers, provided the surgeon's instructions are followed. The advantage of this method is that the surgeon does not waste time and money with unusable or unsatisfactory photographs. However, by passing the photography fee along to the patient, the surgeon increases the patient's total expenses.

THE PHOTO ROOM

It is ideal to use one room for all pre- and postoperative pictures. If this is not possible, a wall should be painted the same color in every examining room where pictures may be taken. The background should be free of doorknobs, light switches, and other clutter. In my studio (Fig. 2-1) I take pre- and postoperative pictures and give computer image consultations. The lighting, cameras, and lenses are always the same. It is impossible to control sun tanning, hair length, or gain and loss of weight, but it is possible to control the background and lighting. Patients should know they are going to be photographed. I have a screen in the room behind which patients change into disposable dressing gowns, which are easy to remove when the pictures are being taken.

BACKGROUND

I prefer a neutral, light, matte background of white or cream because it gives good definition to the subject without interfering with it. Blue can also be used, but it is very difficult to maintain the same tonality in every picture. A black background enhances the subject, giving it a glamorous look. It is easier to alter the contour of a subject on a black background and, unfortunately, this is sometimes done to show a better postoperative result. (There are, of course, easier ways to fake results with new computer programs that can completely change a picture.)

CAMERA

Always use the same brand name SLR camera and the same lens—a 60-mm macro, which avoids the distortions of a 50-mm or a telephoto lens. This works well for close-ups of the face, and for full body pictures with practically no distortion. Any minor distortion will be constant pre- and postoperatively. Always use two cameras, one for slides and one for color prints or black and white. Once the correct light exposure is set and is constant, it is a good idea to stick adhesive tape to the camera aperture and speed controls, so that there are no inadvertent variations. Even with this precaution, it is possible to miss preoperative pictures due to either bad processing or film misplacement. If possible, set the camera on a sturdy tripod, which will ensure that the camera is perpendicular to the ground and to the background at the height of the area being photographed. One of the most common mistakes is to have a different camera position pre- and postoperatively, i.e., the camera was held vertically preoperatively and horizontally postoperatively. When a tripod is used, this can be avoided.

LIGHTS

Hand flashes are unacceptable for a good registration of preoperative photographs. They may be used in the operating room or if one operates in different facilities, but to photograph your own patients in your own office, studio lights will provide a high-quality image. Today's studio flashes are small enough to fit any room and all that is needed is to get a professional to set the flash initially, and the rest is just repetition. Hand flashes leave a dramatic shadow around one side of the subject. This can be avoided by using reflectors and indirect lighting, but the pictures will still lack the quality this type of photograph needs. A professional studio flash with at least three light heads, at a 150-cm distance from the patient at a 45-degree angle, will eliminate the shadows that alter or blur the contour and will allow for good subject detail and uniform background color. Flashes should be set at the height of the area to be photographed. Umbrellas or haze lights smooth the shadows and produce a less dramatic and more realistic image. As long as pre- and postoperative light sources and settings remain the same, it is possible to obtain comparable pictures. To show dramatic shadows, just use the flashes directly on the subject. It is also possible, for special effects—when photographing skin irregularities, for example—to combine the high-temperature flashlight with a lower-temperature floodlight. One lateral light source can increase the shadow effect, if needed.

PATIENT POSITION AND FOCAL DISTANCE

Patients should be photographed standing, with the neck and back straight, at a 50-cm distance from the background. Positions should be standardized for every procedure. Photos should show no clothing whatsoever, and no jewelry, glasses, makeup, wigs or any hairstyle that covers the area to be photographed, unless the purpose of the picture is to show how to disguise a scar. In this case one should take two shots, one with and one without the disguise. When I photograph legs, I ask patients to step onto a stand that places them in a high position so I don't have to get down on my knees. I photograph faces with the patient sitting on a stool. The body is photographed with the patient standing.

In our studio we have a poster with all the standard positions that we follow for preoperative pictures. There is always a certain amount of distortion in position and focal distance (FD), and to help obtain comparable postoperative shots, we have developed a display stand for the preoperative shots with which we can compare when taking the postoperative shots. When I am taking postoperative pictures, I place the preoperative pictures and slides on the display stand in front of me to follow the positions. Sometimes there are special problems that require a picture to be taken in close-up or another nonstandard position, and the display stand makes it easy to follow the sequence postoperatively. We have a separate display for slide shots, because one cannot assume that the slides are taken in the same position as the prints. If the display is not checked often there can be slight differences between pre- and postoperative pictures. The use of an acetate screen grid inside the camera, in conjunction with anatomic boundaries, has been described as a means to achieving accurate, reproducible, standard face and body photographs for aesthetic surgery patients (4). Although we do not use this grid, there should be a standard distance for each different subject. Even very small technical variations in the pictures may cause drastic changes in the value of clinical photography in aesthetic plastic surgery. Unless strict criteria for clinical photography are followed, photographs lose their value with regard to patients and their didactic value for surgeons (5).

Some surgeons find it very difficult to ask their patients to undress for a picture, and end up taking sloppy pictures of patients pulling up their bras and pulling down their panties. One of the common mistakes surgeons make when photographing the face is not to ask patients to remove their blouses and bra straps. Their pre- and postoperative pictures are always messy, with the design of a collar attracting more attention than the result of the surgery. We have solved this problem by establishing the following procedure: One of the nurses takes the patient to the studio, tells them which clothes to take off so the part of the body to be photographed will be nude, and to remove jewelry, glasses, and so on, then hands them a gown, which will be worn until I enter the room. Only then do I enter the studio, turn on the photographic lights, and tell the patient to remove the gown and hand it to the nurse. I then take the pictures as quickly and professionally as possible.

Face

Full Face

The full face should be photographed with the camera vertical, FD 70 cm, with the focus at the eye medial canthus. The head should be straight according to medial and sagittal planes, except for shots with an elevated chin. Eyes should be open, looking forward in the horizontal plane. The mouth should be shut with teeth occluded. The positions on the map should be followed: Left lateral, ¾ left, frontal, ¾ right, right lateral, back of the head (for ear surgery) and frontal with a 45-degree chin elevation (for noses). We always take a full face series on print and slides for facial surgery and, if necessary, one of the other complementing facial sequences described in this chapter. Remember: No earrings, glasses, makeup, or hair accessories, should be seen in the pictures apart from a band to pull the hair back when necessary. Patients should know that they are coming to be photographed and should cooperate and follow instructions (Fig. 2-2).

Upper Face

The upper face should be photographed with the camera horizontal, FD 45 cm, with the focus at the eye medial canthus. For the forehead, eyebrows, and eyelids the same format is followed as for the full face: Left, ¾ left, frontal, ¾ right, right lateral, plus frontal with eyes shut and eyes open looking up without changing the head position (Fig. 2-3). It is easy to spot any changes in head position that can interfere with the result, as Flower and Flower have found: ''Measuring the changes in the intercanthal axis relative to the horizontal plane of the face, shows that each degree of alteration of the axis represents 1 mm of true postural change in the margin of the lower lid, disguised by head tilt or downward gaze'' (6).

Lower Face

The lower face should be photographed with the camera horizontal, FD 45 cm, with the focus at the oral commissure. The mouth and teeth should be shut. For nasolabial folds, ''jowls,'' chin and submental area, left, ¾ left, frontal, ¾ right, right lateral, plus open mouth frontal position should be sufficient (Fig. 2-4).

Nose

The nose should be photographed with the camera vertical, FD 45 cm, with the focus at the labial mental angle. The mouth and teeth should be shut, eyes open and looking forward in the horizontal plane. The following format is followed: Left, ¾ left, frontal, ¾ right, right lateral, plus frontal position and frontal with a 45-degree chin elevation (Fig. 2-5). Life-sized photographs of the face for rhinoplasty preoperative planning have been advocated for many years, and if the surgeon is used to this method, it can help the surgical procedure and can also help the patient visualize a possible result (7–10). One of the advantages of having our flashlights system is that one can measure changes in the light reflexes under very controlled conditions as a method of determining the efficacy of surgical techniques (11).

Body

The patient should wear no jewelry, watches, or underclothes. Ideally there should be no ''elastic marks'' from bras and panties. It is better if the patient can come to be photographed without them, otherwise they will take around forty minutes to disappear, and not everyone can wait that long.

Dorsal Region

Photographs of the dorsal region should be taken with the camera vertical, FD 120 cm. Hair, if long, should be combed to the front. The area should include the shoulders and the gluteal fold. Focus at the waistline. Use two positions: camera horizontal and camera vertical, with the arms above the head and with the arms down, and the hands one-foot away from the body (Fig. 2-6).

Flanks, Thighs and Buttocks

Flanks, thighs, and buttocks should be photographed with the camera vertical, FD 120 cm. The following positions should be followed: Knees separated, focus at the pubis or the intergluteal fold (Fig. 2-7); left lateral, ¾ left, frontal, ¾ right, right lateral, ¾ right back, back, ¾ left back, and the diving position (for abdominal flaccidity).

Abdomen

The abdomen should be photographed with the camera horizontal, FD 100 cm, with the focus at umbilicus. Iliac crests must be symmetrical. Two sequences should be taken: One with the arms down behind the body, and one with the arms above the head, left lateral, ¾ left, front, ¾ right, right lateral (Fig. 2-8).

Breasts

Breasts should be photographed with the camera horizontal, FD 80 cm, with the focus at the medial part of the inframammary fold. Clavicles must be symmetrical. Two sequences are necessary: One with the arms down and behind the body, and one with the arms above the head (Fig. 2-9) in the left lateral, ¾ left, frontal, ¾ right, right lateral positions. The back should be used for scoliosis or axillary breasts.

Calves and Ankles

Calves and ankles should be photographed with the camera vertical, FD 100 cm, with the focus at the edge of the legs. Knees separated, left lateral, frontal, right lateral, back (Fig. 2-10).

Knees

Knees should be photographed with the camera horizontal, FD 80 cm, with the focus at the knees. Knees should be separated and front and back positions should be used (Fig. 2-11).

Arms

Pictures of arms should be taken at 80 cm FD. Each arm should be taken separately, frontal and dorsal, in the same position. Arms should be elevated 90 degrees from the body, forearm bent 90 degrees at the elbows, hands straight (Fig. 2-12).

Hands

Hands should be photographed with the camera horizontal, FD 70 cm. Both hands should be straight, with fingers spread apart. Frontal and dorsal positions should be photographed (Fig. 2-13). A second shot should be taken of the dorsum of the hand with the hands shut.

FILM

Even with all this care there can still be a difference in color either because of a change in the make of the film or even in the date of development of the same make of film. If you always use the same lab, processing solutions might be overused on a Friday and brand new on a Tuesday, and that can produce a change in color.

PREPARING LECTURES AND PUBLICATIONS

There is a tendency to show only the best results, even when we are supposed to show complications. Therefore, in order not to mislead those who are trying to learn, it is very important to state the criteria used to choose the particular pictures for a lecture or article (12). The "random drawing" method has been advocated. Write on a piece of paper the names of all patients whose photographs are complete and have the right follow-up time, shuffle them and draw the names of those whose photographs will be selected. Sometimes the drawn photo does not make the point one is trying to show. In this case it is best to state that the pictures where chosen because they show a specific detail, although it is a result that might not be reproduced constantly by other surgeons.

COMPUTER IMAGES

In 1993 I started saving digital images of my patients obtained through my Mirror Image system with a Sony 3 CCD video camera. The change to digital photography should not be far in the future, and when it comes I want to be ready, with lots of saved images from my patients. I collect these high-quality digital images of my patients with thoughts of future utilization, although presently these pictures do not have the same quality as celluloid. But they do have other qualities, such as easy storage, no susceptibility to fungus, and no color fading.

New computer programs are becoming widely used among plastic surgeons, as a means of filing presurgical photographs and postsurgical projection images (13,14). A comparison of the pre- and postsurgical images can help with the patient's visualization. The surgeon has to be very honest about the proposed modifications, and show a realistic computer image that can be matched surgically. The computer software also provides a tool for creating graphics, 35-mm slides, and, possibly, educational video tapes. Some people predict that celluloid will become absolete and soon all images will be digital. This makes good sense; the color would be constant, the image would not deteriorate as traditional film does, and the information can be stored, reproduced, and accessed easily and quickly. There are two problems, though: It is not as romantic as the film camera, and digitized photos can be easily modified without a trace.

REFERENCES

1. Gilmore J, Miller W. Clinical photography utilizing office staff: methods to achieve consistency and reproducibility. *J Dermatol Surg Surg Oncol* 1988;14:281–286.

2. Rogers BO. The first pre- and post-operative photographs of plastic and reconstructive surgery: contributions of Gurdon Buck (1807–1877). *Aesthetic Plast Surg* 1991;15:19–33.

3. Burns SB. *Early medical photography in America (1839–1883).* New York: The Birns Archive, 1935–1938;1983:789, 1260.

4. Ellenbogen R, Jankauskas S, Collini FJ. Achieving standardized photographs in aesthetic surgery. *Plast Reconstr Surg* 1990;86:955–961.

5. Jemec BI, Jemec GB. Photographic surgery: standards in clinical photography. *Aesthetic Plast Surg* 1986;10:177–180.

6. Flowers RS, Flowers SS. Diagnosing photographic distortion. Decoding true postoperative contour after eyelid surgery. *Clin Plast Surg* 1993;20:387–389.

7. Souza AM. Estudo esquemafico de fotografias em rinoplastias. *Rev Lat Amer Cir Plast* 1964;8:166–184.

8. Souza AM. Planning of rhinoplasties upon natural size photographs. In: Toledo LS, ed. *Annals of the international symposium "Recent advances in plastic surgery (RAPS) 90."* São Paulo, Brazil, March 28–30, 1990. Rio de Janeiro: Marques Saraiva, 1990:573–585.

9. Guyuron B. Precision rhinoplasty. Part I: The role of life-size photographs and soft-tissue cephalometric analysis. *Plast Reconstr Surg* 1988;81:489–499.

10. Guyuron B. Precision rhinoplasty. Part II: Prediction. *Plast Reconstr Surg* 1988;81:500–505.

11. Daniel RK, Hodgson J, Lambros VS. Rhinoplasty: the light reflexes. *Plast Reconstr Surg* 1990;85:859–866; discussion 867–868.

12. Courtiss EH. Photographs: are they misleading? (editorial). *Plast Reconstr Surg* 1992;89:125.

13. Allan JH, Cook TA. A computer-based method of filing photographs and procedures. *Arch Otolaryngol Head Neck-Surg* 1985;111:178–181.

14. Mattison RC. Facial video image processing: standard facial image capturing, software modification, development of a surgical plan, and comparison of presurgical and postsurgical results. *Ann Plast Surg* 1992;29:385–389.

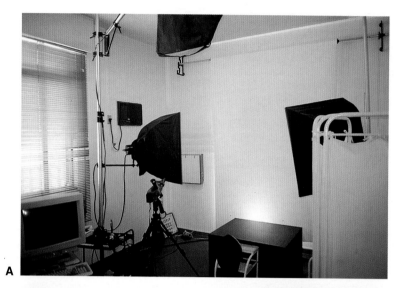

A

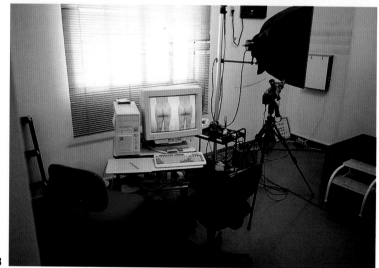

B

FIG. 2-1. A, B: This is the studio/computer imaging/examining room. Patients undress behind the screen and step on a stand to be photographed. I place preoperative slides and photos on the wall in front of me so I can reproduce the same positions. I use four head studio flashlights. The background is white. Digital images are captured by the Mirror Image system. Patients put on a surgical gown and sit by my side to discuss their problems. I can easily reexamine them if I need to.

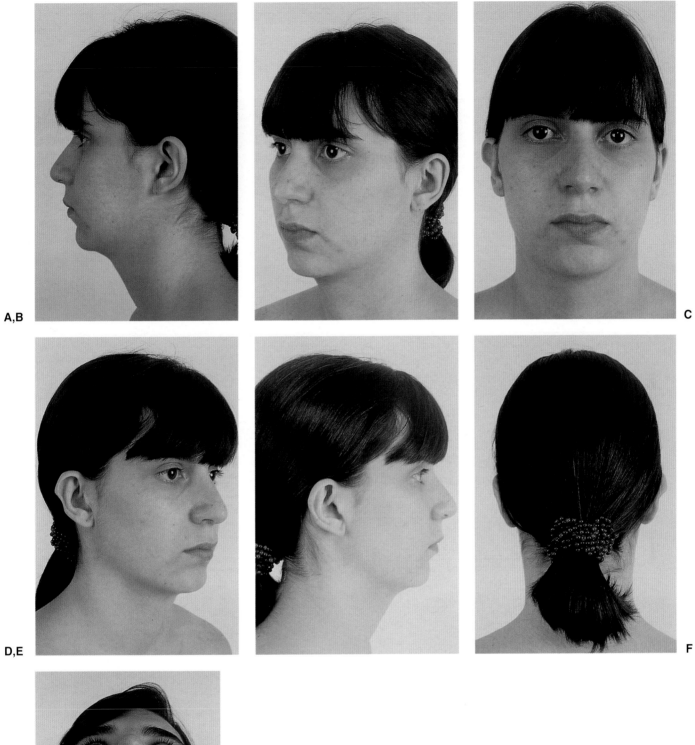

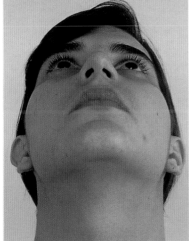

FIG. 2-2. Full face positions. **A:** Left lateral. **B:** Left ¾. **C:** Front. **D:** Right ¾. **E:** Right lateral. **F:** Back. **G:** Chin elevated 45 degrees.

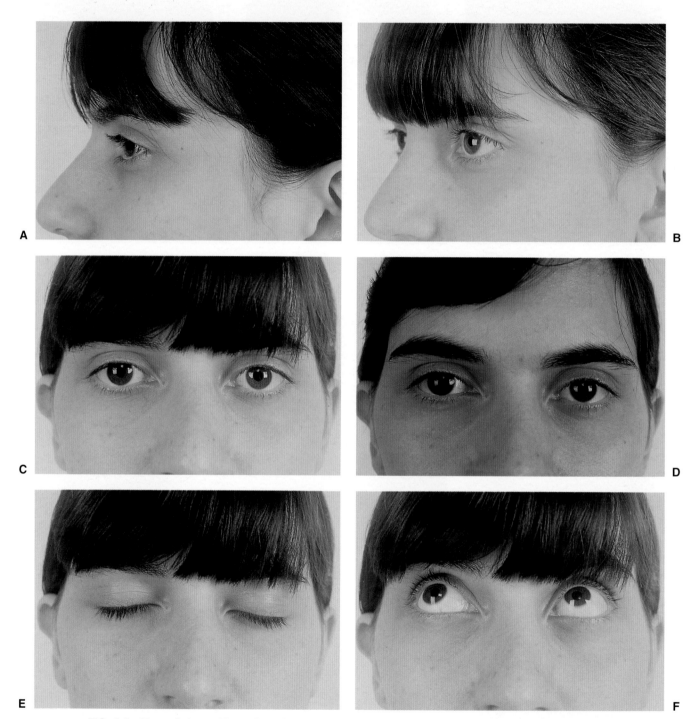

FIG. 2-3. Upper face positions. **A:** Left lateral. **B:** Left ¾. **C:** Front. **D:** Front (hair pulled to the side). **E:** Front (eyes closed). **F:** Front (looking up).

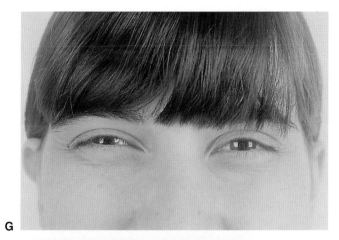

G

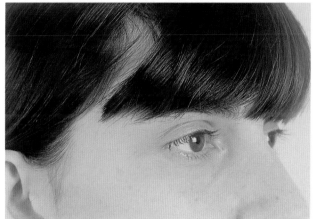

H

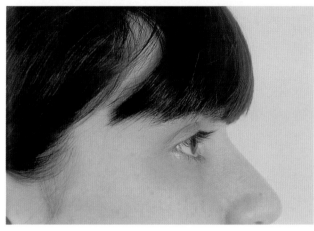

I

FIG. 2-3. *Continued.* **G:** Front (smiling). **H:** Right ¾. **I:** Right lateral.

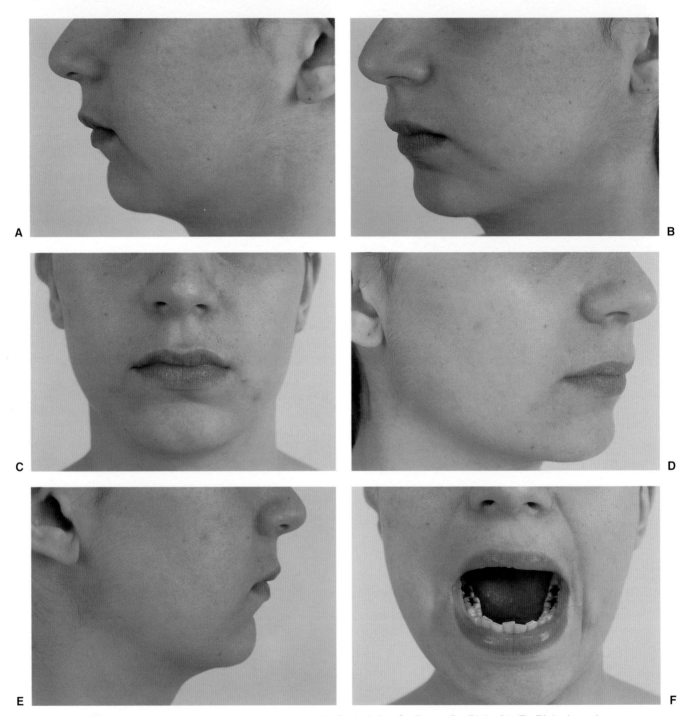

FIG. 2-4. Lower face positions. **A:** Left lateral. **B:** Left ¾. **C:** Front. **D:** Right ¾. **E:** Right lateral. **F:** Front (mouth open).

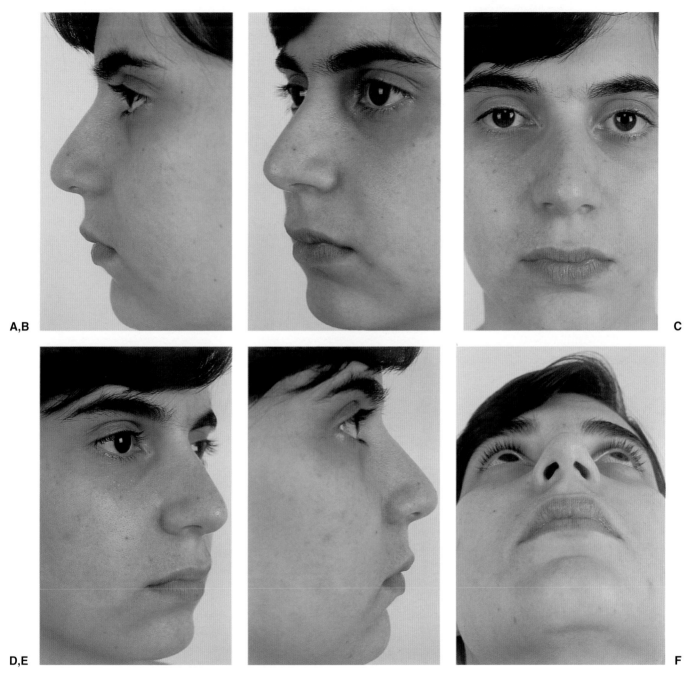

FIG. 2-5. Nose positions. **A:** Left lateral. **B:** Left ¾. **C:** Front. **D:** Right ¾. **E:** Right lateral. **F:** Front (chin elevated 45 degrees).

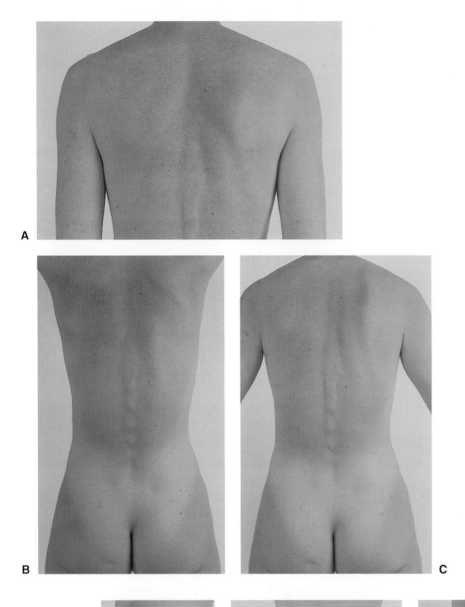

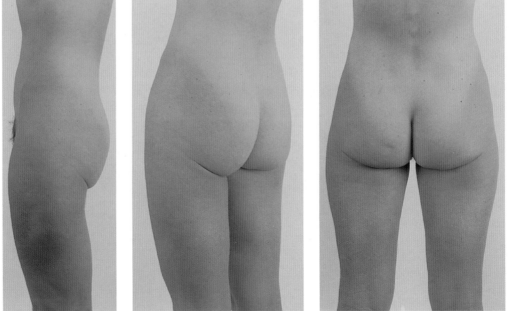

FIG. 2-6. Dorsal region positions. **A:** Back (camera horizontal, arms down). **B:** Back (camera vertical, arms up). **C:** Back (camera vertical, arms down).

FIG. 2-7. Flanks, thighs and buttocks positions (arms up). **A:** Left lateral. **B:** Left ¾ back. **C:** Back.

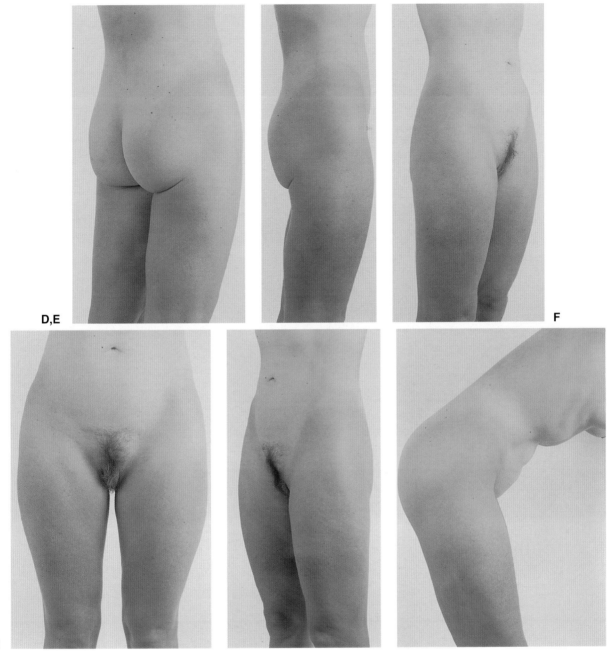

FIG. 2-7. *Continued.* **D:** Right ¾ back. **E:** Right lateral. **F:** Right ¾ front. **G:** Front. **H:** Left ¾ front. **I:** Right lateral (diving position).

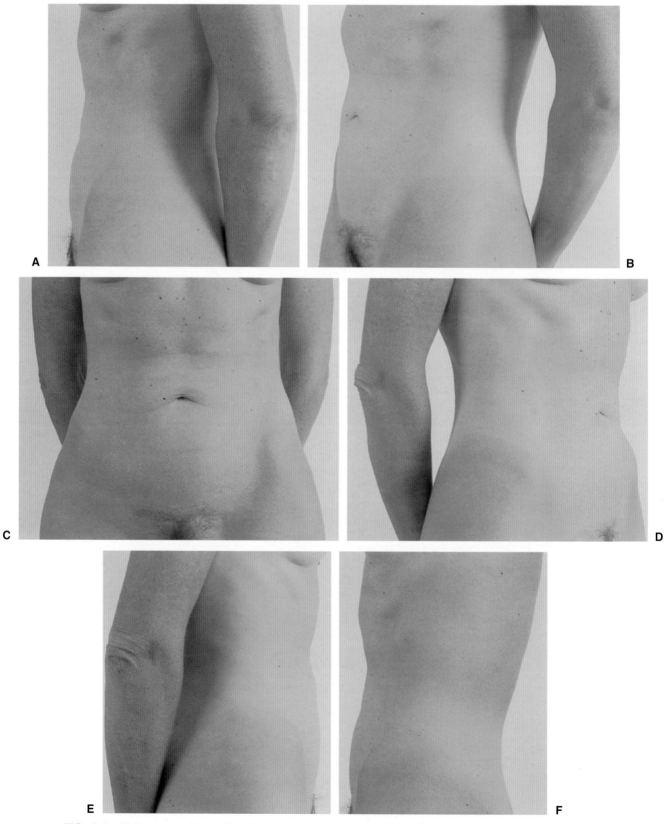

FIG. 2-8. Abdomen positions. (**A–E:** arms down in the back.) **A:** Left lateral. **B:** Left ¾. **C:** Front. **D:** Right ¾. **E:** Right lateral. (**F–J:** arms up.) **F:** Left lateral.

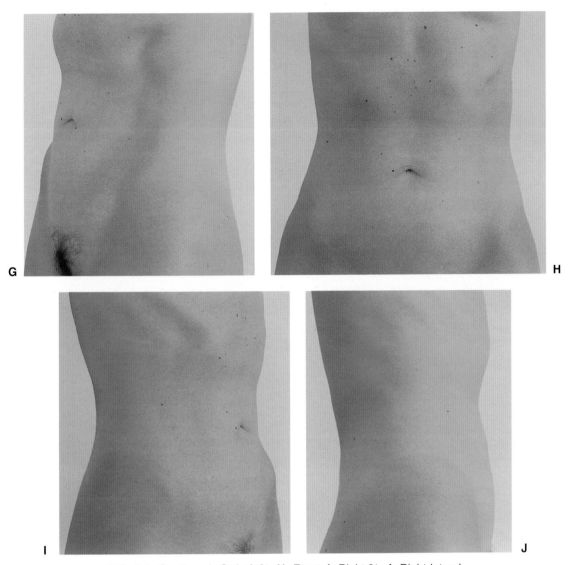

FIG. 2-8 *Continued.* **G:** Left ¾. **H:** Front. **I:** Right ¾. **J:** Right lateral.

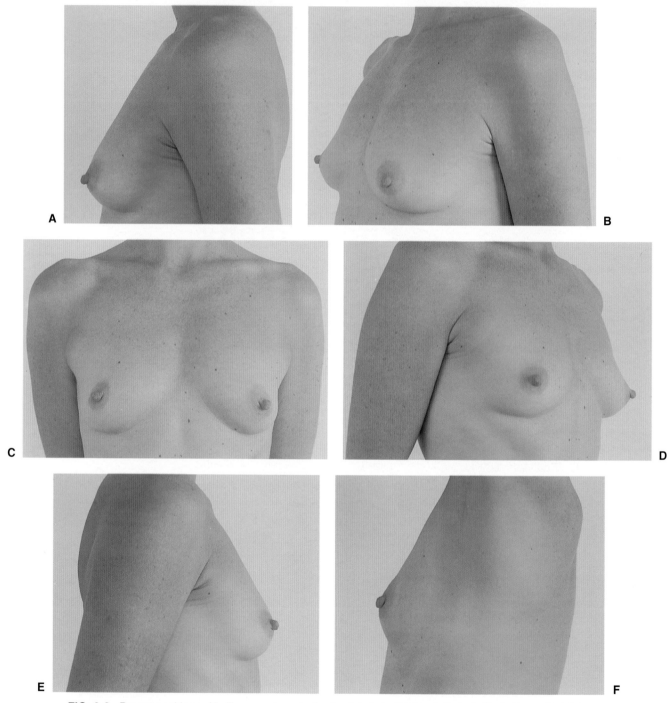

FIG. 2-9. Breast positions. (**A–E:** arms down in the back.) **A:** Left lateral. **B:** Left ¾. **C:** Front. **D:** Right ¾. **E:** Right lateral. (**F–J:** arms up.) **F:** Left lateral.

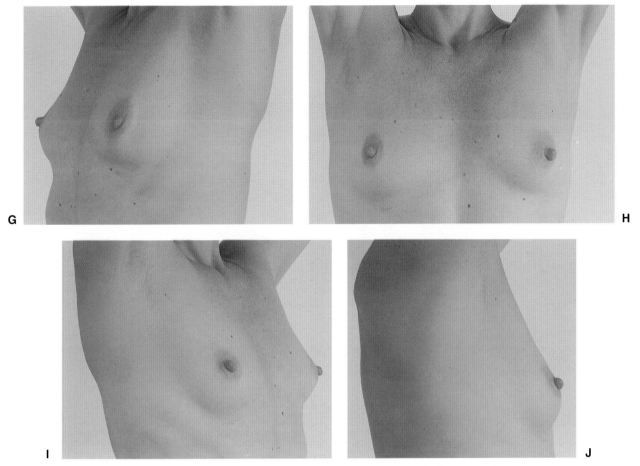

FIG. 2-9. *Continued.* **G:** Left ¾. **H:** Front. **I:** Right ¾. **J:** Right lateral.

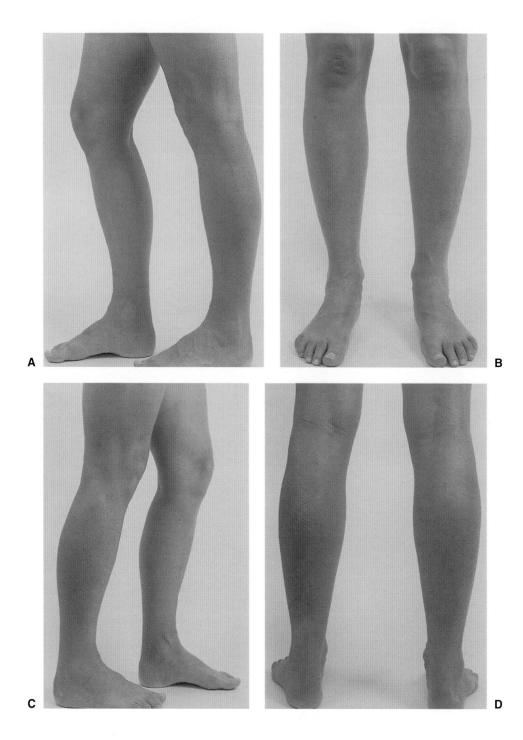

FIG. 2-10. Calf and ankle positions. **A:** Left lateral (right foot forward). **B:** Front. **C:** Right lateral (left foot forward). **D:** Back.

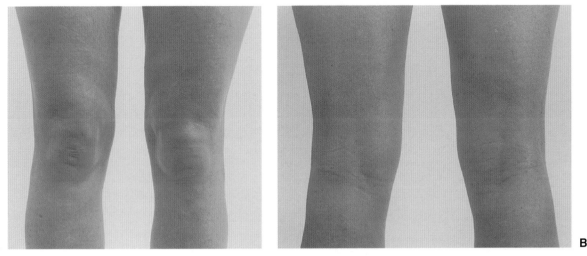

FIG. 2-11. Knee positions. **A:** Front. **B:** Back.

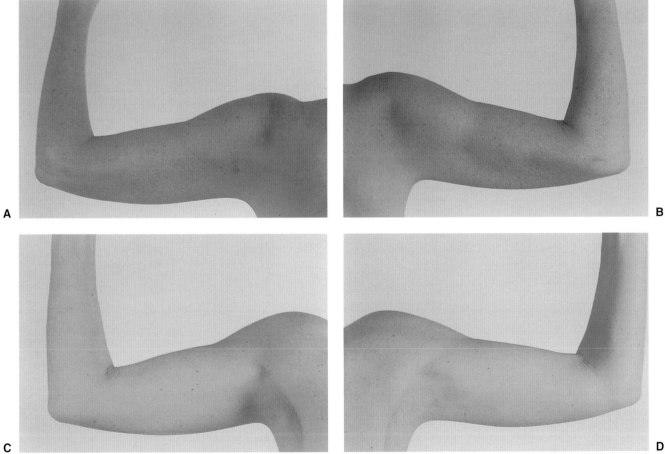

FIG. 2-12. Arm positions. **A:** Left arm back (bent at 45-degree angle at shoulder and elbow). **B:** Right arm back (bent at 45-degree angle at shoulder and elbow). **C:** Right arm front (bent at 45-degree angle at shoulder and elbow). **D:** Left arm front (bent at 45-degree angle at shoulder and elbow).

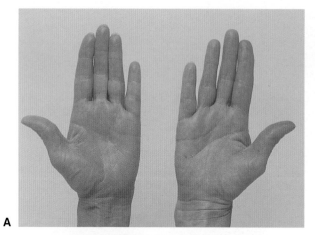

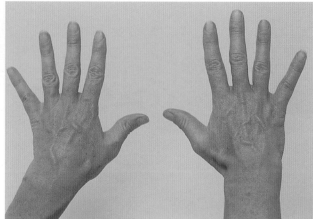

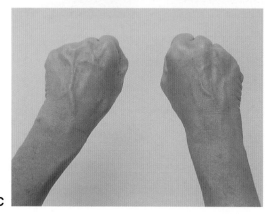

FIG. 2-13. Hand positions. **A:** Palms (fingers together). **B:** Dorsum (fingers apart). **C:** Hands closed.

3

The Preoperative Examination

As plastic surgeons, we must examine patients who come for consultation in a global manner. There is a close relationship between the shape of the body and the overall health of the patient. Internal diseases provoke several disorders, and we should not limit our examination to the specific problem that brings the patient to the office. A complete preoperative examination (1) should be conducted in a rapid manner to screen for possible problems and to avoid mistakes in diagnosis. This will also eliminate patients who ask for impossible improvements.

Since 1992, I have been using computer imaging during my consultations. I use the Mirror Image system. This program helps the doctor and the patient to understand visually the alterations that are possible. This is especially true for the dorsal region. Since patients rarely see themselves from the back, the computer image can help in understanding possible changes in that area.

When patients come for consultation about the shape of their bodies, they usually have very accurate ideas of their problems. They have already compared their bodies with the ''patterns of beauty'' and decided that something has to be changed. But how do we as surgeons identify what is beautiful and what is not? How do we judge if someone needs a change in their body? What do we compare it to?

Beauty is related to function, and it could be said that the beautiful feature is the one that functions well—a beautiful leg, arm, hip, or buttock. The balance between muscle function and the bony frame, combined with the genetic struc-

This chapter is adapted from Hébert G. Muscle et Beauté Plastique Féminine. Librairie Vuibert, Paris, 1919. Georges Hébert was a French Professor of Physical Education at the turn of the last century. He was a great believer that beauty and health are inseparable. Although this seems obvious, modern life tends to separate the two.

ture the person is born with, will produce beautiful body parts, which in the right proportion will form a beautiful body.

THE FIRST CONSULTATION

In the first consultation, when asked the classical opening question ''what can I do for you?'' some patients know exactly the part of the body they want to see improved. They say they want to get rid of the ''love-handles,'' or the inner knees. The diagnosis and treatment are then very straightforward. Others have a complex problem: they want ''everything.'' These are usually people who have neglected their bodies for too long and need work done almost everywhere.

People of the same height can have totally different proportions (Fig. 3-1.) If we analyze the body, we can judge which problems can be fixed through soft tissue remodeling, which need bone surgery, which can be improved with proper diet, muscular exercise, and posture correction, and those that cannot be fixed at all.

Lack of muscle tone can provoke several problems: If the muscles that sustain the column are atrophied, there will be a deviation of the column, either lateral or sagittal. A lordosis can provoke an abdominal protrusion that can only be treated through exercise, not surgery (Fig. 3-2.) A hip deviation, due to one leg being shorter than the other, can show a fat roll in one side of the dorsal region and not the other. If the posture can still be corrected, it is not a case for surgery, but if it is an established defect that will not improve with exercise, liposculpture can help to make the body more symmetrical. As a surgeon I constantly have to remind myself to avoid thinking that every problem has to be corrected through surgery. Many problems do not. The constant use of high heels can provoke atrophy of the calf muscles that can be better treated through exercise than with calf implants (Fig. 3-3.)

The first general exam will show the proportions, shape, and attitude, as well as physical defects and malformations. This first part of the exam can provide an outline of the general conditions, but in order to properly evaluate the relationship between shape and proportions, the following elements should be considered:

1. General appearance.
2. Muscular development.
3. The degree of adiposity.
4. General attitude and posture in front, profile, and back.
5. General appearance and musculature of the trunk.
6. General appearance and musculature of the upper limbs.
7. General appearance and musculature of the lower limbs.
8. General appearance of the skin and complexion.
9. Proportions and measurements of the trunk and limbs.
10. The type of body.
11. Possible defects, malformations, and injuries.

Even when patients come for consultation about a problem on the face, I do not limit the exam only to that area. Usually patients are not prepared to remove their clothes for examination if they have come for a rhytidoplasty, and I don't ask them to do so, but while they are with me in the examining room I am aware of their posture, attitude, body proportions, and the way they carry themselves, because that is usually crucial to understanding patients' problems and needs.

On the first examination, I take into consideration the initial attributes of beauty, the ones directly related to health. I leave aside the secondary attributes, such as the head, facial features, hair, and so on, because they do not play an important role in the patients' health and should be examined separately. The exception is when the facies denotes an internal disease.

Normal Characteristics

General Aspect

Normal characteristics include complete muscular development that is symmetrical, with equal measurements on the right and left sides; the absence of generalized fat, as well as of localized fat accumulation; good skin color and turgor; the look is quick, the eyes are clear.

Proportions and Measurements of the Limbs and Trunk

The average height is between 1.50 m and 1.90 m. The mid-body height is the inferior extremity of the coccyx, the superior part of the pubis, or the more external point of the buttock or of the plane of the external sides of the trochanters. People of the same height can have different proportions between their body and legs (Figs. 3-4–3-7). Although incorrect proportions cannot be corrected through liposculpture, sometimes the redistribution of volume will create an illusion of correction.

People of the same height can have enormous differences in the width of their shoulders and hips (Figs. 3-8–3-10) and between the length of the body and arms (Figs. 3-11, 3-12). On average, the width of the shoulders (external sides of the deltoids) is between 24% and 25% of the height. On average the width of the hips is between 20% and 21% of the height. The width of the waist (the narrowest part of the trunk) is between 13% and 15% of the height. The circumference of the waist is between 38% and 40% of the height. The circumference of the chest is between 55% and 60% of the height, after expiration and complete inspiration. The circumference of the neck, the circumference of the bent arm (contracted biceps), and the circumference of the calf are between 19% and 21% of the height. Generally the neck is slightly larger than the bent arm, and the arm larger than the calf, but the three measurements are sometimes equal.

The abdomen is one of the areas where a complete examination will decide the indication for surgery or not. A protrusion in the abdominal area can be due to lack of muscle tone combined with an excess of volume in the abdominal cavity, or an excess of localized fat on the abdominal wall (Figs. 3-13–3-18). An excess of localized fat that will not disappear with exercise is an indication for abdominal liposculpture. When this excess is combined with muscle flaccidity, we have to consider whether a combination of suction and abdominoplasty is indicated, or only suction with postoperative exercise. When fat from the internal cavity is present, we also have to indicate diet postoperatively. Attempting to solve a complex problem through surgery alone will result in disappointment.

When the abdominal fat excess is combined with a high waist measurement, this problem will have to be addressed separately. Sometimes suction of excess fat is enough, but in many cases the oblique abdominal muscles need some exercise to improve their tone. This cannot be corrected by suction. All of these things must be pointed out to patients during the consultation. They will remember that you have told them the percentage of improvement they could expect from suction alone. I usually write that possible improvement on patients' files. If they complain postoperatively, I point out that I have done my share and now it is their turn to exercise or diet.

Usually a quick look will give the experienced plastic surgeon a general idea of the body, and the problem will be obvious, but the list of considerations presented earlier can be reproduced by all and is the quickest way to check the normal body proportions. Only after this initial examination do I go into detail and examine the specific area of the body that has brought the patient in for consultation.

REFERENCES

1. Hébert G: *Muscle et beauté plastique féminine.* Paris: Librairie Vuibert, 1919.

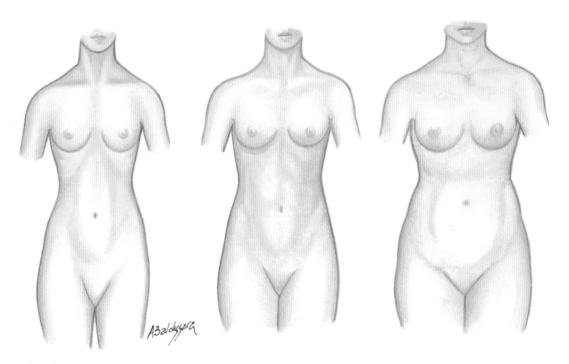

FIG. 3-1. People of the same height can have totally different proportions. **Center:** A person with a balanced shape and weight and normal muscle and fat development. **Left:** A person with lack of muscular and fat development. **Right:** An overweight person.

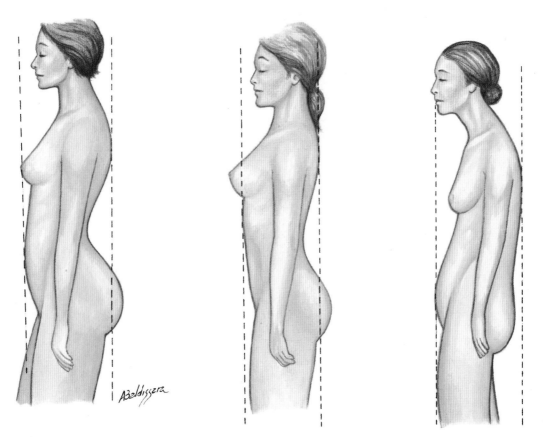

FIG. 3-2. Lack of exercise, together with other problems, can cause muscle atrophy and changes in posture. **Right and left:** Bad posture. **Center:** Normal posture.

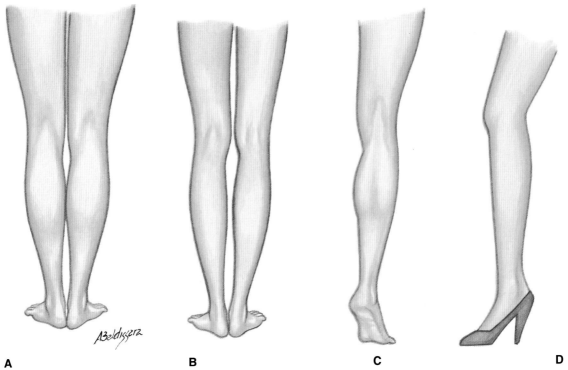

A   **B**   **C**   **D**

FIG. 3-3. A: Fashion also interferes with the legs and calves. The excessive use of high heels can interfere with the shape of legs and calves. Normally developed calves touch at the medial part when the legs are together. **B:** Atrophied calves. The medial borders do not touch each other. There is a depression below the knees, mainly because of lack of muscle. **C:** Normal legs in contraction with the body elevated by standing on the toes. The muscles contract and change aspect. **D:** Atrophied legs develop a cylindrical shape. The constant use of high heels does not stimulate the calf muscles.

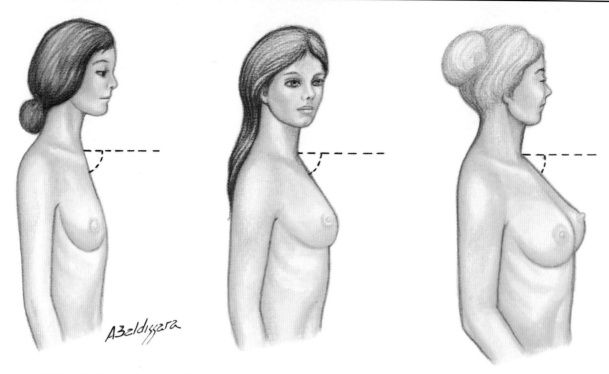

FIG. 3-4. The projection of the chest varies according to muscle development. **Center:** In a normally developed chest, the sternum has an angle of close to 45 degrees. **Left:** In the underdeveloped chest, the sternum angle is almost 90 degrees. **Right:** When the chest is too full, the sternum is elevated and the angle is smaller.

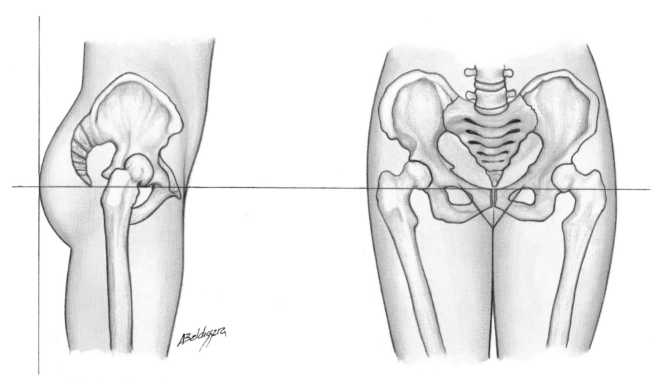

FIG. 3-5. Separation plane between the trunk and lower limbs. The pubis, the coccyx, the lateral trochanter, and the tangency point of a vertical line with the buttocks delimit the plane.

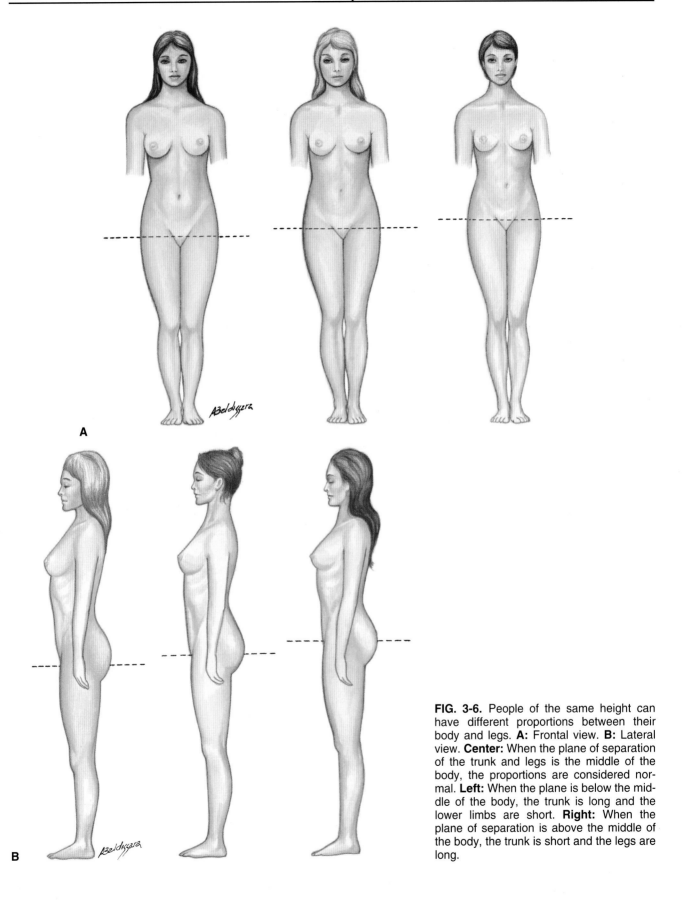

FIG. 3-6. People of the same height can have different proportions between their body and legs. **A:** Frontal view. **B:** Lateral view. **Center:** When the plane of separation of the trunk and legs is the middle of the body, the proportions are considered normal. **Left:** When the plane is below the middle of the body, the trunk is long and the lower limbs are short. **Right:** When the plane of separation is above the middle of the body, the trunk is short and the legs are long.

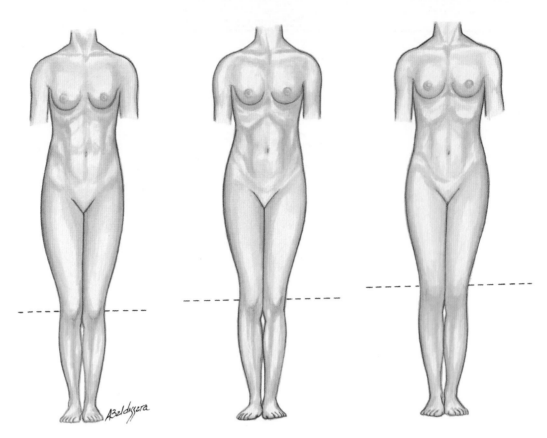

FIG. 3-7. The average proportion between the thighs and lower legs. **Center:** The thighs should be between 5% and 10% longer than the lower legs. **Left:** Short lower legs, long thighs. **Right:** Short thighs, long lower legs.

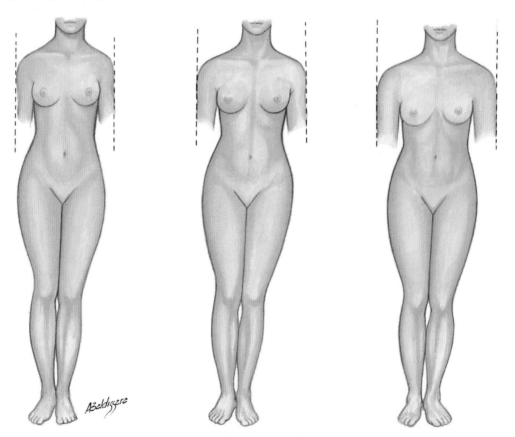

FIG. 3-8. The width of the shoulders is measured by the widest distance that separates the lateral parts of the arms. For a harmonic proportion, the width of the shoulders should be 24% to 25% of the height. **Center:** Normal width. **Left:** Narrow shoulders. **Right:** Broad shoulders.

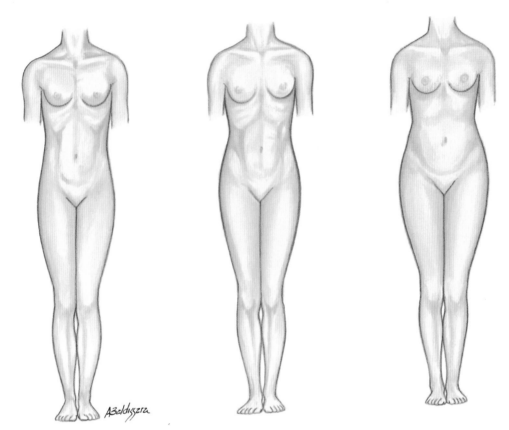

FIG. 3-9. The width of the hips is measured by the widest distance that separates the lateral parts of the thighs. For a harmonic proportion between the hips and chest, the width of the hips should be 20% to 21% of the height. **Center:** Normal hips. **Left:** Narrow hips. **Right:** Wide hips.

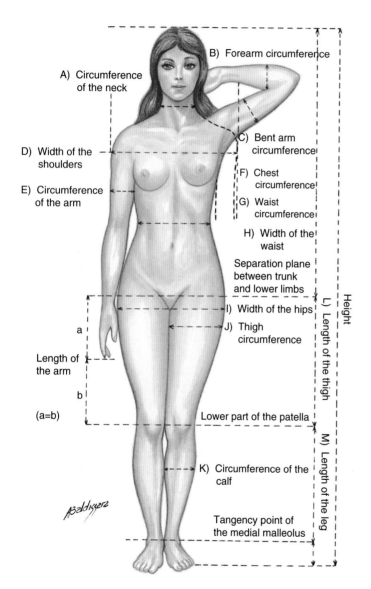

A) Circumference of the neck

B) Forearm circumference

C) Bent arm circumference

D) Width of the shoulders

E) Circumference of the arm

F) Chest circumference

G) Waist circumference

H) Width of the waist

Separation plane between trunk and lower limbs

I) Width of the hips

J) Thigh circumference

a

b

(a=b)

Length of the arm

Lower part of the patella

K) Circumference of the calf

Tangency point of the medial malleolus

Height

L) Length of the thigh

M) Length of the leg

FIG. 3-10. Harmonious proportions of the body. Height = X
A, circumference of the neck = (0.19–0.21)X
B, forearm circumference = (0.14–0.15)X
C, bent arm circumference = (0.20–0.215)X
D, width of the shoulders = (0.24–0.25)X
E, circumference of the arm = (0.18–0.19)X
F, chest circumference = (0.52–0.56)X
G, waist circumference = (0.38–0.40)X
H, width of the waist = (0.13–0.15)X
I, width of the hips = (0.20–0.21)X
J, thigh circumference = (0.31–0.33)X
K, circumference of the calf = (0.19–0.21)X
L, length of the thigh = (0.24–0.25)X
M, length of the leg = (0.21–0.22)X

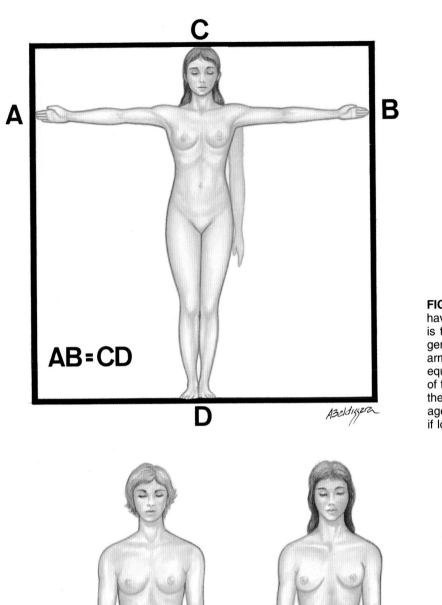

AB = CD

FIG. 3-11. Persons of the same height can have different-sized arms. The width (*AB*), is the distance between the tips of the fingers of the right and left hands with the arms in the horizontal position. The width equals the length of the arms plus the width of the thorax. The harmonious width equals the height (*CD*). 2 cm more is within average. If smaller than that, the arms are short, if longer, they are long.

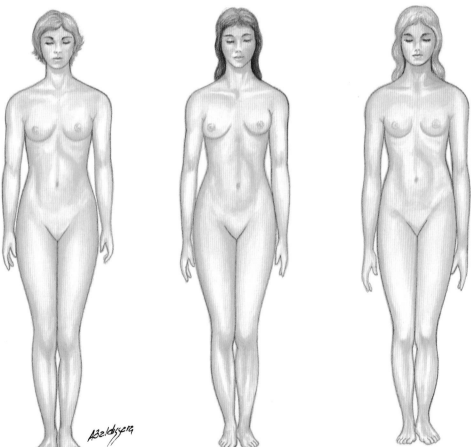

FIG. 3-12. When the arms are held along the body with the shoulders down, the tips of the fingers should touch the middle part of the thighs. **Center:** Normal arm length. **Left:** Short arms. **Right:** Long arms.

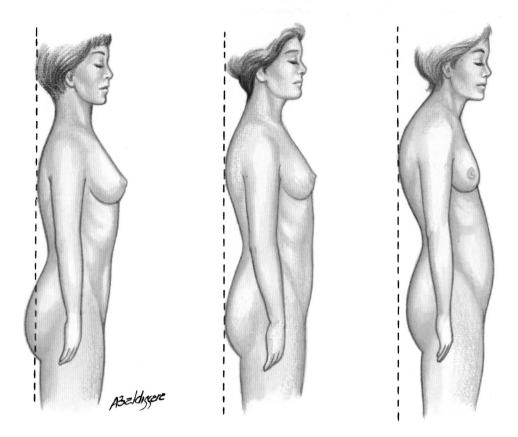

FIG. 3-13. The dorsal posture can show a person's attitude. **Left:** Open chest, shoulders back, vertical neck, good back posture. **Center:** The "couldn't care less" attitude. There is a dorsal and neck curve, the shoulders are forward. **Right:** The dorsal slouch. Flat chest, bent neck, and shoulders forward.

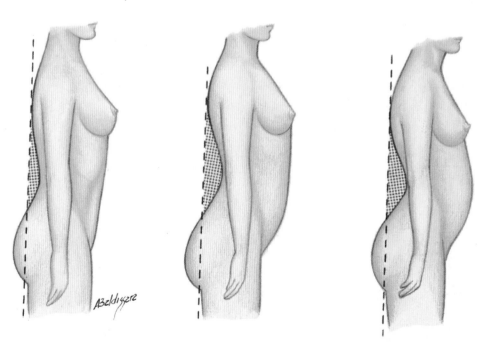

FIG. 3-14. The lumbar posture. **Left:** There is a slight lumbar curve. The chest is open, the neck is vertical. **Center:** Increased lumbar curve. The abdomen is projected. **Right:** A strong lumbar curve with abdominal projection.

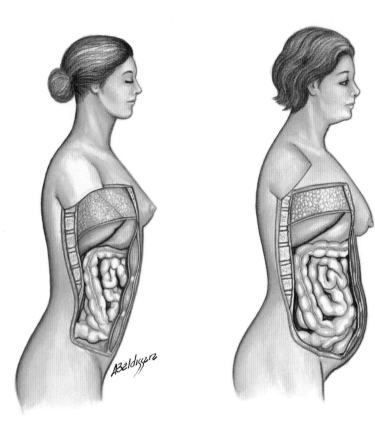

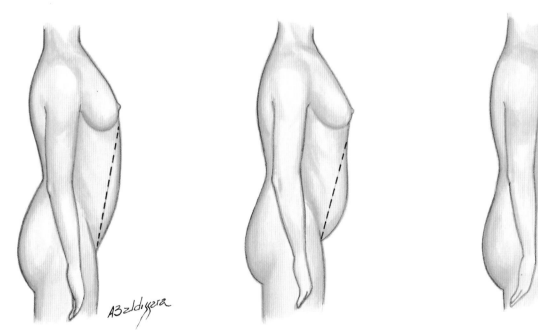

FIG. 3-15. Abdominal muscle weakness can provoke a misplacement of the internal organs. **Left:** Well-developed abdominal wall muscles. The internal organs are in their normal position. **Right:** Loose abdominal muscles. The internal organs are displaced and projected.

FIG. 3-16. The shape of the body can be altered due to abdominal muscle weakness. The dotted line shows the normal line of the abdomen. **Left:** The whole abdominal wall is loose. **Center:** The abdomen is round below the waistline. **Right:** The abdomen is loose and drooping.

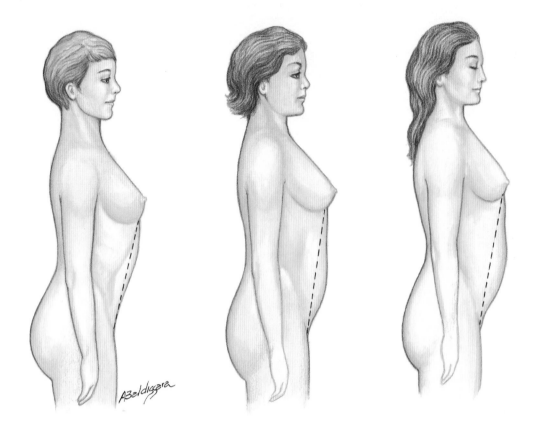

FIG. 3-17. The abdomen can be deformed due to accumulation of fat. The dotted line shows the normal line of the abdomen. **Left:** The abdomen is fat above the waistline. **Center:** The abdomen is globally fat. **Right:** The abdomen is fat around the umbilicus.

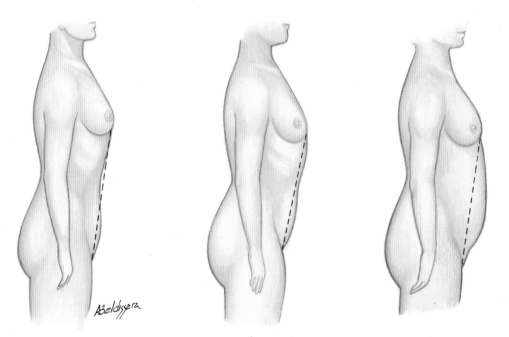

FIG. 3-18. The abdomen can also be deformed by other causes. **Left:** Abdomen marked due to the use of tight clothes. **Center:** Abdomen marked in the waistline due to wearing tight belts. **Right:** Obese abdomen.

4

Instruments

SYRINGES

I use disposable syringes for all face and body contouring procedures, instead of the aspirator. I use four to six 10-cc luer-lock syringes for the face and usually six to eight 60-cc toomey-tip syringes for a body procedure. In 1988, I started using catheter-tip syringes for body work, but they have two main disadvantages over the toomey tip: The tip gauge is too narrow (3 mm), which provokes a slow suction (Figs. 4-1–4-3), and it also breaks easily, because the cannulas are attached only to the tip. The toomey syringes have wider-tipped gauges (8 mm.), and suction time is the same as with the aspirator. Cannulas attach to the body of the syringe instead of the tip, providing a much better grip, and the tip never breaks.

CANNULAS

Infiltration of Anesthesia

I use two 2- or 3-mm-gauge, 35-cm-long, multiholed-tip, blunt needles for local anesthesia infiltration (Fig. 4-4). Always having a duplicate syringe and cannula will eliminate wasting time when changing instruments. If the assistant always has another syringe with the same size cannula ready to change when the first one is full, the reinitiation of suction is almost immediate (Fig. 4-5).

I have seen many devices used to infiltrate the local anesthesia quickly; I prefer to infiltrate with the syringe. It is fast enough, it is comfortable for the patient, and you can always measure the amount of fluid placed in each area. One of the recent problems related to the tumescent technique is the injection of too much fluid, which can easily happen with the infiltrating pumps.

Fat Aspiration

For suction, I use two sets of 2-mm, 3-mm, 4-mm, or 5-mm-gauge, 25- and 35-cm-long, Pyramid-tip cannulas (Fig. 4-6). The Pyramid-tip cannula is very fast and easy to provoke depressions with if one is not used to it. While the

Mercedes tip has three holes in different directions, the Pyramid tip has its three holes facing one side of the cannula, so there is always the possibility of directing the suction, which is not possible with the Mercedes tip. Beginners should start with a one-lateral-hole cannula (Fig. 4-7).

I also use a Toledo 3-mm forked-tip V-dissector cannula, 25 cm to 35 cm long, adapted to the 60-cc syringe for treating skin irregularities, breaking fibrous adhesions, and injecting fat superficially (Fig. 4-8). A two-holed flat-tip 5-mm-gauge cannula is used for suction in difficult areas, such as the dorsal region or secondary procedures (Fig. 4-9). For feathering suction and fat injection, I use a 3-mm gauge cannula with a 45-degree cut tip (Fig. 4-10).

Fat Injection

To inject fat into the body, I use a 25-cm long, one-lateral-hole 2-mm gauge blunt cannula (see Fig. 4-7).

LOCKS

The syringes have locks that maintain a vacuum during suction, closing tips and stands to decant fat. There are two main types of locks: those that go inside the plunger, and horseshoe locks that go on the syringe and bite the plunger to lock (Fig. 4-11). The first ones have the disadvantage of having only one measurement; they can only be regulated to remove 60 cc of fat. With the horseshoe lock, one can regulate the amount of fat to be suctioned beforehand, i.e., the plunger can be locked to aspirate 20 cc only. Syringe locks are used during most of the work; however, there are areas where I prefer pulling the plunger back just a few cc and locking it with my thumb. If I loose the vacuum, I just pull the plunger a little bit more and continue suctioning. Otherwise I would have to stop, remove the cannula from the body, eliminate the air from the syringe, and restart suction. This is especially true when working close to the incision, or when crisscrossing close to another incision.

TRANSFERS

I have transfers of different gauges to transfer fat to another syringe anaerobically (Figs. 4-12, 4-13.) To avoid breaking the fat cells the gauge of the transfer should not be too narrow.

CENTRIFUGE

A centrifuge separates fat from fluid without breaking the fat cells (Figs. 4-14, 4-15). It can be manual or electric, but it must not go faster than 1,500 r/min and must be run for only one minute, otherwise the fat cells will rupture. The fat cells should be kept intact, for a good take of the graft. The electric centrifuge takes only 10-cc syringes, but the manual centrifuge accepts syringes up to 60 cc.

FACIAL INSTRUMENTS

For facial contouring procedures, I use smaller instruments. I prefer 10-cc-luer-lock syringes and fine cannulas (Fig. 4-16).

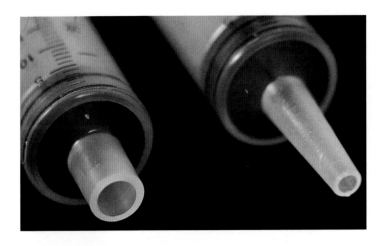

FIG. 4-1. **Left:** A 60-cc toomey-tip syringe. **Right:** A catheter-tip syringe. The toomey tip has two advantages: the tip gauge is 8 mm wide instead of the 3 mm catheter tip, and suction is faster.

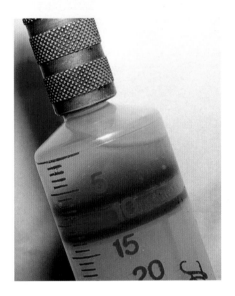

FIG. 4-2. The catheter-tip syringes break easily, because the cannulas are attached only to the tip.

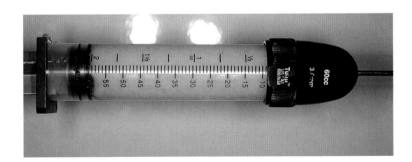

FIG. 4-3. The cannulas attach to the body of the toomey tip instead of only to the tip, providing a much better grip, and the tip never breaks.

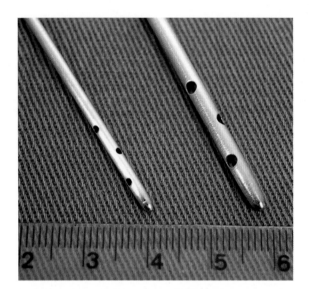

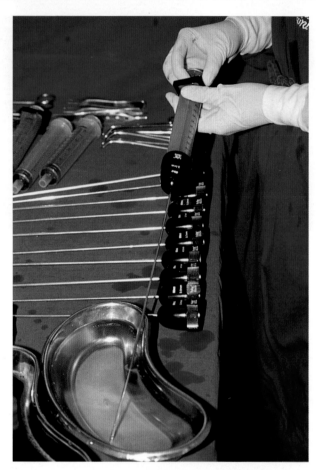

FIG. 4-4. A 2-mm **(left)** A 3-mm **(right)** gauge, multiholed-tip, blunt needle for local anesthesia infiltration, which provides a fast, painless infiltration of our local anesthesia formula and does not provoke unnecessary ecchymosis during infiltration. After a little anesthesia button with a carpule on the dermis, I use the 2-mm gauge for pure local anesthesia when the patient is awake, because the injection of the fluid is slower. I use the 3-mm gauge for faster injection of anesthetic fluid when the patient is under sedation.

FIG. 4-5. I put the anesthesia fluid at body temperature into a recipient on the table, and the assistant refills the syringes. It is a very fast method of injecting a lot of fluid with no pain.

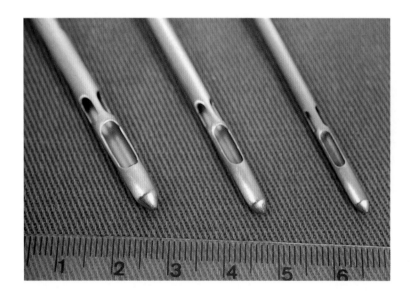

FIG. 4-6. 4.6-mm, 3.7-mm, and 3-mm-gauge Pyramid-tip cannulas used for suction of fat. The Pyramid-tip cannula has three holes facing one side of the cannula, so there is always the possibility of directing the suction.

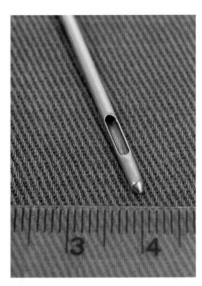

FIG. 4-7. The 2-mm-gauge cannula with one lateral hole is used for delicate superficial suction and fat injection into the body.

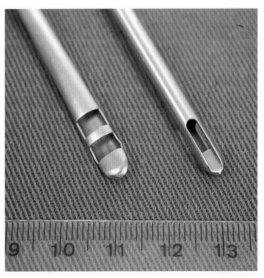

FIG. 4-9. Left: A two-holed flat-tip 5-mm-gauge cannula, used for suction in difficult areas such as the dorsal region, or secondary procedures or liposculpture in men. **Right:** The Tiger-tip cannula, also used for fibrotic areas (Grams Medical).

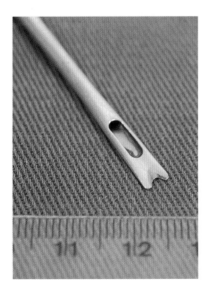

FIG. 4-8. The Toledo 3-mm forked-tip V-dissector cannula is used for treating skin irregularities, breaking fibrous adhesions, and aspirating and injecting fat. The tips of the "V" are blunt and the inside is sharp. This avoids skin perforation.

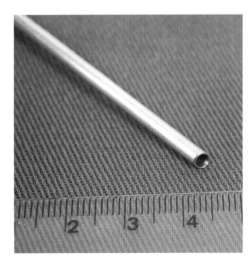

FIG. 4-10. A 3-mm-gauge cannula with a 45-degree cut tip. We use this cannula for feathering suction and also for fat injection. This was the first cannula we used to treat skin irregularities.

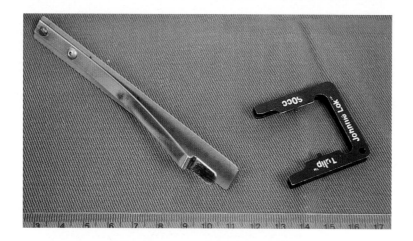

FIG. 4-11. A plunger lock (Byron Medical, Tucson, AZ) and a horseshoe lock (The Tulip Company, San Diego, CA). The plunger lock can only be regulated to remove 60 cc. The horseshoe lock can regulate the amount of fat to be suctioned, i.e., 20 cc or 30 cc.

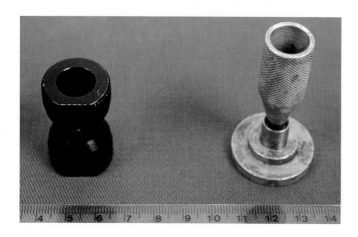

FIG. 4-12. Left: A 60-cc to 60-cc transfer (The Tulip Company). **Right:** a 60-cc to 10-cc transfer with decanting tip stand, used to decant and centrifuge fat.

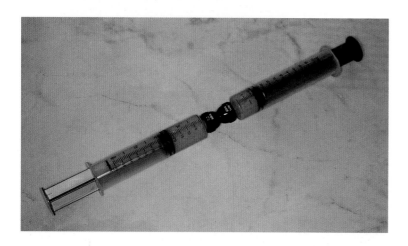

FIG. 4-13. Transfers of different gauges are used to transfer fat from one syringe to another anaerobically.

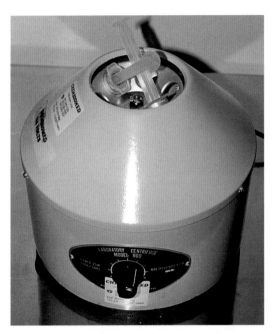

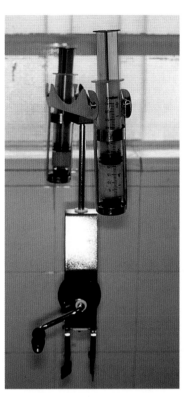

FIG. 4-14. An electric centrifuge is used to separate fat from fluid without breaking the fat cells. It must not go faster than 1,500 r/min and must run for only one minute. It can take only 10-cc syringes.

FIG. 4-15. A manual centrifuge (developed by Dr. Alberto Hodara, Porto Alegre, Brazil) is also used to centrifuge fat for reinjection. It can centrifuge syringes of different sizes, from 10 cc to 60 cc.

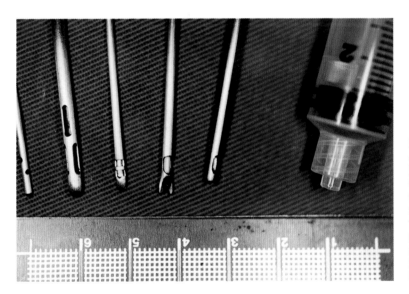

FIG. 4-16. Delicate instruments for facial liposculpture. **From left:** A multiholed, 1-mm-gauge, blunt needle used to infiltrate local anesthesia on the face. A 3-mm-gauge Pyramid-tip cannula for fat aspiration from the deep layer of fat. A 1.5-mm-gauge cannula with a two-holed flat tip, used for superficial suction of the neck and face. A 2-mm-gauge Toledo V-dissector used to free adherences and scars. A 1-mm-gauge, one-lateral-hole, blunt-tip needle for fat injection and a 10-cc luer-lock syringe.

5

Anesthesia

I usually combine local anesthesia with sedation (1–3). There has been an increase in the number of ambulatory procedures in my practice following the improvement of anesthesia methods in the last 10 years. I use the same anesthesia formula when I treat the face and the body. What varies is the sedation, with oral or no sedation for facial treatments and oral or intravenous (IV) sedation for body procedures. The advantages for the patient are a fast recovery to normal activities, protection against hospital infection, less anxiety through avoiding hospital admittance, less waiting for hospital rooms and surgical rooms, and less risk of cancellation of the procedure. There is also a decreased cost.

PREOPERATIVE SCREENING

Preparation for surgery should follow the standards for the size of the procedure, with the appropriate examination of the patient and laboratory tests. I have a very complete questionnaire that my patients fill in, which should identify any possible preoperative problems. The patient should be healthy enough to undergo this type of procedure, not only physically but also psychologically. I ask for a complete blood count, blood sugar level, and coagulation tests, human immunodeficiency virus (HIV) test and, for patients older than 45 years of age, an electrocardiogram (EKG). Patients are evaluated by the anesthesiologist when the tests are completed. If there are any problems, they should be corrected before the surgery. Patients with preoperative anxiety are medicated the day before the surgery.

SEDATION

When we treat only one area, or for small procedures, we use oral sedation with 15 mg of midazolam. For larger areas I prefer IV sedation with midazolam and fentanyl. There is no need for heavy sedation, so recovery is faster. Patients are ambulatory 12 to 24 hours after surgery and return to routine activities in two to three days, depending on the amount of fat treated. Patients who need IV sedation are monitored and prepared to guarantee a safe maintenance of the hydroelectrolitic balance, respiratory function, and hemodynamic stability. Sedation is combined with local anesthesia. The patient is monitored, and the anesthesiologist starts the sedation with midazolam and fentanyl. Midazolam is used in the initial doses of 0.1 mg/kg IV up to a total dose of 0.3 mg/kg, according to the surgical procedure. Although respiratory depression is very low with midazolam it is necessary to have all the conditions to ventilate the patient, especially when fentanyl is utilized. Midazolam's action is antagonized with lanexate (flumazenil) in variable doses from 0.2 to 1.0 mg IV.

ANESTHESIA

The advent of the tumescent technique for local anesthesia has increased the safety of office surgery, not only due to the decrease of peak plasma lidocaine concentrations and, consequently, drug toxicity, but also due to the reduction of blood loss. Studies show that for each 1,000 ml of fat removed, 9.7 ml of whole blood was suctioned (4). The tumescent technique is an exceptionally safe method of liposuction that eliminates the necessity of general anesthesia and blood transfusions. It is safer than liposuction under general anesthesia and results in fewer complications (5). I use general anesthesia for combined procedures or when the patient prefers it.

Drug toxicity in liposuction under local anesthesia, related to the peak concentration in plasma, once the most serious complication and limiting factor of this form of anesthesia, has not been a problem since I've used my anesthesia solution, a modification of the original Klein formula (6). Lidocaine can be administered safely in the tumescent technique in significantly higher doses than recommended (7). The blood loss when using the tumescent technique is dramatically reduced compared with the dry or classical "wet" technique (8).

Local Infiltration

We use 20 cc 2% lidocaine, 1 cc adrenaline, 500 cc Ringer's lactate, 5 cc 3% sodium bicarbonate ($NaHCO_3$.) I inject up to 4 L of this solution with a 60-kg patient. There have been no alterations in hemodynamics or in the conscience of the patient during or after surgery. I use a special blunt needle with several holes on the sides of the tip to inject this solution. Usually the amount of anesthetic solution injected is equal to two times the amount of fat we estimate to remove. Average injection is 2 to 3 L of solution. The tumescent state is reached when the area cannot be filled with more fluid. Palpation shows a typical tension of the injected area. We inject the fluid evenly, without pain. The presence of sodium bicarbonate in the formula neutralizes the acidity of lidocaine and balances the pH, decreasing the discomfort of the injection. The solution is injected at body temperature, approximately 37°C. I do not like to inject cold solution because it is very uncomfortable and the possible vasoconstriction does not last long enough to justify it. I prefer to inject one side and treat that side before we turn the patient, rather than injecting the whole body before suctioning. With this solution, we obtain not only a complete analgesia but also very good bleeding control 10 to 15 minutes after injection. If the whole body is injected, the effect of the anesthesia will have passed by the time some areas are reached. It can take up to four hours to treat a large patient. The usual time is one to three hours. With this technique, I can extract 3 to 4 L of fat safely, with no need for blood replacement. I have aspirated up to 9.5 L of fat from one patient, but we should keep in mind that we should not suction more than 8% of the body weight. One liter of decanted fat usually weighs about 1 kg.

For combined procedures I can associate local anesthesia with sedation, epidural, or general anesthesia, but I prefer not to combine liposculpture with surgeries of other specialties and do it only in special cases.

We have modified the traditional tumescent anesthesia formula by using a larger quantity of lidocaine; this is because we treat a more sensitive layer of fat close to the skin. We have doubled the dose of adrenaline for the same reason, as areas closer to the skin tend to bleed more. Sodium bicarbonate will eliminate the pain of the lidocaine injection by neutralizing its pH. We use Ringer's lactate instead of saline because, as we inject large quantities of the aspirated fat, its osmolarity is better preserved in Ringer's than in saline. This very safe formula has demonstrated its efficiency in providing good anesthesia and good bleeding control, as well as controlling postoperative pain, and it does not interfere with fat injection. The fat is centrifuged at 1,500 r/min for one minute, to separate it from the anesthetic fluid.

DISCUSSION

The advantages of the tumescent technique are many; the most important is the lack of bleeding during suction. This happens not only due to the action of the adrenaline injected, but because of the mechanical act of pressure, which closes the capillaries. After a few minutes it can be easily seen that the skin of the area to be treated becomes whiter due to the vasoconstrictive action of the solution infiltrated. Usually a 10- to 15-minute wait is enough to obtain a good constriction. I prefer to inject the anesthesia formula under normal body temperature, that is, heated to 37°C, instead of 4°C as has been advocated by Fournier, mainly because of the discomfort the low-temperature fluid provokes in the patient under local anesthesia. With this most of the shivering and trembling during and after surgery is avoided. Sometimes, during hot weather, we have to cool the operating room for the surgeon's and crew's comfort and we cannot avoid the patient being exposed to cold air temperature during the two to four hours a total-body liposculpture might take. A heating blanket helps to maintain the patient's temperature. The anesthesia solution is injected into the deep layer of the fat tissue, close to the muscle fascia, to avoid skin distortions and allow for a good tumescence of the fat deposit.

The maximum recommended dose of lidocaine chloride with epinephrine is 7 mg/kg for a total dose of 500 mg. It is possible to pass the recommended doses while maintaining low serum levels. It has been shown that it is possible to inject an average of 70 to 90 mg/kg of lidocaine—10 to 12 times over the traditional maximum limit (9). The highest level of lidocaine in the blood of such patients after 15, 30, and 60 minutes was 1.7 mcg/ml (10). Other studies have shown that the safe dose of lidocaine solution is 55 mg/kg and that rapid injection of the anesthetic solution does not increase toxicity (11,12). The peak level of lidocaine in the blood is reached about 12 hours after the infiltration. Only 5% of the injected lidocaine is removed with the aspirated fat. Patients feel comfortable for the first 24 postoperative hours because there are still residual levels of lidocaine.

REFERENCES

1. Toledo LS. Syringe liposculpture. A two-year experience. *Aesthetic Plast Surg* 1991;321–326.
2. Toledo LS. Superficial liposculpture for total body contouring. In: Gasparotti M, Lewis CM, Toledo LS, eds. *Superficial liposculpture.* New York: Springer-Verlag, 1993:29–51.
3. Toledo LS. Lipoescultura superficial. In: Avelar JM, *Anestesia loco-regional em cirurgia estefica.* ed. São Paulo: Hipócrates, 1993:344–349.
4. Klein JA. Tumescent technique for local anesthesia improves safety in large-volume liposuction. *Plast Reconstr Surg* 1993;92:1085–1098; discussion 1099–1100.
5. Hanke CW, Bernstein G, Bullock S. Safety of tumescent liposuction in 15,336 patients. National survey results. *Dermatol Surg* 1995;21:459–462.
6. Toledo LS. Superficial syringe liposculpture. In: Toledo LS, ed. *Annals of the international symposium "Recent advances in plastic surgery"* (RAPS) 90. São Paulo, Brazil, March 3–5, 1990. Rio de Janeiro: Marques-Saraiva, 1990:446–454.
7. Samdal F, Amland PF, Bugge JF. Plasma lidocaine levels during suction-assisted lipectomy using large doses of dilute lidocaine with epinephrine. *Plast Reconstr Surg* 1994;93:1217–1223.
8. Samdal F, Amland PF, Bugge JF. Blood loss during liposuction using the tumescent technique. *Aesthetic Plast Surg* 1994;18:157–160.
9. Lillis PJ. The tumescent technique for liposuction surgery. In: Lillis PJ, ed. *Dermatolgy clinics,* vol 8. Philadelphia: WB Saunders, 1990;439–450.
10. Lillis PJ. Liposuction surgery under local anesthesia: limited blood loss and minimal lidocaine absorption. *J Dermatol Surg Oncol* 1988;14:1145–1148.
11. Coleman WP. 3rd. Tumescent anesthesia with a lidocaine dose of 55mg/kg is safe for liposuction. Editorial. *Dermatol Surg* 1996;22:919.
12. Ostad A, Kageyama N, Moy RL. Tumescent anesthesia with a lidocaine dose of 55mg/kg is safe for liposuction. *Dermatol Surg* 1996;22:921–927.

6

Preparing the Patient

Preparing the face of the patient for surgery poses no difficulty. However, when we have to prepare the body for a procedure that requires several changes of position during the operation, it is better to have special drapes and to follow some simple steps. With the following prepping technique, the surgeon can treat different areas of the body, changing position to allow for a better access. Many of the techniques I use need constant evaluation, moving the limbs and turning the patient on the operating table.

TECHNIQUE

Double surgical drapes cover the operating table. There is a disposable kit by the Tulip Company (San Diego, CA) especially for body liposculpture, which allows good mobilization of the patient without breaking sterility. A nurse scrubs the patient (Fig. 6-1) in the supine position with the heels elevated or resting on a stand (Fig. 6-2). I use povidone-iodine, 10% (Betadine, Purdue Frederick, Norwalk, CT) solution. The entire area is scrubbed. Sterilized socks cover the feet (Fig. 6-3). After scrubbing, the underlying surgical field is removed and the patient lies on sterile fields (Fig. 6-4). A sterile pillow can be placed under the buttocks during the treatment of the abdomen in the supine position (Fig. 6-5) or between the legs for treating lateral thighs in the lateral position (Fig. 6-6) The groin is covered (Fig. 6-7). The areas that are not being treated are also covered, and the surgeon can treat the whole body in a safe manner (Fig. 6-8).

John Panik, a scrub nurse who assisted me in many surgical demonstrations in the United States, developed this prepping system for the Tulip Company.

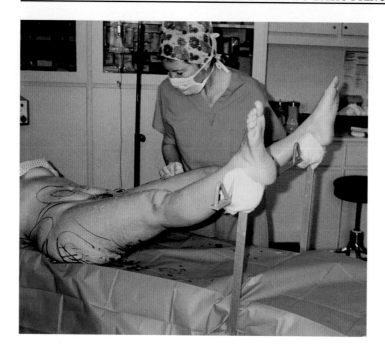

FIG. 6-1. A nurse scrubs the patient in the supine position with the heels elevated or resting on a stand.

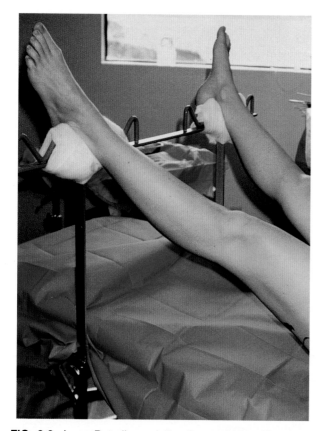

FIG. 6-2. I use Betadine solution for scrubbing. The entire area is scrubbed.

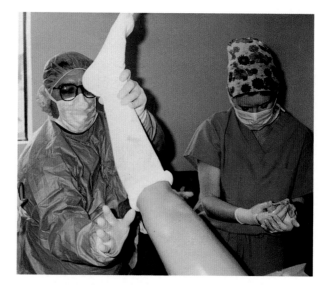

FIG. 6-3. Sterilized socks cover the feet.

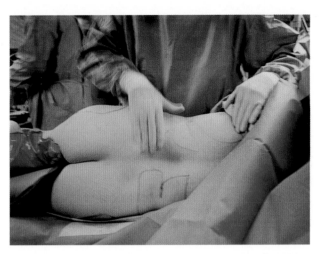

FIG. 6-4. After scrubbing, the underlying surgical field is removed and the patient lies on sterile fields.

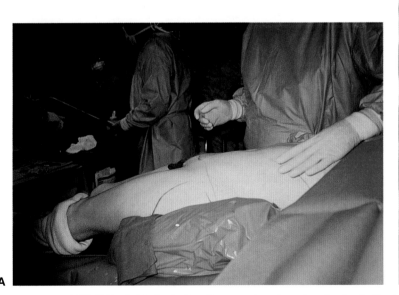

A

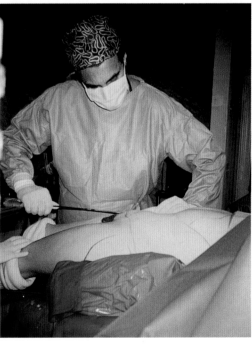

B

FIG. 6-5. A, B: A sterile pillow can be placed under the buttocks during the treatment of the abdomen in the supine position. This increases safety and avoids penetration of the abdominal wall.

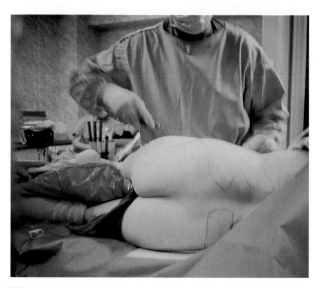

FIG. 6-6. A pillow between the legs helps in treating lateral thighs in the lateral position.

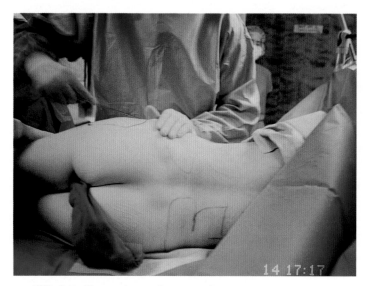

FIG. 6-7. The perineum is covered.

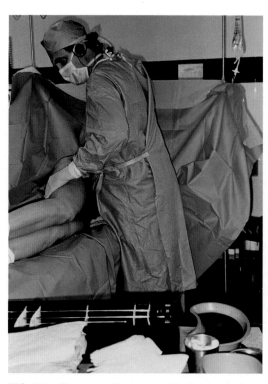

FIG. 6-8. The areas that are not being treated are also covered to treat the whole body in a safe manner.

7

Positioning the Patient

When treating just a single region of the body, the surgery is very straightforward. I just put the patient in the desired position, and operate. However, some patients must be treated in several areas, and need to change positions in the middle of the procedure. The initial difficulty with changing the position of the patient three or four times during a liposculpture procedure is maintaining sterility without having to change too many drapes. If the steps outlined in Chapter 6 for properly prepping the patient are followed, there will be no problem maintaining sterility. The benefits of addressing each area in a specific position are many, particularly to have an immediate view of the treatment result and to avoid sequelae.

POSITIONS

Total liposculpture is when many areas are treated in the same procedure. The following procedure is used for positioning the patient for total liposculpture: First, with the patient in the lateral position (Fig. 7-1), the flanks and the lateral thighs, the buttocks, the gluteal fold, and the "banana" fold (a roll of fat that can form in the subgluteal area) are treated (Fig. 7-2). After treating the other side, the patient is placed in the prone position (Fig. 7-3), and the dorsal region and arms, flanks, dorsal and medial thighs, knees, and calves are treated. In the supine position (Fig. 7-4) the abdomen, breasts, medial thighs, legs, and axyllary region are treated. Bending the patient's knees and spreading the legs helps to complete the treatment of the medial thighs and legs.

Positioning the patient is also important to prevent sequelae and irregularities that can be produced if we do not follow these rules. One of the classical sequelae of liposuction (Fig. 7-5) is a depression that can be produced in the lateral thigh. This is usually due to treating this region in the prone position. When the cannula is inserted through the subgluteal fold to treat the lateral thigh, it is difficult to avoid repeated suction of the subdermal layer during suction. If the patient is placed in the lateral position, it is more difficult to provoke this deformity.

It may be difficult to change positions at first. If a surgeon is used to treating the lateral thighs in the prone position, changing to the lateral position may produce a different evaluation of the amount of fat to be removed. But once the adjustment period is over, it is less likely that a sequela will be produced. During the adjustment it may be useful to put the patient in the standing position in the middle of the procedure, just to make sure one is removing the right amount of fat, and provided that the patient is under local anesthesia. If the patient is too sedated to get up, the action of gravity on the lateral thigh, buttocks, and abdomen can be imitated by pressing the area to see what the adiposity will look like when the patient is standing up (Fig. 7-6).

When treating the abdomen with the patient in the supine position, I hyperextend the abdomen either by bending the table or by placing a pillow under the hips (Fig. 7-7). This is one of the simplest ways to reduce the possibility of abdominal perforation, because if I introduce the cannula into the pubic area it will tend to go through the skin of the epigastrium instead of penetrating the abdominal muscle wall there (Fig. 7-8).

There are other positions in which to treat legs and ankles, adjusting the areas to the best movement of the cannula, depending on the incisions.

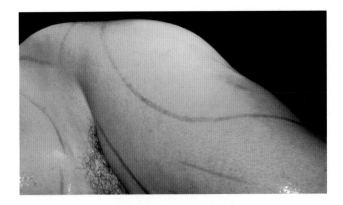

FIG. 7-1. With the patient in the lateral position, the flanks and the lateral thighs are treated. This position gives better access to these two regions, usually through only one incision in the trochanter area.

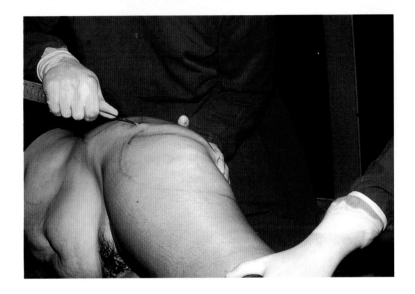

FIG. 7-2. With the patient in the lateral position, the buttocks, the gluteal fold, and the "banana fold" are treated. Sometimes a second incision in the gluteal fold helps with crisscrossing the tunnels from the trochanter incision.

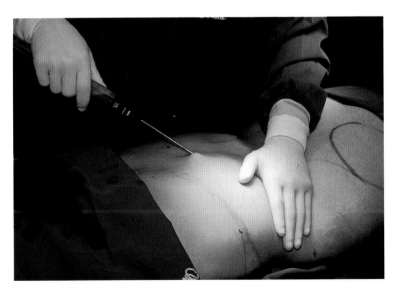

FIG. 7-3. With the patient in the prone position, the dorsal region and arms, flanks, dorsal and medial thighs, knees, and calves are treated. Some regions, such as the arms and dorsal region, can also be treated in the lateral position when the deformity is more lateral, but if it is more medial, depending on the case, the prone position can be used.

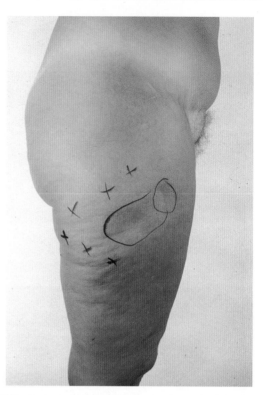

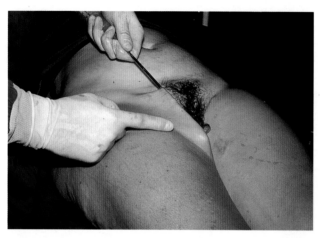

FIG. 7-4. The supine position is ideal for treating the abdomen, breasts, medial thighs, anterior legs, and axillary region.

FIG. 7-5. Liposuction sequela in the lateral thigh produced by treating this region with the patient in the prone position. The cannula is inserted in the subgluteal fold, repeatedly suctioning the subdermal fat layer of the lateral thigh. With the patient in the lateral position it is more difficult to provoke this deformity.

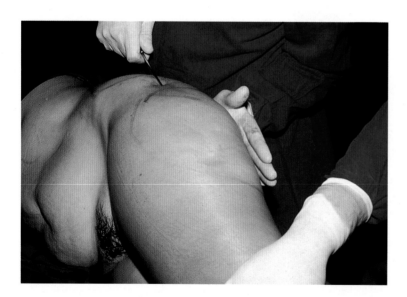

FIG. 7-6. To imitate the action of gravity on the lateral thigh in the standing position, I press the buttocks, protruding the area laterally. This gives an idea of what the adiposity will look like when the patient is standing up.

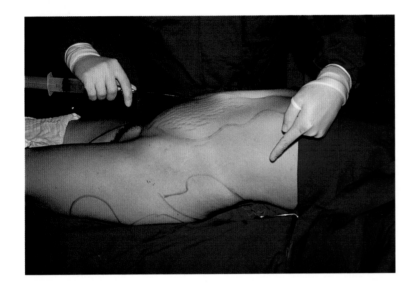

FIG. 7-7. To treat the abdomen with the patient in the supine position, I hyperextend the trunk either by bending the table or by placing a pillow under the hips.

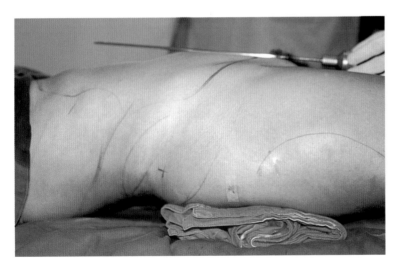

FIG. 7-8. Placing a pillow under the hips is one of the simplest ways to reduce the possibility of abdominal perforation. The cannula introduced into the pubic area will tend to go out through the skin of the epigastrium, instead of penetrating the abdominal muscle wall.

8

Reduction Liposculpture

In the mid 1980s there were a lot of problems associated with liposuction in Brazil and in many other countries. This was before syringe liposculpture was developed, and surgeons were performing liposuction with the aspirator and using mainly the dry anesthesia technique. Consequently, the percentage of blood removed with the aspirated fat was high. Patients would become anemic and very weak in the first postoperative weeks, and would complain of constant headaches; there were a few reported deaths. My patients were afraid of liposuction, and I was looking for an alternative to the liposuction technique. I began using syringe liposculpture and tumescent anesthesia, and realized that this technique was different from traditional liposuction, although I was still aspirating fat. The instruments were different, the method was different, and the results were better. The new method of syringe liposculpture allowed the suction and injection of fat for facial and body contouring. In the cases where I was not reinjecting fat, I was performing reduction liposculpture.

INCISION POINTS

I tell my patients the number of planned incisions, but I also inform them that I will perform as many incisions as necessary to completely treat a deformity. Incisions can be made with a no. 11 blade or with a pokar. Some surgeons claim that the pokar incisions heal better than the ones with the scalpel, but I have seen no difference. The incision must be big enough to allow the cannula to run freely with no friction. This will prevent the occurrence of incisional burns that can cause widening and darkening of the scar. The incision points used for each specific area of the body will be detailed in the text.

CANNULA STROKES

We use long cannulas for large areas of adiposities because the cannula must be at least 10 cm longer than the area to be treated to allow uniform passages and tunnels in the region to be treated. A cannula shorter than the fat deposit can provoke irregularities and makes it difficult to treat the same area uniformly. Surgeons who are beginners in the technique have a tendency to work in short strokes and to treat small areas at a time, because they are not sure of where the cannula should go and how the tissues will behave. Once the initial fear has been overcome, it becomes logical that the deposits should be treated in units, which are finished off before changing to another area. This is because after a certain number of strokes, the area starts bleeding, and one should stop suctioning at that point. Moving to a different site smoothly, one covers the whole area and at the end one gives a final passage with a fine cannula to feather the irregularities.

ASPIRATION OF FAT

Before starting suction, I fill the cannula and 5 cc of the syringe with Ringer's lactate to eliminate the dead space. This will allow a buffering effect when fat gets into the syringe, protecting the fat cells. When the syringe is full, it stops suctioning. With the liposuction machine, suctioning doesn't stop. Fat passes through the tube and gets to the vial. The machine keeps suctioning, and there are sudden variations of negative pressure that can cause breakage of the capillaries and can increase bleeding.

I start with deep suction to improve body contour using 5-mm or 4-mm-gauge cannulas. The number of incisions will depend on each area to be treated. I start suctioning the deep layer in a fan shape, making parallel tunnels. As I get closer to the skin, I change to a smaller-gauge cannula. This will provoke an even retraction of the skin. It is often necessary to crisscross, which means inserting the cannula at a different port or incision and making tunnels perpendicular to the first ones.

After reducing the volume by deep suction, I treat the superficial layer of fat only if there are superficial irregularities (1). This is a continuation of the aspiration of the deep layer, but closer to the skin and using finer cannulas (Fig. 8-1). I treat the areolar layer of fat using fine gauge—2 mm to 3 mm—cannulas. Superficial suction causes skin retraction. Even suction causes even retraction. Irregular suction will cause superficial irregularities. It is very important to use fine cannulas superficially, controlling skin thickness either with the "pinch test" or the outstretched hand. The amount of fat suctioned or injected is recorded on a map.

Depth Control

The pinch test is done with dry skin, but we can run the outstretched hand easily on the skin when we wet the skin surface with an antiseptic solution. That helps not only to slide the hand easily despite the latex glove, but also to observe skin irregularities through the changes of light reflex. We call this "the panel beater trick" because this is a common maneuver when fixing irregularities in the bodies of crashed cars. The other instrument to control regularity is the "pizza roll." It is a 1-cm-thick steel bar with two handles that can be passed over the wet skin of the treated area. An old, thick cannula will do the job. When there is an irregularity, a little bump is felt; it can be corrected by going back with a fine cannula.

"Keep Your Eye on the Ball"

In tennis, the most important thing is to keep your eye on the ball, and in liposculpture, it is to keep your eye at the cannula tip. One should always know where the cannula tip is going. That will prevent many of the secondary problems and sequelae. Although it sounds obvious, there is a tendency to forget the cannula tip and pay attention only to the area being treated.

Treatment of Superficial Irregularities

I also break fibrous adhesions with the 3-mm Toledo V-tip dissector cannula, and inject fat superficially (2) (Fig. 8-2). This layer of injected fat will prevent the adhesions from reattaching, which is what usually happens if one does not inject fat after freeing the adhesions. Very often with superficial liposculpture, a pinch test shows a layer less than 1 cm thick, so it is very important to accommodate this skin in the right place.

OPERATING UNDER TUMESCENT ANESTHESIA

The area is tumescent when it will not retain any more fluid and expels it through the incision. There is a distinct feeling when the area, is palpated like a balloon completely full of water. We pretunnel the marked area with the cannula, to make it easier for suction. Initially the surgeon has to get used to the feeling of treating the infiltrated area, which is different from the noninfiltration dry technique. But generally, the result at the end of the procedure is what we want as a final result, before the area gets swollen. If there is a residual fat deposit, it will have to be treated before the surgery is over, because it will not disappear by itself.

REFERENCES

1. Gasparotti M. Superficial liposuction for flaccid skin patients. In: Toledo LS, ed. *Annals of the second international symposium ''Recent advances in plastic surgery (RAPS) 90.''* São Paulo; Brazil, March 28–30, 1990. Rio de Janeiro: Marques-Saraiva, 1990:441–445.
2. Toledo LS. Secondary liposculpture. In: Gasparotti M, Lewis CM, Toledo LS, eds. *Superficial liposculpture.* New York: Springer-Verlag, 1993:107–121.

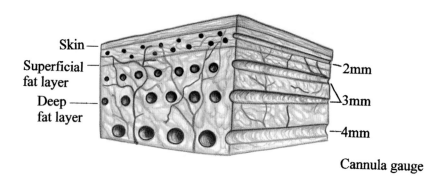

Skin

Superficial fat layer

Deep fat layer

2mm

3mm

4mm

Cannula gauge

FIG. 8-1. A drawing of the fat deposit being treated by liposculpture. The deep layer is treated with the thickest cannulas, following the tunnels principle. As I get closer to the skin, I will change to a smaller-gauge cannula. The superficial layer is treated as a continuation of the deep, producing tunnels of regular suction to provoke a uniform skin retraction.

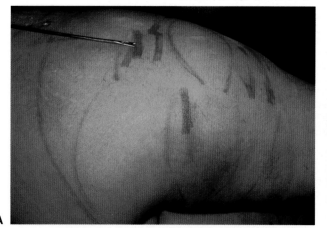

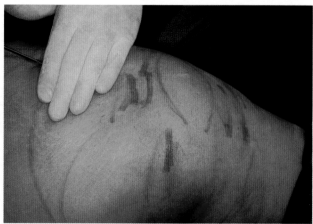

A

B

FIG. 8-2. A: The superficial irregularities are marked with the patient in the standing position. After improving the contour with liposculpture, I will break the fibrous adherences that pull the skin down with the 3-mm Toledo V-tip dissector cannula. **B:** The left hand compresses the area, imitating the effect of gravity. A layer of fat is then injected to prevent the adhesions from reattaching.

9

Contour Augmentation Liposculpture

Fat injection has been a controversial subject for many years (1). After the advent of liposuction made the procedure possible, it became widely practiced. The technique of fat grafting is by far the simplest and most straightforward among the different techniques used for correcting the soft tissues of the facial contour (2–5) and to correct various problems involving buttocks augmentation and re-shaping (6,7), trochanteric depressions (8), breast augmentation, scar depressions, thighs and legs (calf and ankle augmentation), small wrinkles and depressions of the face (9,10) (Romberg's disease), nasolabial fold, and fingers and hands (11). Our findings also allow us to treat superficial irregularities or depressions, "cellulite," and liposuction sequelae (12). Autogenous graft tissue is better than homologous and heterologous tissue for the improvement of body contour to eliminate deep defects in the skin surface (13).

Several papers have been published recently (14,15), on topics including ex-periments in surgery of the lumbar spine (16), using fat grafts thicker than 5 mm applied to prevent postoperative peridural fibrosis followed by computed tomography (CT) scanning (17), and a 40-month postlaminectomy case report (18).

There were also experiments in animals (19–22) showing results in agree-ment with those of Peer consistent with his cell-survival theory. Fat is injected into the subcutaneous tissue or into the muscle, depending on the area and the problem to be corrected, although some reports state that there is a better take of fat cells injected into the muscle (23). Sometimes there is no available muscle to inject fat where it is needed. Reports of experimental studies with rats, state that the fat cells should be previously mixed (24,25), with either basic fibroblast growth factor (bFGF) alone or dextran beads pretreated with bFGF. These findings suggest that the addition of cell-specific bioactive pep-tides, which affect either the preadipocyte cell line and/or the fibroblastic components of the recipient site, improves postoperative fat graft weight maintenance. Insulin was also mixed with fat cells in an attempt to improve cell take (26), but the method was abandoned and the efficacy of insulin treatment remains unproven (27).

Future research endeavors include the growing and multiplying of fat cells *in vitro,* development of preadipocyte transplants, and hormonal manipulation of fat grafts, which will perhaps improve results of transplantation (28). Some surgeons have successful follow-ups after five years (29) and advocate the technique; others find it disappointing (30). Severe complications are rare and are usually due to the use of inappropriate instrumentation (31), or bad technique (32). Fat grafting has also been used successfully in ophthalmology for treatment of enophthalmos (33), and in urology for treatment of sphincteric incontinence (34). Some results suggest that greater long-term soft tissue augmentation and graft survival is obtained with insulin-treated free fat ''pearl'' grafts (35–37). We think the fat graft's viability decreases if the graft diameter is greater than 3 mm because the fat's ability to obtain nutrition through plasmatic imbibition occurs approximately 1.5 mm from the vascularized edge (38).

Most of my patients have one of two types of bodies. The first type, the ''V''-shaped (android obesity), concentrates localized fat from the waistline up, and usually has thin, even masculine, legs and buttocks. The second type, the ''A''-shaped (gynoid obesity), with a very lean upper body, concentrates fat below the waistline. Both types need reshaping of the buttocks.

The first body type usually needs suction of the arms, dorsal region, flanks, upper abdomen, breasts, axilla, neck, and face, and fat injection on the buttocks, thighs, and ankles. I inject fat in the trochanter area and on the upper part of the buttocks. The medial thighs are injected in the middle part. Fat is aspirated from the upper third of the thighs, close to the inguinal region, and from the knee area. People with thin legs, calves, and ankles can have some improvement through fat injection. This is a simpler procedure than calf prosthesis, and the best procedure for the ankles, because there are no good prostheses for the ankles. Fat injection can recontour the calves and ankles in a natural way, improving the contour and adding centimeters to these areas.

The second body type usually needs suction of flanks, lateral thighs, medial thighs, and abdomen, and injection on the buttocks. These patients usually need fat suction in the lower part of the buttocks and injection on the upper part, which, combined with aspiration of the lower third, will give the impression of a buttock lift. If I inject in the lower third, the buttock will get heavier and will drop with the weight.

I schedule facial liposculpture in three stages, the second two months after the first and the third injection four months after the first, because, where the face is concerned, I do not overcorrect. However, I prefer to treat the body, if possible, in one stage. To do that, I can overcorrect by approximately 50%. I do not inject fat in the breasts because of the possibility of microcalcification and confusion in the diagnosis of a possible breast cancer.

Even if I do not plan injection, I always reserve a few syringes of suctioned fat in case it is needed. I have injected up to 500 cc of fat on each side of the buttocks into the muscle, into the fat, and into the subcutaneous tissue, when needed. In the medial thigh I have injected from 100 cc to 300 cc, from 50 cc to 150 cc in the calf, and 50 cc to 80 cc in the ankles (39). These procedures will be explained more fully in the chapters discussing those areas of the body.

FAT INJECTION

I will harvest fat from wherever I can find it. I do not believe that some types of fat are better for reinjection than others—at least not as far as injection into the body is concerned, where one needs great quantities.

I inject my tumescent anesthesia formula to aspirate fat (Fig. 9-1). The diluted anesthesia formula will not damage the fat cells, and Ringer's lactate is more similar to body fluids than saline. I have sent samples of fat cells removed with different samples of my anesthesia formula to be analyzed, removing one of the components per sample, and the number of fat cells viable for reinjection was the same. Cell destruction occurs through excessive manipulation, hence manipulation of aspirated fat should be performed with great care. To avoid oxidation, I do not expose the fat cells to air (Fig. 9-2). I do not sieve fat. If fat cells are mixed with blood, I gently wash them with Ringer's lactate. Then I decant the syringes (Fig. 9-3) and use a transfer to pass fat from one syringe to the other anaerobically (Fig. 9-4). If possible, I centrifuge the syringes for one minute at 1,500 r/min. Normal centrifuges will take only 10-cc syringes (Fig. 9-5), but my manual centrifuge can take the 10-cc and the 60-cc syringes. Centrifuging at this speed and time just separates the anesthesia fluid without breaking the cells (Fig. 9-6). To inject small amounts of fat, I use a 10-cc syringe adapted to a gun (based on a veterinary gun used to administer injections) for precision (Fig. 9-7). For larger amounts I use the 60-cc syringe. The blunt cannula used for injection varies from a 1.5-mm gauge to a 3-mm gauge, depending on the gauge the fat was aspirated with. I inject fat with the same gauge that I have used for aspiration in order to avoid cell destruction. I anesthetize the recipient area with the tumescent anesthesia formula. The injection of the anesthesia helps me estimate the amount of fat to be grafted.

I do not inject lakes of fat. I inject threads in tunnels—the opposite of liposuction—to give the grafts the opportunity of neovascularization (Fig. 9-8). If the grafts are thicker than 3 mm, there will be necrosis at the center of the graft. The other possibility of injection is in 2-mm-thick layers. I use this type of graft for hand rejuvenation.

I prefer not to store fat for reinjection in the future. It is quick, safer, and simpler to obtain more fresh fat when needed. The exception to this rule is for patients who do not have much excess fat but who undergo fat aspiration in the body and will need this fat for injection on the face in the future. There are companies who are now storing fat at a yearly or monthly rate. The patient deposits the fat, and it will be stored under ideal conditions. I prefer to store fat separated into 10-cc syringes.

"CELLULITE"

"Cellulite" is a special type of fat with fibrous adhesions that pull the skin down, producing an effect similar to the buttons of a mattress (40). Deep liposuction alone will not solve this problem and can sometimes make it worse. I use a combination of superficial liposculpture and breaking the fibrous adhesions, plus fat injection to improve superficial skin irregularities. I can obtain a 40% to 50% improvement in skin irregularities in the first procedure, depending on the age and skin type of the patient.

LIPOSUCTION SEQUELAE

Liposuction sequelae patients can be treated by aspirating fat from the areas that were undertreated and injecting it into the depressed areas. I use the Toledo

V-tip dissector cannula to free the fibrous adhesions and inject fat under the depression. These patients are advised that they will need two or more treatments per affected area. The amount of fat to be injected depends on each case. I often perform small procedures under local anesthesia if the patient needs correction in only one region of the body. These procedures are fast, and the patient can return to social activities soon afterwards.

REFERENCES

1. Peer LA. The neglected "free fat graft": its behavior and clinical use. *Am J Surg* 1956;92: 40.
2. Toledo LS. Liposculpture of the face and body. In: Toledo LS, ed.; Pinto ES, coord. *Annals of the international symposium "Recent advances in plastic surgery (RAPS) 89."* São Paulo, Brazil, March 3–5, 1989. São Paulo: Estedão, 1989:177–192.
3. de la Fuente A, Tavora T. Fat injections for the correction of facial lipodystrophies: a preliminary report. *Aesthetic Plast Surg* 1988;12:39–43.
4. Levy S, Pitombo V. Facial graft. In: Toledo LS, ed.; Pinto ES, coord. *Annals of the international symposium "Recent advances in plastic surgery (RAPS) 89."* São Paulo, Brazil, March 3–5, 1989. São Paulo: Estedão, 1989:163–169.
5. Pitombo V, Levy S. Fat graft in the face (evolution). In: Toledo LS, ed.; Pinto ES, coord. *Annals of the international symposium "Recent advances in plastic surgery,"* São Paulo, Brazil, Mar. 28–30 1990. Rio de Janeiro: Marques-Saraiva, 1990:204–211.
6. Matsudo PK, Toledo LS. Experience of injected fat grafting. *Aesthetic Plast Surg* 1988;12: 35–38.
7. Gonzalez R. Buttocks contouring: prosthesis and fat grafting. In: Toledo LS, ed.; Pinto, ES, coord. *Annals of the international symposium "Recent advances in plastic surgery (RAPS) 90."* São Paulo, Brazil, March 28–30 1990. Rio de Janeiro: Marques-Saraiva, 1990:263–272.
8. Lewis CM. Correction of deep gluteal depression by autologous fat grafting. *Aesthetic Plast Surg* 1992;16:247–250.
9. Moscona R, Ullman Y, Har-Shai Y, Hirshowitz B. Free-fat injections for the correction of hemifacial atrophy. *Plast Reconstr Surg* 1989;84:501–507; discussion 508–509.
10. Chajchir A, Benzaquen I. Liposuction fat grafts in face wrinkles and hemifacial atrophy. *Aesthetic Plast Surg* 1986;10:115–117.
11. Aboudib JH, Jr., de Castro CC, Gradel J. Beautifying the hands. In: Toledo LS, ed.; Pinto ES, coord. *Annals of the international symposium "Recent advances in plastic surgery,"* (RAPS) 90; São Paulo Brazil, March 28–30 1990. Rio de Janeiro: Marques-Saraiva, 1990: 197–203.
12. Toledo LS. Syringe liposculpture: a two-year experience. *Aesthetic Plast Surg* 1991;15:321–326.
13. Chajchir A, Benzaquen I. Fat-grafting injection for soft-tissue augmentation. *Plast Reconstr Surg* 1989;84:921–934; discussion 935.
14. Chajchir A, Benzaquen I, Wexler E, Arellano A. Fat injection. *Aesthetic Plast Surg* 1990;14: 127–136.
15. Carraway JH, Mellow CG. Syringe aspiration and fat concentration: a simple technique for autologous fat injection. *Ann Plast Surg* 1990;24:293–296; discussion 297.
16. Deburge A, Benoist M, Lassale B, Blamoutier. [The fate of fat grafts used in surgery of the lumbar spine]. *Rev Chir Orthop* [French] 1988;74:238–242.
17. Van Akkerveeken PF, Van de Kraan W, Muller JW. The fate of the free fat graft. A prospective clinical study using CT scanning. *Spine* 1986;11:501–504.
18. Weisz GM, Gal A. Long-term survival of a free fat graft in the spinal canal. A 40-month postlaminectomy case report. *Clin Orthop* 1986;205:204–206.
19. Wetmore SJ. Injection of fat for soft tissue augmentation. *Laryngoscope* 1989;99:50–57.
20. Matthews RD, Christensen JP, Canning DA. Persistence of autologous free fat transplant in bladder submucosa of rats. *J Urol* 1994;152:819–821.
21. Kononas TC, Bucky, LP, Hurley, C, May, JW, Jr. The fate of suctioned and surgically removed fat after reimplantation: a volumetric and histologic study in the rabbit. *Plast Reconstr Surg* 1993;91:763–768.
22. Curi MM, Singer MJM, Iaconelli LM, Naccache FA, Vianna MR. Autologous fat graft: experimental study. In: Toledo LS, ed.; Pinto ES, coord. *Annals of the international symposium "Recent advances in plastic surgery,"* (RAPS) 90 São Paulo, Brazil March 28–30 1990. Rio de Janeiro: Marques-Saraiva, 1990:213–229.
23. Eppley BL, Smith PG, Sadove AM, Delfino JJ. Experimental effects of graft revascularization and consistency on cervicofacial fat transplant survival. *J Oral Maxillofac Surg* 1990;48:54–62.

24. Eppley BL, Snyders RV, Jr, Winkelmann T, Delfino JJ. Autologous facial fat transplantation: improved graft maintenance by microbead bioactivation. *J Oral Maxillofac Surg* 1992;50:477–482; discussion 482–483.
25. Eppley BL, Sidner RA, Platis JM, Sadove AM. Bioactivation of free-fat transfers: a potential new approach to improving graft survival. *Plast Reconstr Surg* 1992;90:1022–1030.
26. Bircoll M. Autologous fat transplantation. *Plast Reconstr Surg* 1987;79:492–493.
27. Silkiss RZ, Baylis HI. Autogenous fat grafting by injection. *Ophthal Plast Reconstr Surg* 1987;3:71–75.
28. Boyce RG, Nuss DW, Kluka EA. The use of autogenous fat, fascia, and nonvascularized muscle grafts in the head and neck. *Otolaryngol Clin North Am* 1994;27:39–68.
29. Asaadi M, Haramis HT. Successful autologous fat injection at 5-year follow-up. *Plast Reconstr Surg* 1993;91:755–756.
30. Ersek RA. Transplantation of purified autologous fat: a 3-year follow-up is disappointing. *Plast Reconstr Surg* 1991;87:219–227. See comments in: *Plast Reconstr Surg* 1991;88:543–544; *Plast Reconstr Surg* 1991;88:736; *Plast Reconstr Surg* 1991;88:1110–1111; *Plast Reconstr Surg* 1991;87:219–227; discussion 228.
31. Egido JA, Arroyo R, Marcos A, Jimenez-Alfaro I. Middle cerebral artery embolism and unilateral visual loss after autologous fat injection into the glabellar area. Letter. *Stroke* 1993;24:615–616.
32. Trockman BA, Berman CJ, Sendelbach K, Canning JR. Complication of penile injection of autologous fat. *J Urol* 1994;151:429–430.
33. Hunter PD, Baker SS. The treatment of enophthalmos by orbital injection of fat autograft. *Arch Otolaryngol Head Neck Surg* 1994;120:835–839.
34. Santarosa RP, Blaivas JG. Periurethral injection of autologous fat for the treatment of sphincteric incontinence. *J Urol* 1994;151:607–611.
35. McFarland JE. The free autogenous fat graft. A comparison of the fat "pearl" and fat "cell" graft in an animal model. *Ophthal Plast Reconstr Surg* 1988;4:41–47.
36. Shorr N, Christenbury JD, Goldberg RA. Free autogenous "pearl fat" grafts to the eyelids. *Ophthal Plast Reconstr Surg* 1988;4:37–40.
37. Loeb R. Naso-jugal groove leveling with fat tissue. *Clin Plast Surg* 1993;20:393–400; discussion 401.
38. Carpaneda CA, Ribeiro MT. Percentage of graft viability versus injected volume in adipose autotransplants. *Aesthetic Plast Surg,* 1994;18:17–19.
39. Toledo, LS. Superficial syringe liposculpture. In: Toledo, LS, ed. *Annals of the second international symposium "Recent advances in plastic surgery (RAPS) 90,"* São Paulo, Brazil, March 28–30 1990. Rio de Janeiro: Marques-Saraiva, 1990:446–453.
40. Illouz Y-G., de Villers YT. The Anatomy of Subcutaneous Fat. Dankoski E, ed. *Body sculpturing by lipoplasty.* New York: Churchill Livingstone, 1989:34–38.

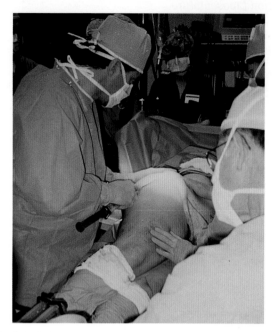

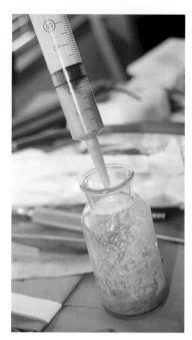

FIG. 9-1. Injecting my tumescent anesthesia formula to aspirate fat. The diluted anesthesia formula will not damage the fat cells. This is a surgical demonstration by Dr. Luis Vasconez at the University of Alabama, Birmingham.

FIG. 9-2. I do *not* keep the fat cells for reinjection in an open vial like this.

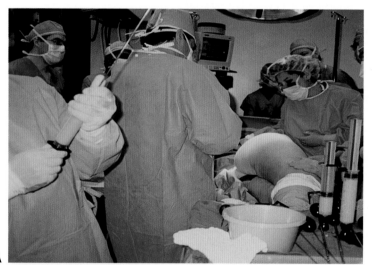

A

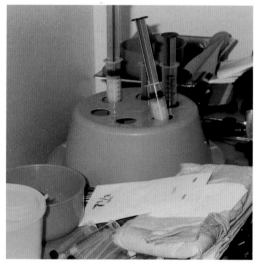

B

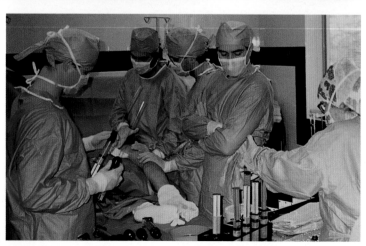

C

FIG. 9-3. A: The syringes with fat are decanted and kept with no air. Manipulation of the fat is kept to a minimum. If the fat is not mixed with blood, it will not be washed. **B:** Fat being decanted in a special stand for 60-cc syringes. **C:** Another stand for 60-cc syringes. Demonstration in Toronto with Dr. Lloyd Carlsen.

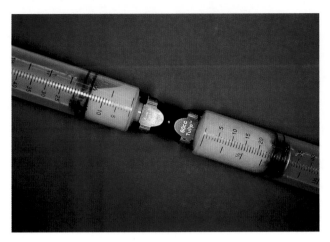

FIG. 9-4. A transfer from a 60-cc syringe to 60-cc syringe being used to pass fat anaerobically.

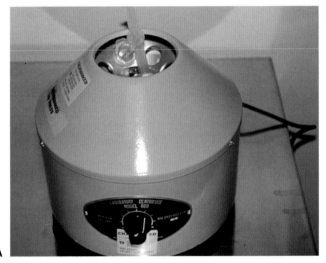

A

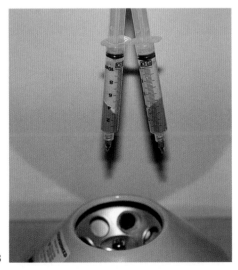

B

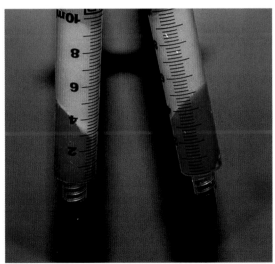

C

FIG. 9-5. A: Normal centrifuges will take only 10-cc syringes. **B:** I centrifuge the syringes for one minute at 1,500 r/min. More time or a faster speed will destroy fat cells. **C:** Centrifuging at this speed and time just separates the anesthesia fluid without breaking the cells.

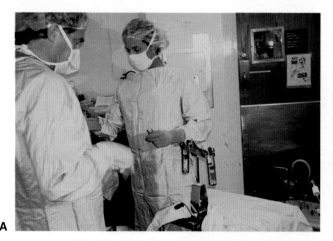
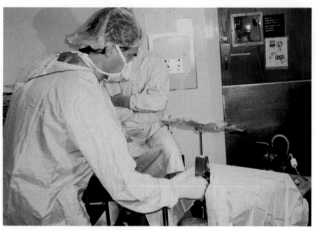

A   B

FIG. 9-6. A, B: The manual centrifuge idealized by Dr. Alberto Hodara, from Porto Alegre, Brazil. It is a simple, low-tech machine that can be sterilized and takes 10-cc and 60-cc syringes. Here it is being used in Baltimore at a surgical demonstration at Johns Hopkins University with Dr. Oscar Ramirez.

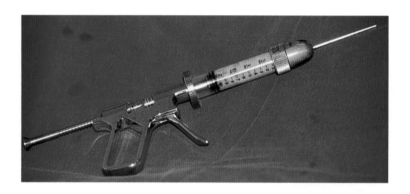

FIG. 9-7. To inject small amounts of fat, I use a 10-cc syringe adapted to a gun for precision.

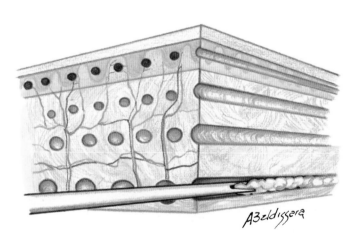

FIG. 9-8. Fat is injected in threads in tunnels—the opposite of liposuction—to give the grafts the opportunity of neovascularization. Grafts thicker than 3 mm will have a central zone of necrosis. The layer that can survive is between 1 and 1.5 mm thick. Grafts that are 3 mm thick have a good chance of taking.

10

Dressings

There are always different opinions about whether or not to use dressings. Even with face-lifts, some surgeons prefer to use the compressive dressing for three days, while others use no dressing at all. It is the same with facial and body contouring techniques. I always use a dressing when I need compression, when I want the skin to retract, or when I want to hold the excess of anesthetic fluid that leaks after the tumescent anesthesia.

TYPICAL POSTOPERATIVE DRESSINGS

I usually apply only a Micropore tape dressing over the incisions for five days, until the stitches are removed. This tape is covered with gauze dressing in the first 24 hours because of leaking of the tumescent anesthesia fluid on the first postoperative day. If I treat superficial irregularities, I apply elastic adhesive tape, usually Microfoam, for five days. Although it is not a rule, I can use suction drains for two to three days to avoid too much bruising, depending on the amount of fat treated. After 24 hours patients can shower but not take a bath. If they have drains, they will have to wait for them to be removed before they shower.

Patients usually wear a girdle day and night for one month. This controls edema and bruising, and secures skin in place to retract to its normal position. But if after 24 hours the dressing is folding and marking the skin, or the girdle is provoking a depression on the treated area, I remove the dressing and girdle and start manual lymphatic drainage to avoid permanent marks. After a few days I reintroduce the girdle.

We have designed special girdles[1] (Fig. 10-1) (1) with triple reinforcements in the abdomen (Fig.10-2), buttocks, and subgluteal area (Fig. 10-3). The girdle fastens with hooks and zippers for the sake of hygiene (Fig 10-4), and tightness

---

[1] Girdle manufactured by Design Veronique/My True Image Mfg. Inc., Oakland, CA. I have no commercial interest in any of the products mentioned.

at the legs can be adjusted with Velcro (Fig. 10-5). There are different models for different procedures, and we advise patients to buy at least two for the initial recovery period. When the swelling starts to disappear, the patient can have the girdle adjusted or just buy a smaller one.

Some patients complain of itching in the first few postoperative days. This must always be checked; if erythema is present, there might be an allergy to the dressing or girdle material (Fig. 10-6). We remove the girdle and start treating the problem seriously before it gets to the point where it can leave permanent marks on the skin. I believe the use of the girdle is especially important after superficial treatment. It is not as important for deep liposculpture, especially during summer in the tropics. Some surgeons don't prescribe girdles, but most of my patients say they feel much more comfortable in the postoperative period while they are wearing girdles.

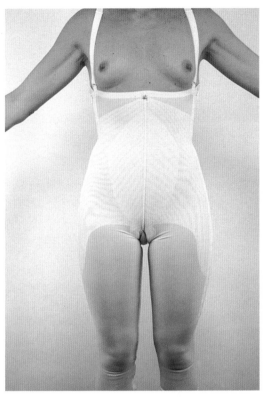

FIG. 10-1. This is a special long girdle used for patients who undergo total liposculpture with treatment from the abdomen and trunk to the knees.

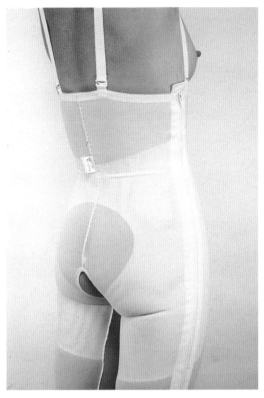

FIG. 10-3. The reinforcement at the buttocks and subgluteal area helps retraction there.

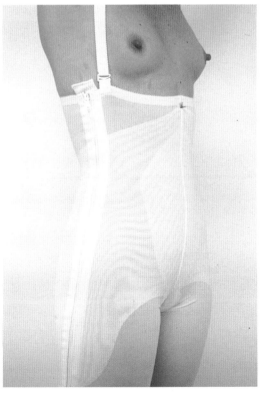

FIG. 10-2. Triple reinforcements in the abdomen will help protect the areas where more retraction is needed.

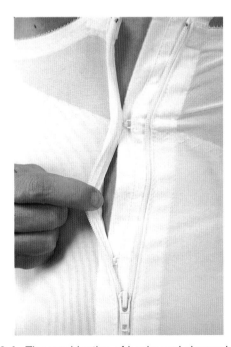

FIG. 10-4. The combination of hooks and zippers improves hygiene and makes it easier for the patient to get dressed independently in the first postoperative days, when it is a bit difficult to move.

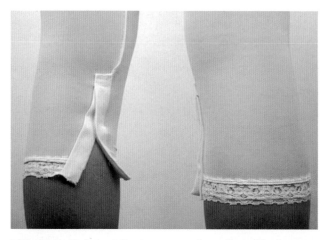

FIG. 10-5. Velcro at the knees can be adjusted to improve comfort when the area is swollen.

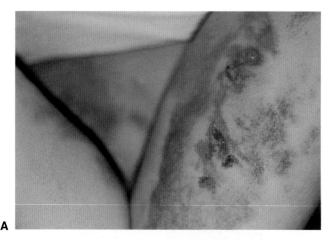

A

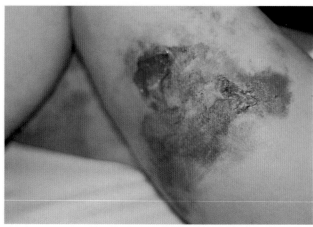

B

FIG. 10-6. A, B: A serious case of allergy to the girdle material. We saw this patient 24 hours after the surgery and she was fine, but 48 hours later there were blisters. The patient wore the girdle for 48 hours more before she came back to the clinic on the fifth postoperative day to remove stitches.

11

Scar Release

During a body contour procedure, the surgeon may find a scar from a previous surgery or accident and will have to deal with it in the procedure. Patients sometimes mention the scar and ask if it will pose any problem during the surgery. Scars can be released during a facial or body contour procedure without the traditional open scar revision (1). Scars in the abdominal area pose a danger in that they can hide an incisional hernia and, therefore, should be examined properly during the physical examination. If there are any clinical doubts about the presence of hernias, a preoperative ultrasound or computed tomography (CT) scan should be performed.

I use the Toledo V-tip dissector cannula as a closed method for the treatment of retracted scars (2,3). By introducing the cannula under the retracted scar, I can release its attachments without reopening and resecting the old scar (4), which in many cases is a mature and inconspicuous scar. This technique is most commonly utilized on a retracted Pfannenstiel incision from a cesarean section combined with superficial suction of the elevated flap. It is also used to treat abdominoplasty scars as well as other scars such as those related to complications of infection and subsequent retraction. Scars on the face and neck and acne scars can be improved using this technique in combination with other techniques.

INSTRUMENTS

The Toledo V-tip dissector cannula is made in different gauges and lengths, and is selected according to the specific problem. For work on the face and in more delicate areas, I use a 1.5- to 2-mm-gauge, 15-cm-long, Toledo V-tip dissector cannula connected to a 10-cc syringe. A 3-mm-gauge, 20 to 35-cm-long version can be connected to a larger 60-cc syringe to treat larger areas on the body. The tips of the V are blunt, and the cutting edge of the cannula is in the inner part of the V. The blunt tips prevent perforation of the skin when working in the superficial layers of fat.

TECHNIQUE

First the cannula is introduced under the scar to break the fibrous adhesions either close to the dermis or deeper, depending on the area of the body. Following the tunnel principle, the cutting action is with in-and-out movements, not laterally. Sharp instruments should not be used for suction, but this cannula, with its blunt protection, works well and does not damage the tissues. Once the cannula has freed the adhesions, the skin depression "pops up." Smoothness is monitored by the constant wetting of the skin with an antiseptic solution, running a hand along the surface of the skin, and changing the angle of the operating table and the lights (Fig. 11-1).

Often I need to suction fat from the surrounding elevated areas; this fat is centrifuged manually at 1,500 r/min for one minute and used for reinjection. I inject a fine layer of fat superficially under the freed scars and, if possible, I build up a depression by injecting threads of fat to elevate it. This helps to prevent the adhesions from reattaching (5). Patients are informed that, depending on the severity of the case, repeated treatments may be necessary. Finally, it is very important to tape the treated area, and I do so with elastic adhesive tape that the patient will wear for five postoperative days.

A word of caution: When treating the abdomen, be aware that there might be unsuspected hernias, usually in the *linea alba* at the epigastrium, even if the normal preoperative exam was done. This area should be avoided.

REFERENCES

1. Almeida RH. Correcting a stairstep deformity secondary to lower abdominal scars by the use of a decorticated hypogastric flap. *Plast Reconstr Surg* 1990;86:1004–1007.
2. Toledo LS. Superficial syringe liposculpture. In: Toledo LS, ed. *Annals of the international symposium "Recent advances in plastic surgery" (RAPS) 90.* São Paulo, Brazil, March 3–5, 1990. Rio de Janeiro: Marques-Saraiva, 1990:446–453.
3. Toledo LS. Syringe liposculpture. A two year experience. *Aesthetic Plast Surg* 1991:321–326.
4. Toledo LS. Secondary liposculpture. In: Gasparotti M, Lewis CM, Toledo LS, *Superficial liposculpture.* New York: Springer-Verlag, 1993:107–121.
5. Verardi G. Fat graft for the prevention of scar formation after laminectomy (macroscopic and microscopic findings in a case report). *Chir Organi Mov* 1990;75:147–51.

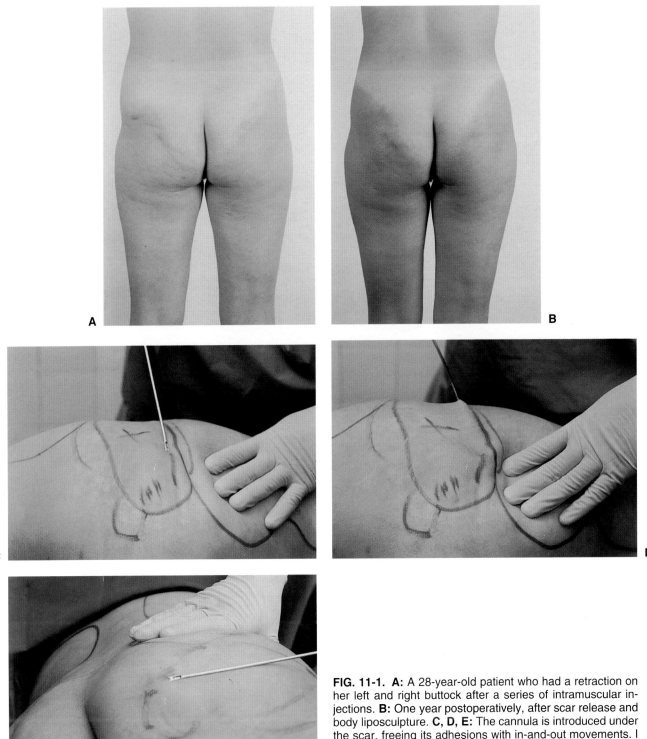

FIG. 11-1. A: A 28-year-old patient who had a retraction on her left and right buttock after a series of intramuscular injections. **B:** One year postoperatively, after scar release and body liposculpture. **C, D, E:** The cannula is introduced under the scar, freeing its adhesions with in-and-out movements. I aspirated 460 cc of fat from the left flank and 320 cc from the right and prepared it for reinjection. I injected 280 cc on the left buttock and 210 cc on the right after freeing the scar tissue.

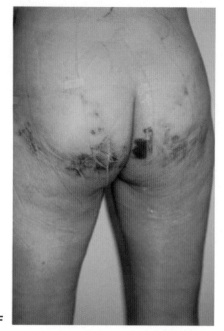

F

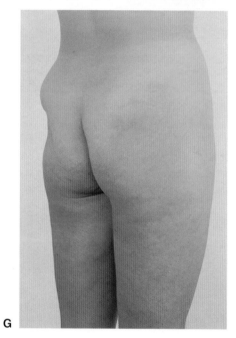

G

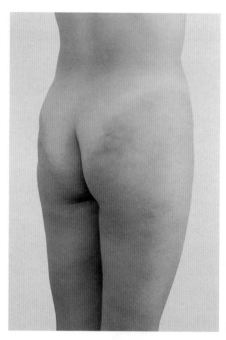

H

FIG. 11-1 *Continued.* **F:** Twenty-four hours postoperatively. **G:** Pre-operative picture with excess fat on the flanks and lateral thighs and a depression on the buttocks. **H:** One year postoperatively, with a good correction of the defect. The patient has been informed of the possibility of a second procedure and she has decided to have it soon to improve the result even more.

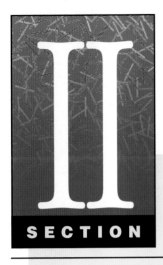

SECTION II

Body Contouring

12

The Flanks
and Lateral Thighs

I usually treat the flanks and lateral thighs as a unit in body contour procedures; it makes sense to me to address them together. Most of the body work I perform requires some treatment in these areas, and it is probably here that the results are most apparent, with or without clothes.

Overweight and exaggerated fat deposits can appear in early adolescence. I usually perform liposculpture on patients over 16 years; there might be exceptions depending on the circumstances of each case. The lateral thighs become heavy during the childbearing years, the mid-twenties to mid-thirties (Figs. 12-1–12-4). This can be related to lack of exercise, hormonal disturbances, or genetic vulnerability. Differences in size between the upper and the lower parts of the body can make buying clothes a problem (Figs. 12-5, 12-6). The contour of the lateral thigh is allied to that of the buttock, and recontouring procedures usually involve both areas. For the sake of clarity, and to define the specific problems of these regions, we have separated the lateral thigh from the buttock in this text.

After menopause, beginning in the mid-forties (Fig. 12-7), the hips have a tendency to become boxy, and the contouring of this area is like a body rejuvenation procedure. Patients are measured, weighed, and photographed pre- and periodically postoperatively. I work with a picture of the patient standing, so that I can observe the changes. The preoperative examination is carried out with the patient in the standing position and lying down. By bending the patient's legs when they are lying down, the contour changes that will take place in the areas to be operated on can be seen (Figs. 12-8, 12-9).

INSTRUMENTS

We use 60-cc toomey-tip syringes, Pyramid-tip cannulas that range from 25 to 35 cm long, with gauges varying between 3.5 and 5 mm. Locks and transfers must be available, and we always store some of the aspirated fat in the syringe for reinjection.

ANESTHESIA

Procedures involving the flanks and lateral thighs are usually performed in conjunction with other areas of the body; I use local tumescent anesthesia combined with sedation. Sedation is not normally necessary for those patients undergoing small corrections, (see anesthesia formula in Chapter 5).

POSITION

After prepping, the patient is turned to the lateral position (Figs. 12-10, 12-11). This is a good angle for seeing the deformities to be treated in the flank and lateral thigh area. Before 1988, patients were placed in either the supine or prone position and it took some time to adapt to the different approach, but the irregularities are more clearly visible and a much better access is obtained to these areas. It is also a safer position with less risks of causing sequelae. The possible initial difficulty in turning the patient three times during the procedure is made easier by the specific prepping that does not require changing the drapes every time the patient is moved. The use of local anesthesia with sedation is also helpful because I can ask the patient to turn on the operating table.

INCISIONS

Through one trochanter incision we can reach most of the lateral thigh and the "banana fold" area. A second incision in the infragluteal fold and a third incision in the midfemoral lateral area might be necessary for crisscrossing purposes. The sacral incision is used when there is excess fat to be removed from the upper buttock (Fig. 12-12).

FAT ASPIRATION

Deep Suction

The procedure can begin 10 to 15 minutes after the anesthesia infiltration. With a young patient with moderate-sized fat deposits and good skin tone and elasticity, good results can be obtained through deep liposculpture alone. The body contour is improved with deep suction. I usually first start suctioning the lateral thighs, because this is usually more difficult and time-consuming than the flanks. Deep liposculpture will reduce the volume of the adiposities and improve the contour. The amounts of aspirated fat, injected fat, and the anesthetic fluid are recorded, and it is possible to know exactly how much was removed from each area.

Superficial Suction

After deep plane liposculpture to reduce the volume of the deformity, I treat the superficial (areolar) layer of fat if there is an indication. The indications are the presence of flaccidity and superficial irregularities, which are more common in older patients. If there is flaccidity and only the deep layer of fat is treated, the area becomes heavy and irregular. There will be a tendency to form skin irregularities because the skin cannot retract uniformly (Figs. 12-13, 12-14). To treat the superficial layer of fat, we use Pyramid or one-lateral-hole tipped cannulas with a 2-mm to 3-mm gauge and 25 to 35 cm long. With the use of these fine cannulas superficially, the thickness of the flap can be controlled, and the outstretched hand technique guides the tip of the cannula (Fig. 12-15). The more superficial the suction, the better the retraction, and the more even the suction, the more even the retraction of the skin will be. If the suction is irregular, the defects will show, and superficial irregularities will be created. The wet skin also aids in following the passage of the cannula (see Fig. 12-15C).

Superficial irregularities can also be treated by breaking the fibrous adhesions with our 3-mm-gauge Toledo V-tip dissector cannula and injecting fat superficially, as previously mentioned (Fig. 12-16). Molding the injected area with the fingertips to finalize a uniform result can also help break the remaining adhesions. To check the irregularities, I like to work with the skin wet, with a mixture of Ringer's lactate and povidone-iodine 10% (Betadine, Purdue Frederick, Norwalk, CT). This solution also helps with sterilization, and the hand is much more sensitive on the wet skin. By changing the position of the operating lights and by moving the patient I can see the changes in the irregularities using the light's reflection on the skin (Fig. 12-17). Pressing the buttock tissues to imitate gravity makes the lateral thigh defects more evident, and I treat them individually with a 2-mm gauge and with the V-tip dissector cannula (Fig. 12-18). Figures 12-19 through 12-24 show examples of liposculpture of the flanks and thighs.

At the termination of the surgery, some patients, especially those with flaccid skin, will have a very fine layer of fat attached to the skin. This flap covers the final sculptured shape and should be treated carefully and secured well in its correct place. Patients should be careful not to provoke permanent folds or marks on the treated areas. This can happen if, for example, a patient returns to work too soon and sits for hours on end at a desk. The girdle will likely fold at the waistline and cause some folding of the skin that can be difficult to treat. A girdle that is too tight can also cause these problems. Loose clothing is recommended, and if the girdle is too tight, it should be replaced with one of a larger size.

FAT INJECTION

Usually suction and injection of fat are combined when treating the flanks and lateral thighs (Fig. 12-25). The augmentation of the buttock and trochanter areas improves the contour of the flanks and thighs, giving a more uniform curve to the body (Figs. 12-26, 12-27). I keep the aspirated fat in the syringes in case it is needed for reinjection. When planning the injection of large amounts of fat, the fat will be centrifuged to separate it from the anesthesia fluid, which will be decanted while I am still aspirating. Then it will be injected into the trochanter area, the buttocks, or under superficial irregularities. I usually overinject by about 50%.

POSTOPERATIVE CARE

Elastic adhesive tape usually stays on for five days, but it is removed if there are marks on the skin (Fig. 12-28), as is the girdle. Usually patients have to wear a girdle for one month to control edema and bruising. If the dressing or the girdle starts provoking folds, I tell the patients to stop wearing it and indicate only manual lymphatic drainage.

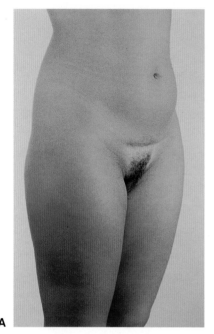
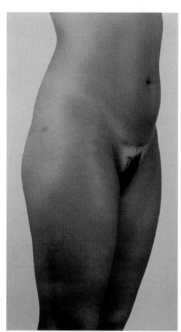

A   **B**

FIG. 12-1. **A:** A 30-year-old patient with a mild excess of fat in the abdomen, lateral thighs, and flanks. **B:** One month postoperatively, after deep liposculpture of the abdomen, lateral thighs, and flanks. No superficial suction was needed. She had a weight reduction of only 1 kg. The measurements were much smaller than preoperatively. The patient is still swollen.

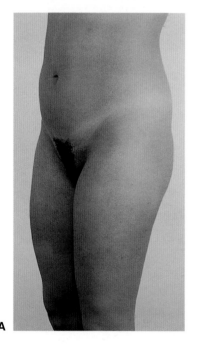
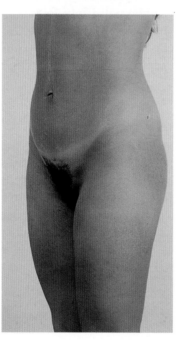

A   **B**

FIG. 12-2. **A, C:** Preoperative photo of a 34-year-old patient with excess fat in the flanks and abdomen. **B, D:** Three months postoperatively, after deep liposculpture of the abdomen and flanks, with a reduction of several centimeters in the patient's measurements.

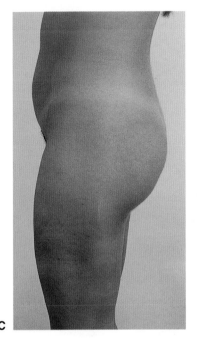

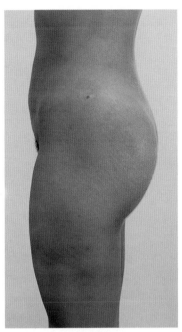

D **FIG. 12-2.** *Continued.*

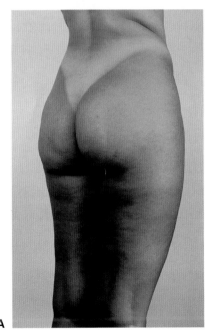

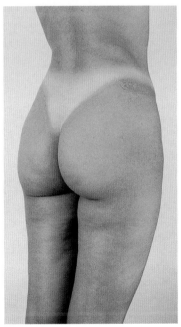

A **B**

FIG. 12-3. A: Preoperative photo of a 29-year-old patient with excess fat in the flanks and lateral thighs. Even with her arms up it is possible to see the folds in the flanks. **B:** Three months postoperatively, after deep liposculpture of the lateral thighs and superficial liposculpture of the flanks.

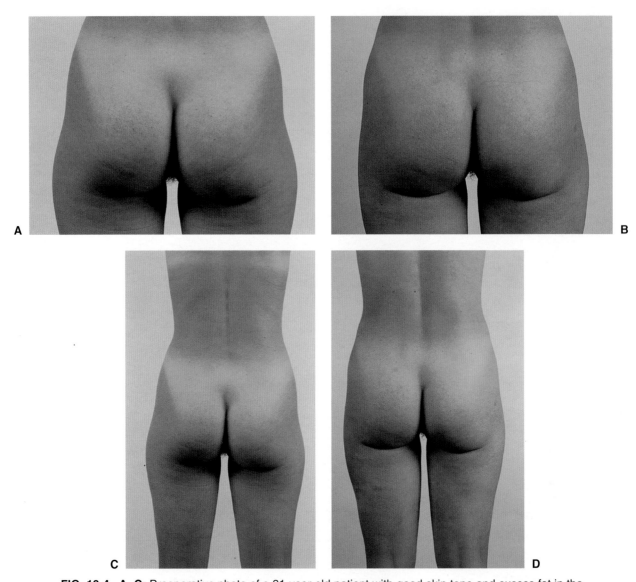

FIG. 12-4. A, C: Preoperative photo of a 31-year-old patient with good skin tone and excess fat in the flanks and lateral thighs. **B, D:** One month postoperatively, after deep liposculpture removing 100 cc of fat from each flank and 300 cc from each lateral thigh.

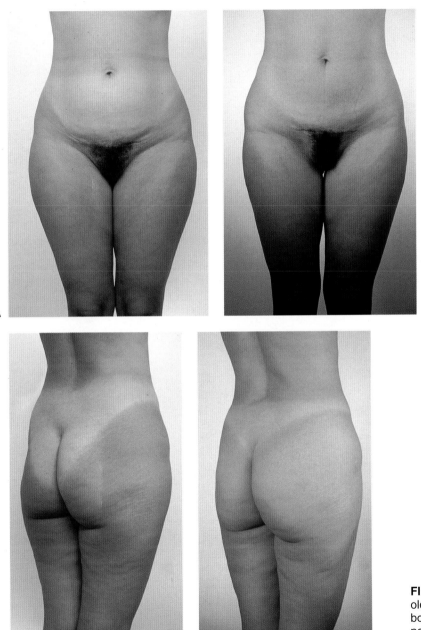

A

B

C

D

FIG. 12-5. A, C: Preoperative photo of a 35-year-old patient with thighs disproportionate to her upper body. **B, D:** Three months postoperatively, after superficial liposculpture of the lateral thighs with the removal of 760 cc of fat per side.

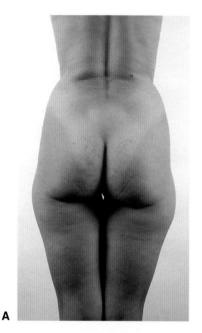
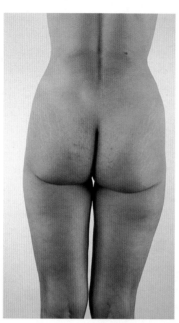

FIG. 12-6. A: Preoperative photo of a 42-year-old patient with excess fat in lateral thighs and a little excess on the flanks. **B:** Four-months postoperatively, after superficial liposculpture of the lateral thighs with the removal of 400 cc of fat per side, plus removal of 60 cc from each flank.

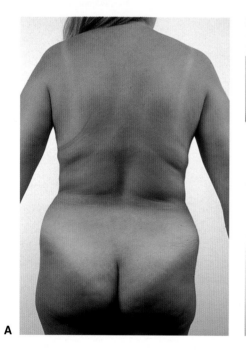
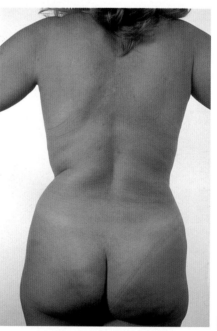

FIG. 12-7. A, C: Preoperative photo of a 48-year-old patient who complained that her body had become "boxy" after she entered menopause. There was excess fat in the flanks and dorsal region. **B, D:** One year postoperatively, after superficial liposculpture of the flanks and dorsal region. She has developed a younger shape.

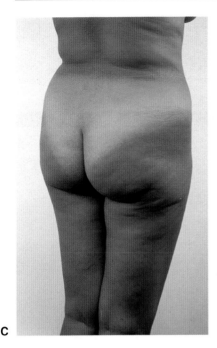
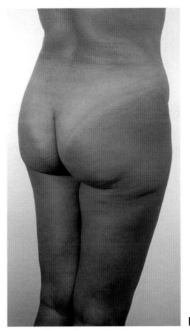

C   D   **FIG. 12-7.** *Continued.*

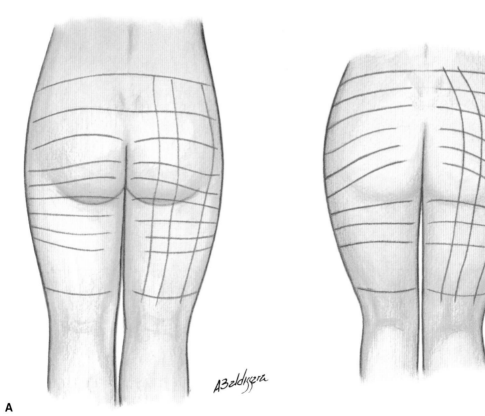

A   B

FIG. 12-8. A: How patient position changes the markings. The patient standing up. **B:** The patient bending over. The markings on the gluteal fold become wide apart.

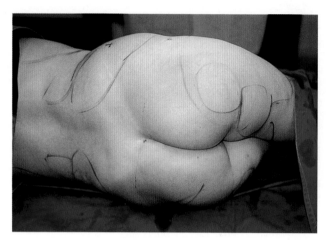

FIG. 12-9. Intraoperative picture of superficial liposculpture with the patient's markings being affected by bending the patient's legs.

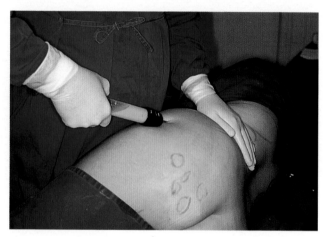

FIG. 12-10. Suctioning fat from the flanks with the patient in the lateral position.

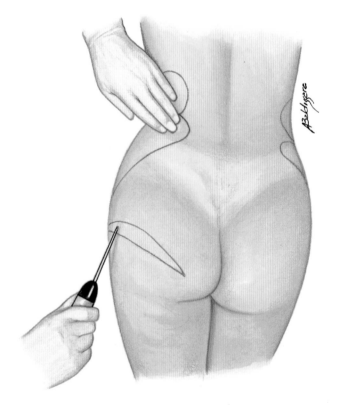

FIG. 12-11. Aspiration of fat from the flanks in the lateral position. There is easy access to the whole area. It is also a good position for treating the lateral thighs and buttocks.

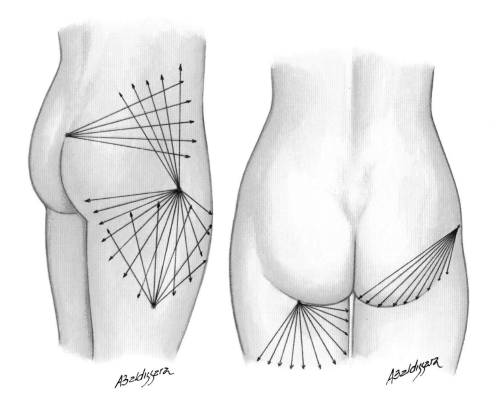

A

B

FIG. 12-12. A, B: Through the trochanter incision I treat the lateral thigh and the "banana fold." Sometimes a second incision in the infragluteal fold and a third incision in the midfemoral lateral area might be necessary for crisscrossing. The sacral incision is used when there is too much excess fat in the upper buttock.

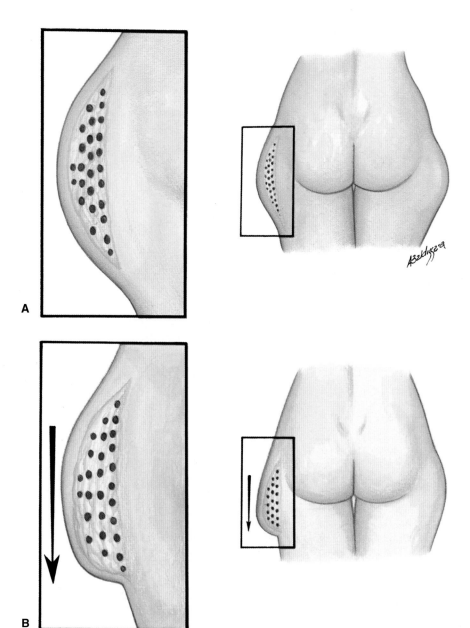

FIG. 12-13. A: If there is flaccidity and only the deep layer is treated, the superficial flap gets too heavy. **B:** There will be a tendency for skin irregularities to form because the skin cannot retract uniformly.

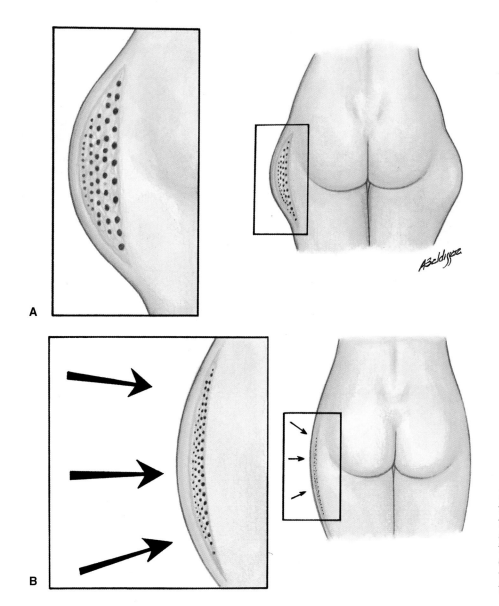

FIG. 12-14. A: If the deformity is treated with superficial liposculpture using fine cannulas, we obtain a lighter superficial flap. **B:** The flap treated uniformly with superficial liposculpture will be lighter and will retract better and more uniformly.

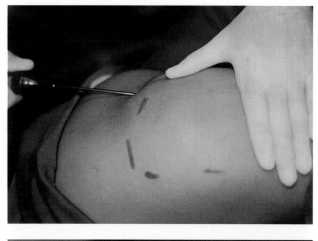

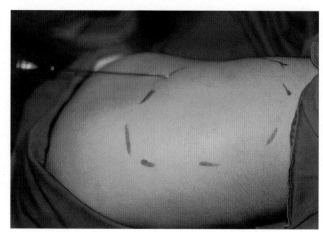

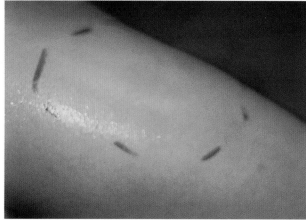

FIG. 12-15. A, B: I control the thickness of the flap and where the tip of the cannula is going with my outstretched hand. An even superficial suction will result in an even retraction. **C:** The wet skin, together with reflections from the lights, help the surgeon find irregularities.

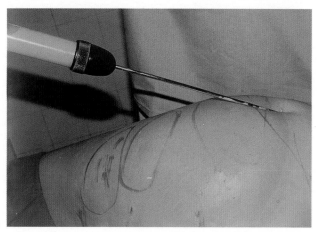

FIG. 12-16. A: Treatment of superficial irregularities on the lateral thighs. I aspirate fat from the elevated areas and prepare them for reinjection.

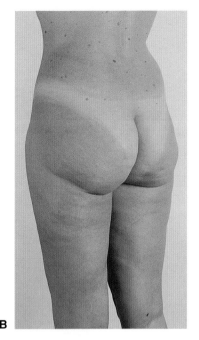
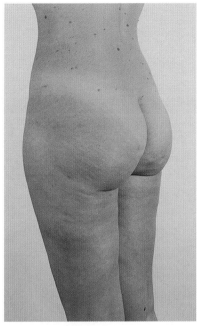

B **C**

FIG. 12-16. *Continued.* **B:** Preoperative photo of the same patient with small irregularities on the lateral thigh. **C:** Six months postoperatively, with improvement of the area.

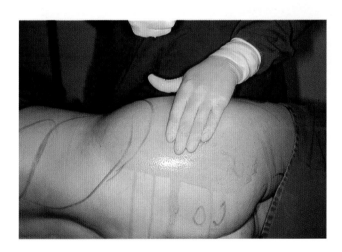

FIG. 12-17. By changing the lights or by moving the patient I can assess the changes in reflections of light on the skin. I also run my hand on the wet skin to feel any elevations or depressions.

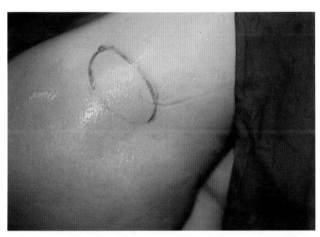
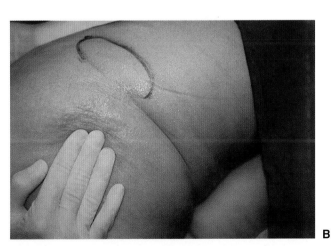

A **B**

FIG. 12-18. A, B: Pressing the buttock tissues to imitate gravity makes the lateral thigh defects more evident. I treat them individually with a 2-mm gauge and with the V-tip dissector cannula.

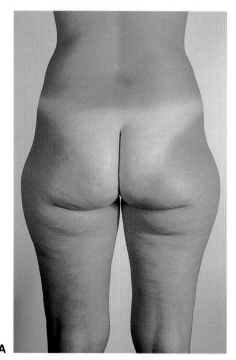

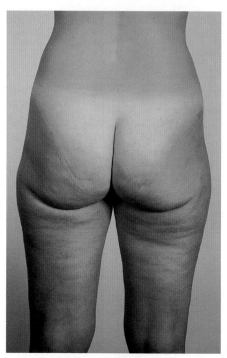

A

B

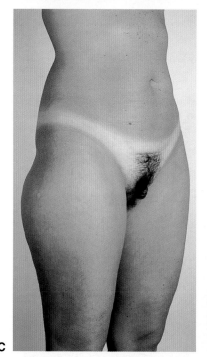

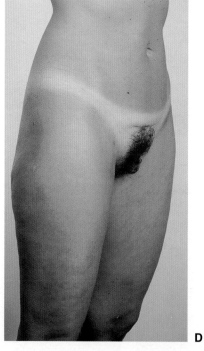

C

D

FIG. 12-19. A, C: Preoperative photo of a 28-year-old patient with excess fat in the flanks, buttocks, lateral thighs, and "banana fold." **B, D:** Three months postoperatively, after body liposculpture. The patient had lost 3 kg. I removed 300 cc from each flank and 650 cc from each lateral thigh, including the buttock. It is important not to remove too much fat from a patient with flaccid skin like this one. It is very easy to overdo it and end up with a dropped buttock. I stopped when I thought I had reached a limit. There is still some excess in the "banana fold," but she has had some improvement there. The patient rated the contour as "much better."

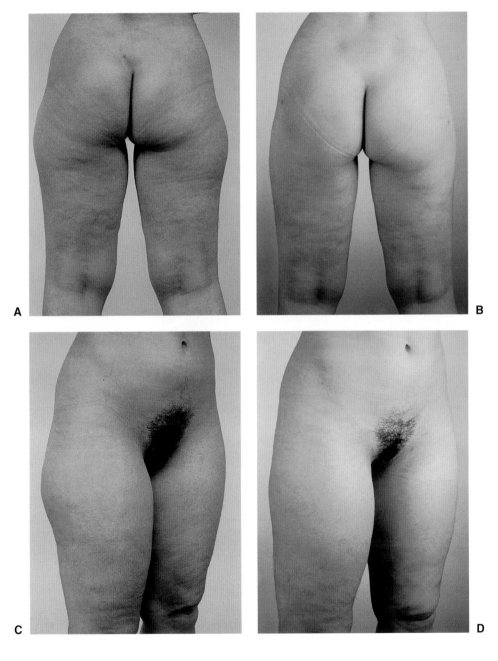

FIG. 12-20. A, C: Preoperative photo of a 37-year-old patient with circumferential excess fat in the thighs. **B, D:** Four months postoperatively, after circumferential liposculpture of the thighs. I removed 260 cc from each medial thigh, 240 cc from the anterior thigh, 105 cc from the medial knees, 530 cc from the lateral thighs, and 60 cc from the posterior thigh.

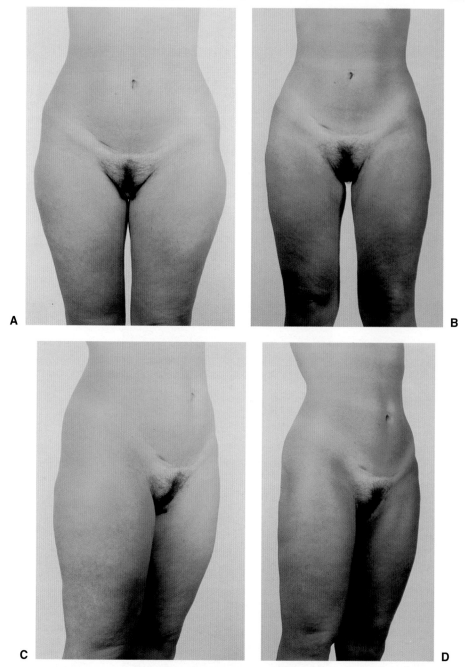

FIG. 12-21. A, C, E: Preoperative photo of a 33-year-old patient with excess fat in the flanks, medial thighs, and lateral thighs. **B, D, F:** Six months postoperatively, after the removal of 140 cc per side from the flanks, 350 cc from the lateral thighs, and 120 cc from the medial thighs. I injected 135 cc on each buttock and 20 cc on the irregularities of the left thigh. The patient weighed 51 kg preoperatively and 48 kg postoperatively. She lost 3 cm on the waist, 4 cm on the hips, and 4 cm on each thigh.

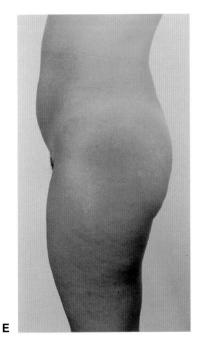

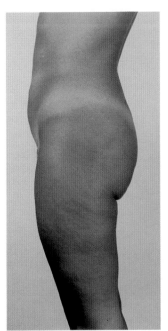

E   F   **FIG. 12-21.** *Continued*

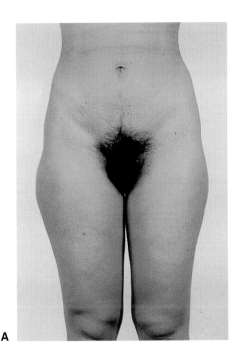

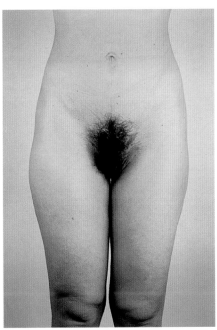

FIG. 12-22. A, C: Preoperative photo of a 35-year-old patient with flaccid skin and excess fat on the lateral thighs. **B, D:** One year post-operatively, with a good retraction of the lateral thigh skin. There was a 6-cm reduction on each thigh. The weight of the patient was not altered. *Figure continues on next page.*

A   B

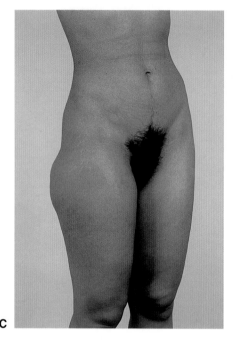

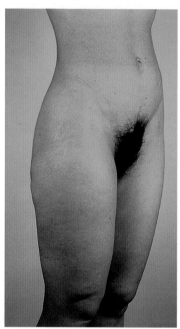

C   D   **FIG. 12-22.** *Continued*

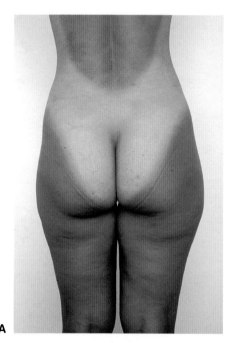

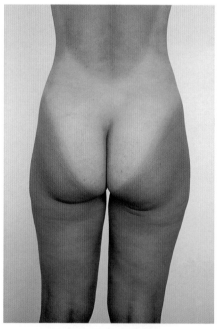

A   B   **FIG. 12-23. A:** Preoperative photo of a 36-year-old patient with flaccid skin and excess fat on the lateral thighs and "banana fold." **B:** Four months postoperatively, with a moderate improvement. This is a type of buttock that I would rather suction less, even if it necessitated a second procedure, than provoke a sequela by oversuctioning.

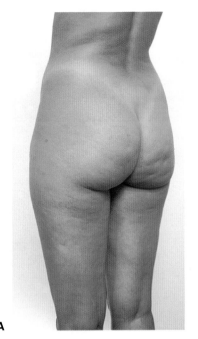
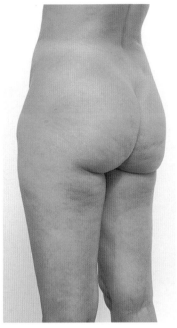

FIG. 12-24. A: Preoperative photo of a 29-year-old flaccid-skin patient with excess fat on the flanks, buttocks, and lateral thighs. My evaluation of improvement in the superficial irregularities of this patient was about 50%. **B:** Analyzing this six-month postoperative photo I would confirm that, in my evaluation, this patient had a 50% improvement.

A   B

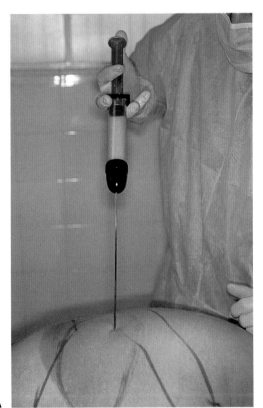
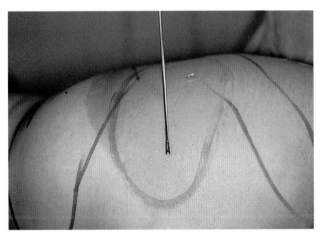

A   B

FIG. 12-25. A, B: Injection of fat into the trochanter and buttock regions. The areas marked in *blue* are areas of fat suction. The area in *red* is where fat is injected. Fat is injected into the gluteal muscle and the subcutaneous tissue in 3-mm threads. The take of the graft in this area is usually between 30% and 50%.

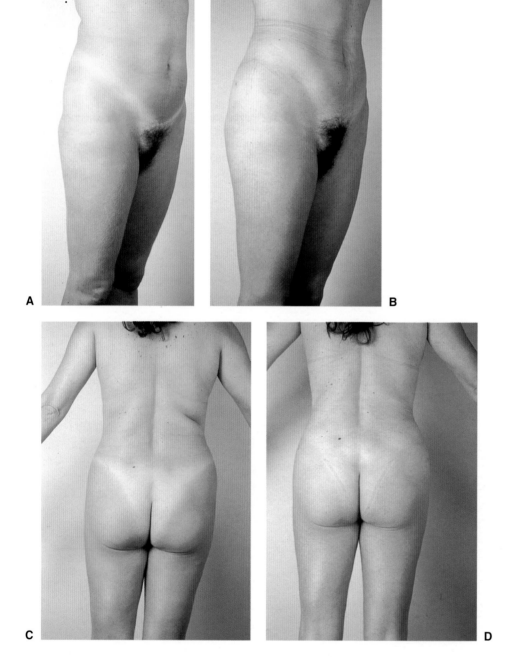

A

B

C

D

FIG. 12-26. A, C, E, G: Preoperative photo of a 28-year-old patient with excess fat in the abdomen, dorsal region, and flanks, and lack of fat on the buttocks. **B, D, F:** One year postoperatively, after liposculpture, suctioning fat from the abdomen, flanks, and dorsal region, and injecting 300 cc on each buttock. There was a lasting contour improvement. **H:** 6½ years postoperatively, still maintaining the contour.

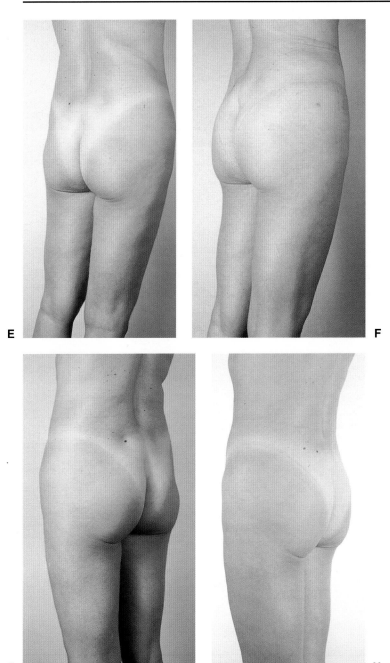

E

F

G

H **FIG. 12-26.** *Continued.*

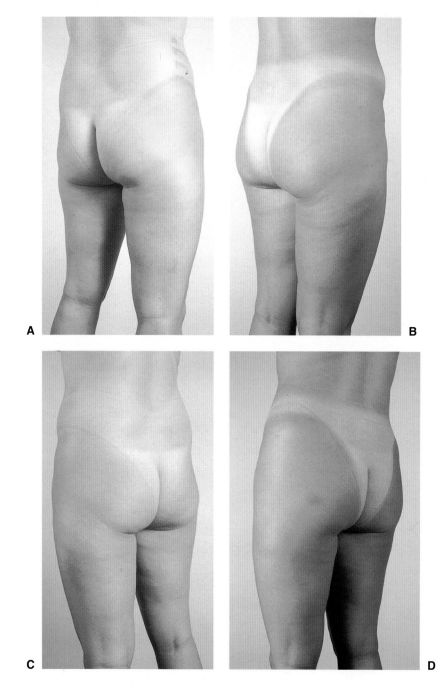

A

B

C

D

FIG. 12-27. A, C, E: Preoperative photo of a 27-year-old patient with excess fat in the abdomen and flanks, and lack of fat on the buttocks. **B, D, F:** One year postoperatively, after suction of fat from the abdomen and flanks and injection of 480 cc of fat in each buttock. There was a contour improvement that produced a complete change of lifestyle and habits in this patient, as demonstrated by her bathing suit marks.

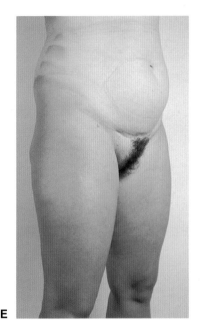
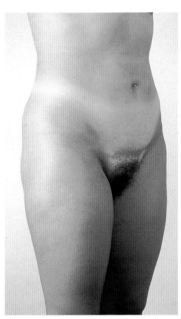

E   F   **FIG. 12-27.** *Continued.*

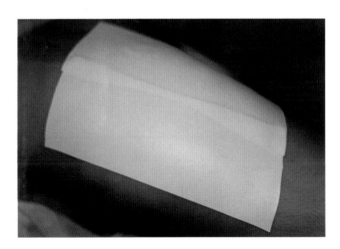

FIG. 12-28. A dressing with Microfoam can stay for one to four days after superficial liposculpture to keep the tissues in place.

13

The Medial Thighs

The medial part of the thighs is a region that requires special treatment. Skin tone in that area is usually more flaccid than on the lateral thigh, especially close to the inguinal region. The adiposities can be divided into three areas: the upper or cephalic part, close to the groin, the middle part, and the knee area (Fig. 13-1). Each of these areas has its peculiarities. The skin thickness also varies between these parts, and scraping dermis of the thin-skinned areas should be avoided. It is common to see a deformity where there is excess fat in the upper third and knee and a depression in the middle part (Fig. 13-2). Other thighs are uniformly thick, without the middle depression (Fig. 13-3). The treatment of the medial thighs is rarely isolated; it is usually combined with treatment of other areas of the body during a body liposculpture.

The choice of the procedure always depends on the patient's needs. The younger the patient, the better the skin tone should be, and liposculpture should be the technique of choice (Fig. 13-4). Some patients who have a more flaccid skin tone but who will accept an improvement in shape with the same flaccidity can also be operated on through superficial liposculpture alone (Fig. 13-5). Although there are some exceptions, with older patients, we have to think more about dermolipectomies and less about liposculpture if we want to achieve a good contour. Patients with very flaccid skin who want to get rid of excess skin and fat are candidates for a thigh lift. I will perform the thigh lift dermolipectomy either combined with liposculpture or without it.

The difficult indication is with the borderline cases. Because I am known for minimally invasive procedures, patients often want to ''stretch'' my indications, trying to ''force'' me to perform superficial liposculpture where there is a clear indication for a thigh lift. Depending on the case, I will propose a reduction in the volume of the medial thigh area with around 50% improvement in contour, try not to worsen the flaccidity, and postpone the thigh lift. Through computer imaging I can show the type of improvement they can expect (Fig. 13-6).

Some older patients are obvious candidates for thigh lift but do not want to undergo open surgery. They do not wear bathing suits, do not have too much time to recover from open surgery, want a cheaper procedure, and prefer liposculpture. It has to be established beforehand that the result in these cases will never be the same as thigh lifts—there will always be flaccid skin if it is not removed (Fig. 13-7). Finally, there are cases where there is the indication for aspiration of fat in the upper part of the thigh and knees and fat injection in the middle part of the thigh (Fig. 13-8). I also treat some patients with poliomyelitis sequelae who need fat suction from a different part of the body and fat injection in the atrophed muscles to try to even out deformities (Fig. 13-9).

INSTRUMENTS

For liposculpture, I use a Tulip system (The Tulip Company, San Diego, CA), with 60-cc toomey-tip syringes and 2-mm to 3.7-mm-gauge Pyramid-tip cannulas for superficial liposculpture. For fat injection in the middle part I use a 3-mm-gauge, one-lateral-hole cannula or a 3-mm-gauge, 45-degree cut blunt tip. For the thigh lift dermolipectomy, I use general plastic surgery instruments.

ANESTHESIA

For liposculpture, I usually use a combination of IV sedation and local tumescent anesthesia. When dermolipectomy is also performed, I use general anesthesia combined with local tumescent infiltration. First I suction and then I do the dermolipectomy. If the syringe is used in combined procedures, it is always necessary to aspirate first and then do the resection, to keep the vacuum in the syringe.

POSITION

I treat the medial thighs with patients in the supine position (Fig. 13-10). The knees can be straight or bent, depending on the area (Fig. 13-11). Sometimes during the procedure it is necessary to move the legs to assess the deformity. When it is necessary to treat the posterior part of the medial thighs, it might be necessary to put the patient in the prone position (Fig. 13-12). The scheme for turning the patient on the operating table is established before I start operating, and I simply follow the sequence.

INCISIONS

I use one or two incisions to treat the anterior area of the upper part of the thighs, depending on the problem—one in the inguinal region and one in the mid-part of the medial thigh (Fig. 13-13). When the treatment of the posterior upper part of the thighs is combined with the anterior, another incision in the gluteal fold is necessary. The medial knees are usually treated with one or two incisions in the medial part.

FAT ASPIRATION

Superficial Suction

The medial thigh is one of the best areas for superficial suction. The suction, however, cannot be subdermal (1 to 2 mm), because the skin is too thin to be scraped. Suction 4 mm to 5 mm below the dermis will provide a good retraction without causing any irreversible irregularities. If a depression is inadvertently caused, I use the Toledo V-tip dissector cannula to free the lateral parts of the depression and inject some of the preserved fat under it. Wetting the skin and palpating constantly, together with changing the position of the legs, gives a good idea of the changes produced in the area.

Using very fine cannulas makes it possible to stop suctioning before a serious defect is caused. Uniform suction will produce uniform retraction. Changing the angle of the lights also helps to obtain a uniform result. It is better to be conservative here; it is always possible to remove a little bit more later in a smaller procedure if there is a residual deposit, than to risk provoking a serious defect. When using superficial aspiration, we have to remove less fat to reach the desired result than we would if using deep aspiration. Be conservative (Fig. 13-14).

Avoid using the same tunnel close to the incisions. Do not remove the cannula before stopping suction. Passing a cannula aspirating fat unnecessarily close to the incision is one of the most common causes of depressions. When using the syringe, unlock the plunger to stop the vacuum before removing the cannula. If the aspirator is being used, turn it off before removal.

POSTOPERATIVE CARE

As with every area treated by superficial liposculpture, patients have to avoid folds and depressions in the early postoperative period—they can stay marked permanently. Light, uniform compression will help to control swelling, and manual lymphatic drainage will reduce discomfort (Fig. 13-15).

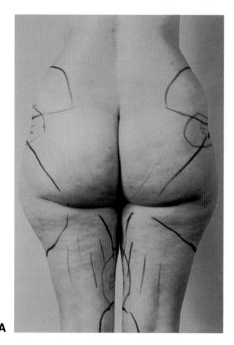
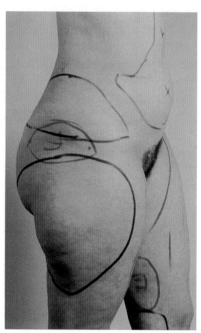

A

B

FIG. 13-1. A, B: The medial thigh adiposities can be divided into three areas: There is excess fat in the upper or cephalic part close to the groin and in the knee area (marked in *blue*), and a depression in the middle part (marked in *red*). Treatment of the medial thighs is combined with treatment of the flanks, lateral thighs, trochanter, and abdomen.

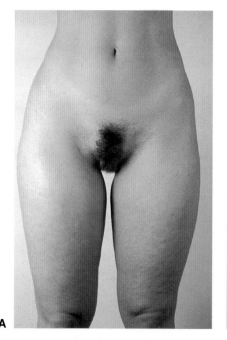
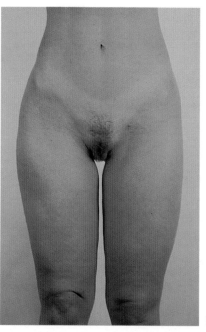

A

B

FIG. 13-2. A, B: Pre- and six-year postoperative photos of medial thighs with excess fat in the upper third and knees and a depression in the middle part. I suctioned fat from the upper part and knee and injected it into the middle.

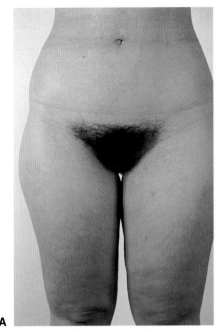

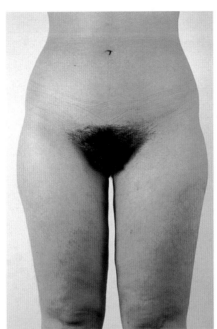

A

B

FIG. 13-3. A, B: Pre- and one-month postoperative photos of uniformly thick medial thighs with excess fat in the three thirds.

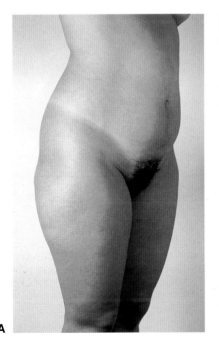

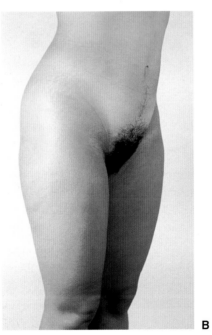

A

B

FIG. 13-4. A: Preoperative photos of a 28-year-old patient with good skin tone. **B:** One-year postoperative photo of superficial liposculpture with a good reduction, not only on the medial thighs but also in the lateral thighs, flanks, and abdomen.

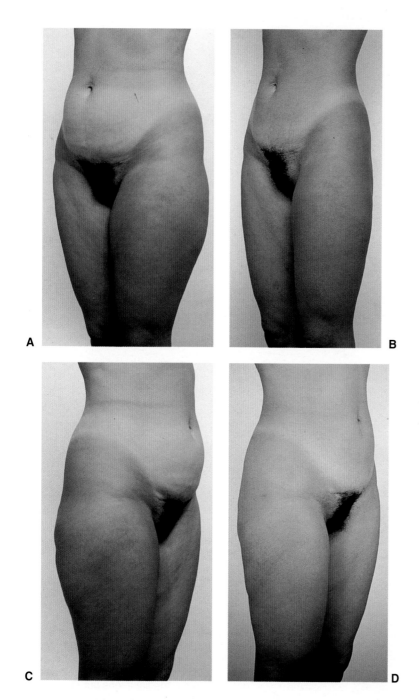

A　　B

C　　D

FIG. 13-5. A, C: Preoperative photo of a 38-year-old patient with flaccid skin tone. **B, D:** One-year postoperative photo of superficial liposculpture alone. The patient accepted an improvement in shape without improvement of the flaccidity.

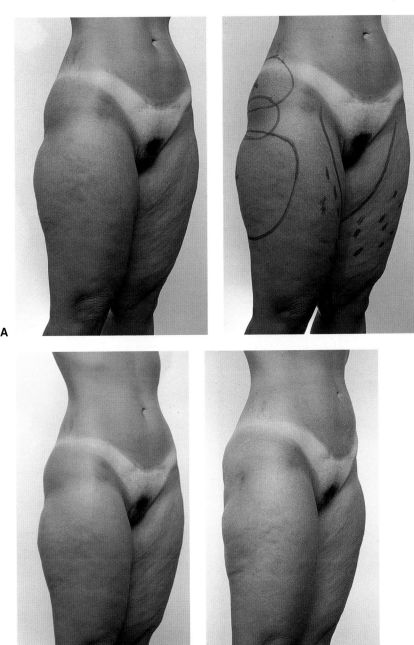

A

B

C

D

FIG. 13-6. **A:** Preoperative photo of a 41-year-old patient with disproportional thighs and upper body. There was too much flaccidity and excess fat. Even with dermolipectomy, it would be difficult to improve her thighs. I proposed an improvement of around 50% in contour and superficial irregularities. **B:** The patient marked for surgery. In *blue* are the areas of suction and in *red,* the areas of fat injection. The little blue marks correspond to superficial irregularities that were treated individually. **C, D:** Pre- and six-month postoperative photos with some improvement in contour and superficial defects. The patient already looks better in clothes and can have a second procedure in the future.

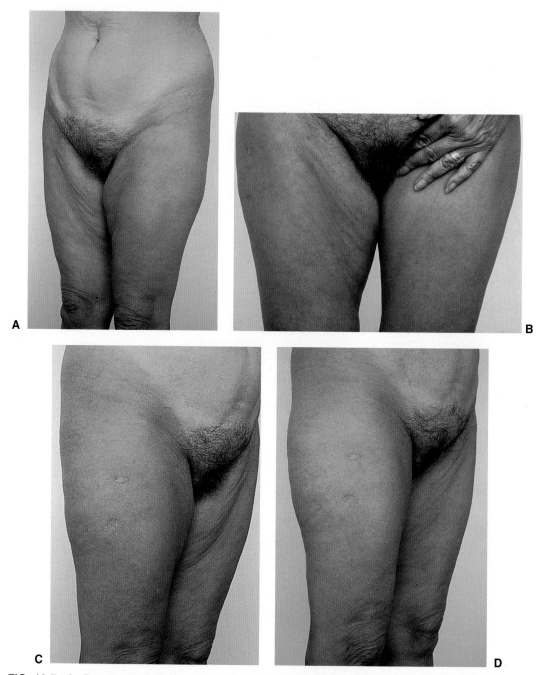

FIG. 13-7. A: Preoperative photo of a 60-year-old patient with flaccid medial thighs, an obvious candidate for a thigh lift. **B:** The patient showed me the improvement she would like. I told her she needed a thigh lift to get that result, but she did not want to undergo open surgery. She said she did not have time to recover from the open surgery and wanted a cheaper procedure. She was informed the result would never be the same, but she said she wanted to look good in clothes. **C, E:** Preoperative photo. **D, F:** Two months postoperatively, with a reduction in the mid-thigh volume, without increasing the flaccidity.

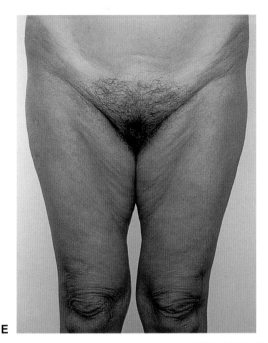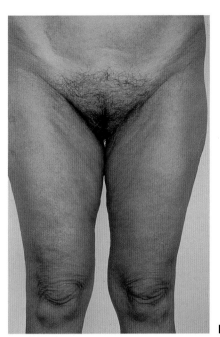

FIG. 13-7. *Continued*

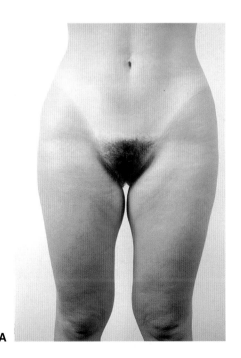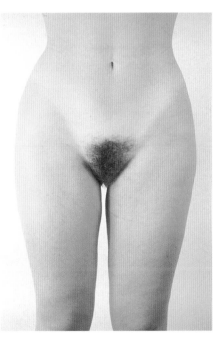

FIG. 13-8. **A:** Preoperative photo of a 32-year-old patient who needed aspiration of fat from the upper part and knees and fat injection in the middle part of the thigh. **B:** One year postoperatively. I injected 150 cc of fat on each middle thigh.

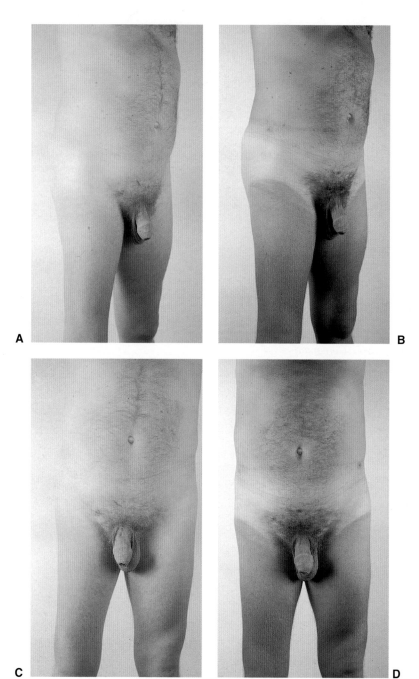

FIG. 13-9. A, C: Preoperative photo of a 45-year-old patient who had the right thigh thinner than the left due to a poliomyelitis sequela. **B, D:** Six months postoperatively. I aspirated fat from the flanks and abdomen and from the upper part of the medial thighs. I injected fat circumferentially in the right thigh intramuscularly and subcutaneously, a total of 850 cc in one stage.

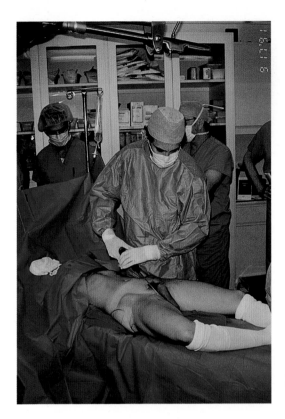

FIG. 13-10. A surgical demonstration at the La Jolla Surgicenter with Dr. Carson Lewis in 1991. The patient's medial thighs are being treated in the supine position with bent knees.

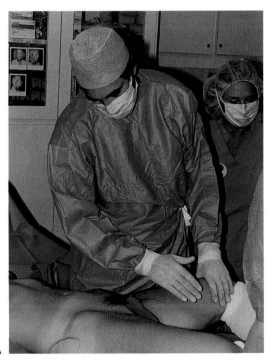

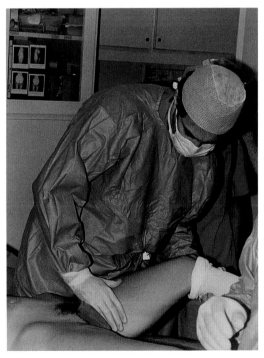

FIG. 13-11. A: I treat the medial thighs with the knees straight or bent, depending on the problem.
B: Sometimes during the procedure it is necessary to move the legs to assess the deformity.

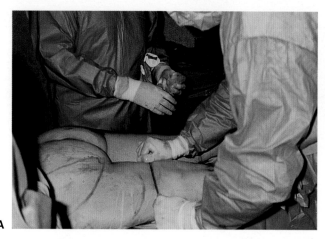
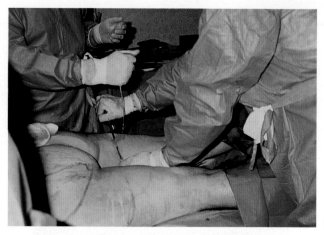

FIG. 13-12. A, B: A surgical demonstration in Dr. Frederick Grazer's clinic in Newport Beach, in 1990. When it is necessary to treat the posterior part of the medial thighs, it might be necessary to put the patient in the prone position. The assistant wets the skin, and I use the "pizza roll," a thick cannula that is passed over the surface to find small irregularities.

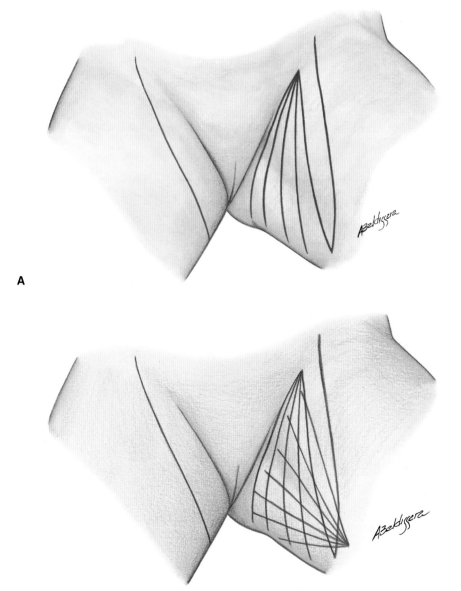

FIG. 13-13. A, B: The incision points and the direction of the tunnels. To treat the anterior area of the upper part of the thighs, I use one or two incisions, depending on the problem: one in the inguinal region and one in the mid-part of the medial thigh, for criss-crossing.

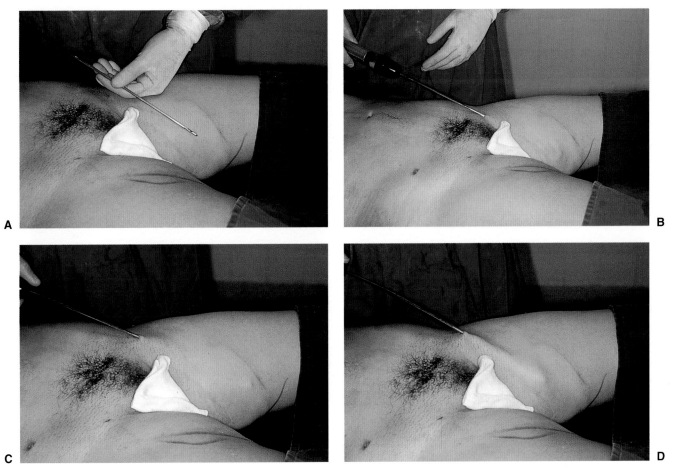

FIG. 13-14. A: The cannula direction when introduced through the inguinal incision. **B:** The cannula introduced deeply into the medial thigh through the inguinal incision. **C:** By elevating the tip of the cannula we can always check where the tip is going. **D:** The cannula introduced superficially in the anterior thigh through the inguinal incision. By elevating the whole cannula, we can see the depth of the tunnels.

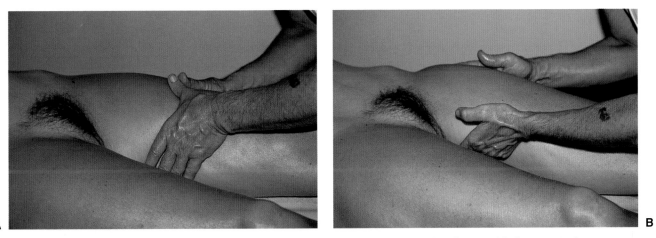

FIG. 13-15. A, B: The French method of manual lymphatic drainage will reduce and help to control swelling discomfort.

14

The Anterior Thighs

Together with the abdomen, the anterior thigh is one of the most difficult areas of the body to treat. Luckily, it is not often that I have to treat anterior thighs, but when the patient needs local or circumferential liposculpture of the thighs, we have to be very careful not to create defects there, because they are very difficult to correct. The worst defects are depressions, irregularities, and loose skin.

Some patients accumulate too much fat in the anterior thigh, and it can get too heavy and irregular. The problem is usually difficult to see and photograph, and when patients complain about their anterior thighs they usually mention that the problem only shows with special lights or that they have to pinch the fat layer with their hands to show the excess (Fig. 14-1). This is one of the areas where the superficial irregularities from ''cellulite'' show, and patients complain that they see them when they look down at their thighs or when they pinch them, but they cannot see the problem in the mirror.

The only type of ''cellulite'' I treat with liposculpture is when I see superficial irregularities when the patient is standing up, not sitting down. The defects must be visible without the pinch test. For the incipient type of ''cellulite,'' I have started the use of endermology, but my results are too preliminary to have a serious evaluation.

The two problems I usually treat in the anterior thighs are excess volume of fat and superficial irregularities. Both of these problems have to be treated with very fine cannulas, even if it takes longer, to allow for a very uniform retraction of the tissues.

Patients must be marked in the standing position, and it is necessary that they mention all the areas where they see deformities, even if they seem small to the eye. After I mark, I place the patient on a table to see what the deformities will look like when the patient is on the operating table and, if necessary, I do some extra markings. I like to mark every small irregularity so I do not forget to treat them (Fig. 14-2).

INSTRUMENTS

I like to use 2- and 3-mm-gauge, 35- to 45-cm-long cannulas with 60-cc toomey-tip syringes. The cannulas I prefer are the Pyramid-tip cannulas, although I can use a 2-mm one-lateral-hole tip. For freeing the irregularities I use the 3-mm-gauge Toledo V-tip dissector cannula.

ANESTHESIA

I usually perform all my body contour work under local anesthesia, and the anterior thighs are no exception. I infiltrate a proportion of 1:1 of my local anesthesia formula at body temperature, and wait 10 minutes before I start suctioning.

POSITION

I usually treat the anterior thighs with the patient in the supine position (Fig. 14-3) and with the knee bent at 90 degrees. In these two positions it is possible to address most of the defects. If I have to remember what the defect looked like in the standing position, I look at the preoperative pictures on the wall (Fig. 14-4).

INCISIONS

The incision points will vary according to the areas of treatment, but usually one incision at the inguinal region and one or two at the knee are enough (Fig. 14-5). For circumferential aspiration other incisions are used, such as the trochanter, the gluteal fold, and the two popliteal incisions. From these points we can address almost any defect in the thigh area.

FAT ASPIRATION

Deep Suction

When there is a large fat deposit, I start suctioning deep, with a 3-mm-gauge long cannula in the area marked preoperatively, trying to aspirate fat uniformly to thin down the defect. I always save some fat for reinjection, especially when there are superficial irregularities. Even when I do not plan reinjection, I save some fat for a possible immediate correction.

Superficial Suction

After I reach a point when I think I have removed enough from the deep layer, I change to a 2-mm-gauge cannula and aspirate fat closer to the skin. I try to avoid reaching the point where a subdermal groove can form because of a too-superficial suction. I like to stay 4 to 5 mm deep. This superficial suction will improve the skin retraction in that area. If after this treatment I notice skin irregularities when I wet the skin with an antiseptic liquid, I introduce the V-tip dissector cannula and, with in-and-out movements, treat each marked irregularity, freeing them from their attachments and injecting some fat underneath. With my other hand I pull the skin down, imitating the effect of gravity to check if there are irregularities that have not been treated (Fig. 14-6).

FAT INJECTION

After I free the superficial irregularities, I always inject some of the stored fat to prevent the adhesions from coming back. Fat injection is also used in secondary cases when there are depressions that need to be filled up with fat.

SECONDARY LIPOSCULPTURE

The anterior area, being very unforgiving, is one of the areas where the irregularities of bad liposuction become evident. When I receive patients with many irregularities, I tell them I will have to perform several procedures to obtain the estimated improvement. The improvement will depend on several factors, including skin type and age. I usually remove fat from areas that still have excess, and inject it into the depressions after freeing them (Fig. 14-7).

ABOVE THE KNEES

One of the most difficult parts of the body to treat is the anterior thigh just above the knees. There are usually some fat deposits in that area that some women find so ugly they completely stop wearing skirts and shorts because of it and live their lives in slacks and trousers to hide ''ugly knees.'' To aspirate these fat deposits, is to risk provoking folds and wrinkles in this area due to the excess skin needed to cover the knee joint when the knee is bent. This problem is worsened in patients who sunbathe too much because their skin gets dry and wrinkled. I have seen young patients with knees that looked like old patients' knees. I have always been against proposing skin resections on the knees, although I have seen the technique performed in patients who lose to much weight. One patient complained so much about her wrinkled knees that I ended up peeling her anterior thighs with trichloroacetic acid (TCA). She had a long recovery period with sensitive red skin on her legs, but after a few months, the redness cleared up and her legs became much better (Fig. 14-8). I have never repeated the procedure, but it is an option to be remembered in extreme cases.

DEEP VERSUS SUPERFICIAL SUCTION

One of the difficulties when indicating a technique is to know when to perform deep and when to choose superficial liposculpture. Two different examples are shown (Figs. 14-9, 14-10). Two patients of the same age, both in their mid-twenties, can have totally different indications. One has firm fat deposits with a good skin tone, a candidate for only deep liposculpture. The other has flaccid skin and superficial irregularities, so superficial liposculpture is the technique of choice.

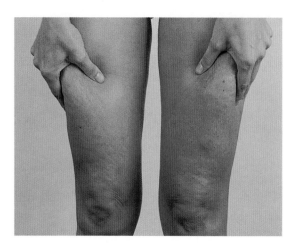

FIG. 14-1. A patient with excess fat on her anterior thighs. This degree of "cellulite" is visible only when the patient presses the fat. I cannot improve this problem through liposculpture.

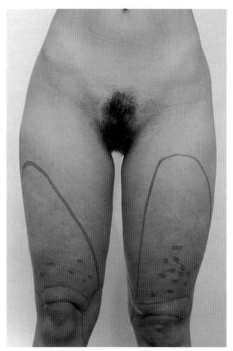

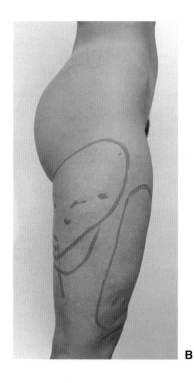

A

B

FIG. 14-2. A, B: Front and profile of a 32-year-old lean patient with very heavy thighs, especially anteriorly. We have marked the areas for deep suction. The small marks correspond to small depressions to be treated individually.

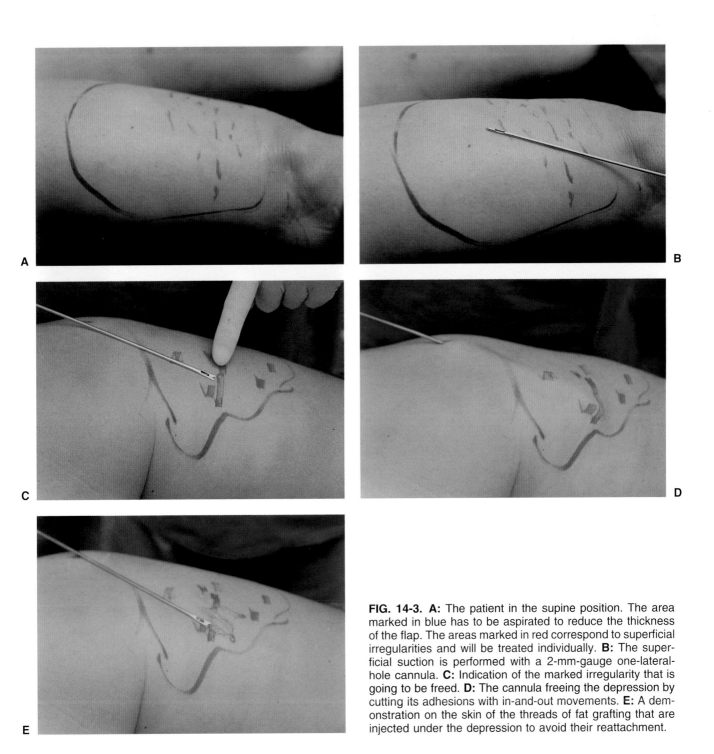

FIG. 14-3. A: The patient in the supine position. The area marked in blue has to be aspirated to reduce the thickness of the flap. The areas marked in red correspond to superficial irregularities and will be treated individually. **B:** The superficial suction is performed with a 2-mm-gauge one-lateral-hole cannula. **C:** Indication of the marked irregularity that is going to be freed. **D:** The cannula freeing the depression by cutting its adhesions with in-and-out movements. **E:** A demonstration on the skin of the threads of fat grafting that are injected under the depression to avoid their reattachment.

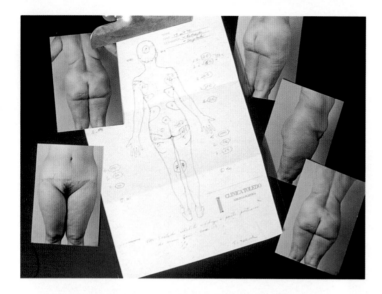

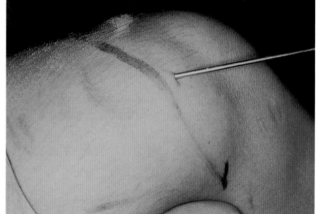

FIG. 14-4. In order to remember what the defect looks like in the standing position, I look at the preoperative pictures on the wall. The map will show the amounts of fat aspirated or injected.

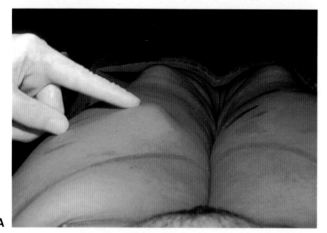

A

B

FIG. 14-5. A: The Toledo V-tip dissector cannula being used in the anterior thigh through the inguinal incision. B: Through a small, 3-mm incision we can complement the access to most of the anterior thigh. Sometimes another incision in the other side of the knee is necessary.

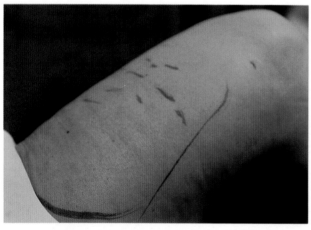

A

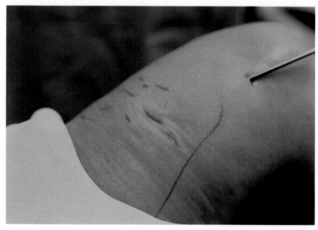

B

FIG. 14-6. A, B: The treatment of the skin irregularities of the anterior thigh. We imitate the gravity effect by pulling the skin down.

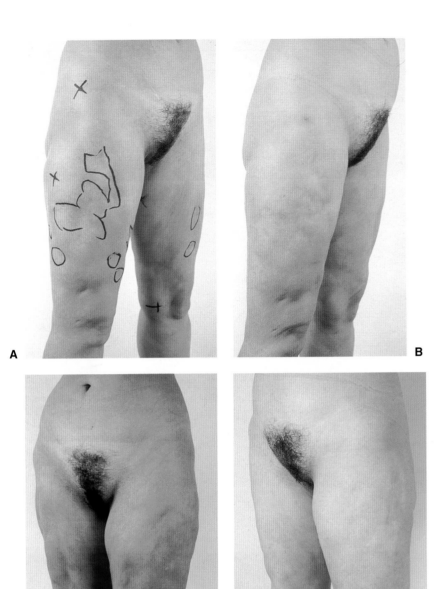

FIG. 14-7. A, C: Preoperative photo of a 37-year-old patient who had irregular circumferential liposuction on her thighs, with several sequelae, two years after the procedure. The areas surrounded in blue are the areas of depression, the crosses are areas with too much fat. Some of the anterior thigh depressions were so deep I could palpate the muscle just under the skin. B, D: Fourteen months after three procedures to aspirate the excess fat from the elevated areas, free the adhesions, and inject fat in the depressed areas.

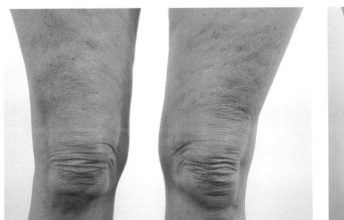
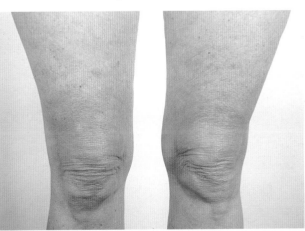

FIG. 14-8. A: Preoperative photo of a 39-year-old patient with very old-looking knees. B: Four months after a 35% trichloroacetic acid peel of the anterior-thigh knees area, with a good improvement of the skin excess and wrinkles.

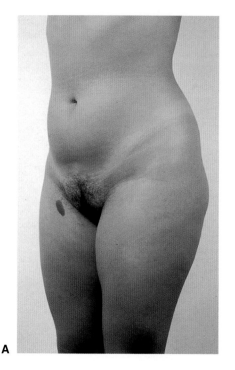
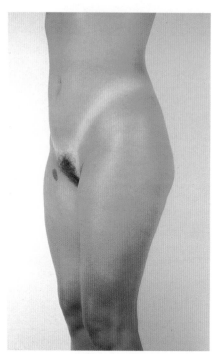

A   B

FIG. 14-9. **A:** Preoperative photo of a 23-year-old patient with excess fat on the abdomen, flanks, and thighs. **B:** One year postoperatively, after deep liposculpture with a good skin retraction and good contour improvement. Her type of fat and skin allowed us to do only deep liposculpture.

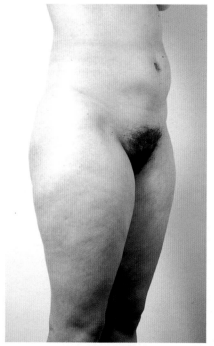
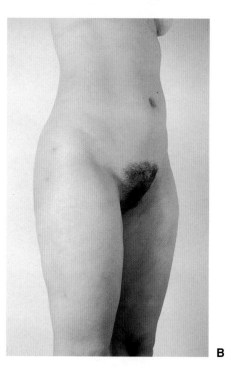

A   B

FIG. 14-10. **A:** Preoperative photo of a 26-year-old patient with excess fat on the abdomen, flanks, and thighs. **B:** One year postoperatively, after superficial liposculpture with a good skin retraction and good contour improvement. The superficial irregularities have also been improved. Her type of fat and skin allowed us to perform only superficial liposculpture.

15

The Buttocks

Beginning in the 1980s and peaking in the '90s, the world witnessed a trend toward exercising. Running and aerobics became fashionable, and the search for a more athletic-looking body influenced the aesthetic pattern, especially for the thighs, legs, and buttocks.

When we started liposuction in 1982 we would use Illouz's trick of turning the hole of the cannula towards the dermis, scraping the surface to create a new subgluteal fold. Today this maneuver is rarely needed, as many patients now prefer the buttock to blend smoothly, as though a continuation of the thigh, without the definition of the subgluteal fold separating the buttock from the thigh (Fig. 15-1).

Brazilian bikinis become smaller every summer, and most of our patients who come for body contour procedures are looking for some improvement in this area, usually augmentation and remodeling. We cannot forget the importance of exercise to improve the gluteal area, and this is always pointed out to the patient. Recontouring with fat, although a great technique, is limited by the amount of available fat. *In vitro* fat growth studies are in progress, but we still have not reached the point where harvested fat cells can be grown and reproduced in a lab for reinjection to remodel the body. This reality is not far away, and it will change the indications of many procedures we perform today. It is well known that we lose fat from our face as we grow older, and a "fat bank" could store our cells for future rejuvenation procedures. Today we are limited by the amount of fat we can harvest for reinjection, and some patients just do not have enough cells to complete their reshaping. The use of silicone buttock prostheses is very common in Argentina and in some parts of Brazil; the surgeons who insert these prosthesis are wonderful technicians and can obtain good results. On the other hand, I have seen too many complications related to displacements and contracture, possibly caused by less experienced hands. But there are complications and specific problems to every implant surgery, and I refer my patients who need buttock prosthesis to those more experienced in the procedure, reminding them that they will not be able to have an intramuscular gluteal injection once the prosthesis is in place.

INSTRUMENTS

The instruments used are basically the same as those used in other areas of the body: 60-cc syringes and cannulas varying in gauge between 2 mm and 4.6 mm. Depressions and fibrotic areas can be treated with a 3-mm-gauge Toledo V-tip dissector cannula. Fat can be injected into the buttock with a blunt-tip 3-mm-gauge one-lateral-hole cannula.

ANESTHESIA

The anesthesia used is usually local anesthesia in the same formula as for other areas of the body and combined with sedation.

POSITION

The buttock is treated in the lateral position; however, depending on the problem and on whether other areas are to be treated simultaneously, the prone position can also be used. But generally the lateral position allows for a good visualization of the problems and helps when we have to imitate gravity. One of the difficulties in body contour surgery is that a patient will show you a defect that is usually visible in the standing position. During surgery the patient is lying down and under different lights, and it is often difficult to see where the problem was. To help avoid this uncertainty, there are a few tricks that can be employed.

There are expensive operating tables developed to turn the patient into the orthostatic position during surgery to check the irregularities. Patients under general or epidural anesthesia can develop serious problems with such a dramatic change of position during surgery; this has to be taken into account. A safer method could be to operate under local anesthesia and to ask the patient to stand up when checking the deformities. In my experience, this tactic has never worked well. Patients often get dizzy because of the quick change in position, the effect of sedation, or simply because they are uncomfortable in a surgical environment. I once even tried to operate while the patient was standing, but it didn't work.

The easiest and safest method is to utilize some tactics that imitate the effect of gravity during the orthostatic position. I use them for the face and jowls, for the abdomen, and especially for the buttocks and lateral thighs (see Fig. 15-15). By pushing the buttock down, we elevate the lateral thigh; this is similar to what would happen in the standing position. With the other hand we can suction superficially the cephalic and caudal parts of the gluteal fold until the area has the desired shape. Usually after this superficial suction, the fold tends to be shortened.

INCISIONS

The buttock region can be treated through three incisions, one in the trochanteric area, one in the subgluteal fold and, if necessary a third in the sacral region. These incisions allow good access to the whole area.

FAT ASPIRATION

Deep and Superficial Suction

The buttock is an area where the limit between deep and superficial suction is crossed in almost every procedure. It is almost impossible to treat the buttock with one of these two techniques alone.

I have many patients who come for minor alterations and corrections, and these are probably my most demanding patients. They often have good body shapes and want them even better (Figs. 15-2, 15-3). Some patients ask for a reduction in the volume of the buttock itself, and in these cases I prefer to perform a uniform superficial suction of the dorsal area of the buttock, provoking a retraction of the tissues (Figs. 15-4, 15-5).

Patients with the tendency to accumulate fat below the waistline can present the buttocks in continuation with the thigh, but it can be in a slightly deformed manner (Fig. 15-6). Usually there will be a lack of definition between the two areas, and the accumulation of fat, together with the absence of a subgluteal fold, makes the deformity look even bigger. In these cases I will remove the excess fat from the lateral and posterior thigh; this will also lengthen the fold just a little, to create a more graceful look.

FAT INJECTION

The buttock is also an area where I most often combine fat injection with fat aspiration. I find that to obtain the result that I want, it is necessary to add fat injection to the procedure. An existing longer fold with flaccidity of the tissues will provoke a depression in the gluteal trochanteric area, and the accumulation of fat in the lower third of the buttock, above and below the gluteal fold, is the so-called "banana fold" (Fig. 15-7). This defect can be primarily due to tissue flaccidity and the weight of the buttock, or secondary to deep liposuction in the subgluteal area (Figs. 15-8, 15-9). Patients with good skin tone will be treated with superficial liposuction of the lower third of the buttock and the "banana fold," combined with fat injection of the gluteal depression (Fig. 15-10). I aspirate the flanks and lateral thighs, keeping the syringes of fat for reinjection. The area cephalic to the gluteal fold is treated using superficial suction to remove some of the weight of the buttock and provoke a slight retraction of the skin. This procedure, combined with fat injection (Fig. 15-11) in the trochanteric area, will produce the illusion of elevation of the buttock (Figs. 15-12, 15-13). Treating these delicate areas with deep suction can accentuate the problem, as you will destroy the fibrotic support that keeps the buttock in place. The buttock will drop, and the fat deposits will become more evident (Fig. 15-14, A-F). There is a limit to what can be accomplished with liposculpture in these cases, because too much suction, even superficial, can accentuate the defect (Fig. 15-14, G-K). Deep suction of the "banana fold" area can break the fibrous structures that hold the buttock in place; this will increase the length of the fold and the "banana" adiposity. Strangely enough, when the patient elevates the thigh, a depression can appear in the same place that will show a fat deposit in the standing position (Fig. 15-14 L,M). There comes a point when suction is ineffective due to the extent of the skin's flaccidity, and results in too much excess skin. (Fig. 15-15). The problem is no longer the fat deposit, but the excess skin that cannot retract (Fig. 15-16). The indication is for dermolipectomy (Fig. 15-17). The procedures should be discussed to decide what will be more acceptable to the patient: a scar along with a good shape and less flaccidity, or flaccidity with no scar. Each case is examined and evaluated individually, taking into consideration the patient's age, social activities, habits, and preferences. An older woman who no longer wears bathing suits and wants to look better in her clothes will probably think differently from a younger patient who wears small bikinis and spends a lot of time at the beach.

Superficial irregularities and depressions are very common in the buttocks. Some are provoked by cellulite (Figs 15-18–15-20), others by injections (Fig. 15-21) or trauma (Fig. 15-22), and some depressions are caused by the ischium pressure while sitting (Fig. 15-23). Patients who wear tiny bikinis usually ask for improvement of these depressions. We treat them with our V-tip dissector cannula (Fig. 15-24), freeing the fibrous attachments that pull the skin down and injecting a few cc of fat to fill the depression. We overinject up to 50% more than needed, counting on some reabsorption of the injected fat (Fig. 15-25). Computer imaging is good in these cases, first to point out the problem to the patient, and second to show the expected degree of improvement, i.e., 30% to 50%, depending on the skin tone and the gravity of the depression. We advise our patients that fat injection in the ischium depression has a high reabsorption percentage due to the constant pressure in this area. Even so, some patients want fat injected in this depression not necessarily for aesthetic reasons, but because they feel pain when they sit for too long. We perform the procedure allowing for repeated fat injections in accordance with the patient's reabsorption rate.

Patients who have a bony sacral region also need fat injected in this area to protect this region against trauma and also to refer local pain (Fig. 15-26). Fat is usually aspirated from the flanks and injected into the sacral area. The technique of fat injection in parallel threads is described in Chapter 9.

POSTOPERATIVE CARE

One of the main concerns of patients who undergo buttock contouring is the postoperative period. This is especially true in combined procedures, when patients may think that they will not find a comfortable position in which to recuperate.

I prescribe girdles to support the area in place. The girdle provides comfort and a sense of security. The time this girdle should be worn varies according to the severity of the problem and the flaccidity of the skin. A patient with a good skin tone who had only fat aspiration can wear the girdle only for a week, while someone with flaccid skin who underwent superficial liposculpture and fat injection will feel safer wearing the girdle for 30 days, until there is a good recovery and skin retraction.

Patients should lie in bed in the prone or lateral position for the first days, but if they have had other procedures they can rest in the supine position. Sitting should be limited to a minimum on the first postoperative days, to avoid displacement of the injected fat. Walking is prescribed after the second postoperative day, driving after a week, and exercising after a month.

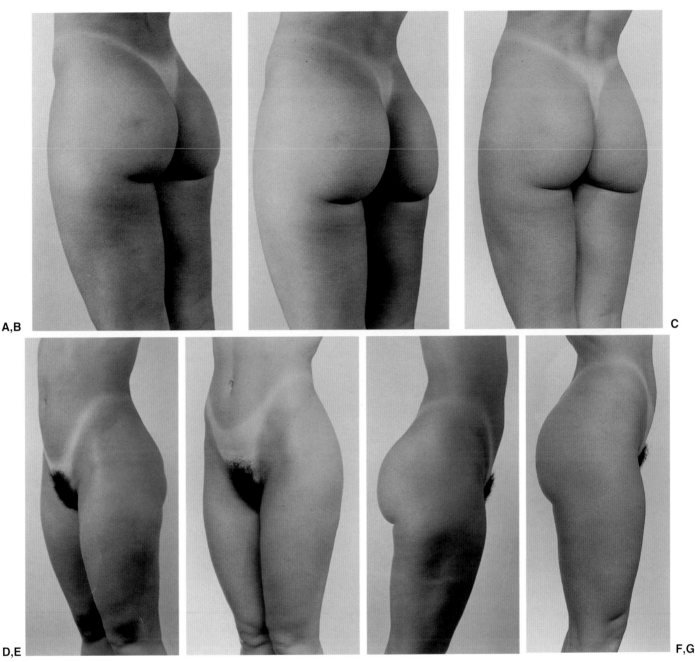

FIG. 15-1. A: Preoperative picture of an 18-year old patient who wanted to augment her buttocks, reduce her thighs and hips, and improve the small depression on her left buttock. Syringe liposculpture was performed, fat was aspirated from the lateral thighs and flanks and 100 cc was injected into each buttock, plus 20 cc under the irregularity. **B:** The same patient two years postoperatively, with the same weight. **C:** The same patient four years postoperatively with a weight loss of two kilos. There is a good improvement of the thigh and buttock shape and a lasting result from one session of fat grafting. **D:** A ¾ preoperative view of the same patient showing a irregular contour of the flank buttock and lateral thigh. **E:** Four years postoperatively, showing the improvement in the contour of the waist, buttock, and lateral thigh. **F:** Preoperative profile of the same patient showing the lateral thigh deformity and the heavy buttock that was starting to fall because of excess fat in the lower third. **G:** Four years postoperatively, showing the new contour of the buttock and lateral thigh. The injection of fat in the upper part and suction in the lower gives the impression of elevation of the buttock.

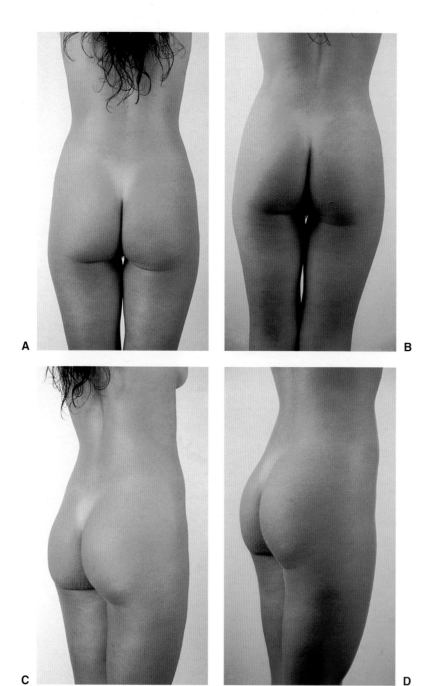

A

B

C

D

FIG. 15-2. A, C, E: Preoperative photos of a 23-year-old patient who wanted to improve her waist and buttocks. **B, D, F:** One year postoperatively, after aspiration of fat from the flanks and waist and injection into the upper part of the buttocks. This is a very slight improvement, but there is a difference in measurements and a change in the contour that can be appreciated particularly in the ¾ view. This patient entered and won a beauty contest after this procedure.

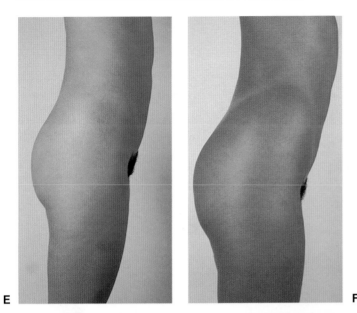

E   F   **FIG. 15-2.** *Continued.*

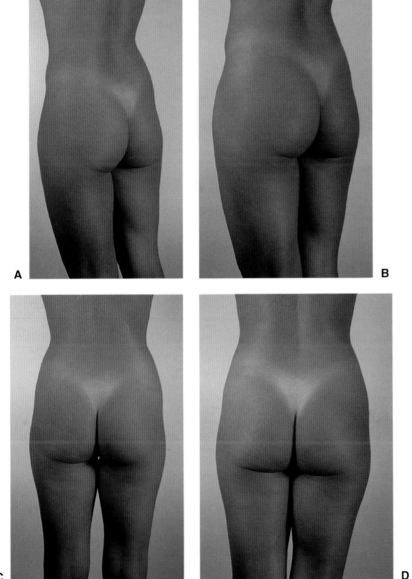

A   B

C   D

FIG. 15-3. A, C: Preoperative photos of a 32-year-old patient who needed only small improvements to her flanks and body contour. **B, D:** Fat was aspirated from the flanks and injected into the buttocks. The waistline is narrower and the buttock rounder.

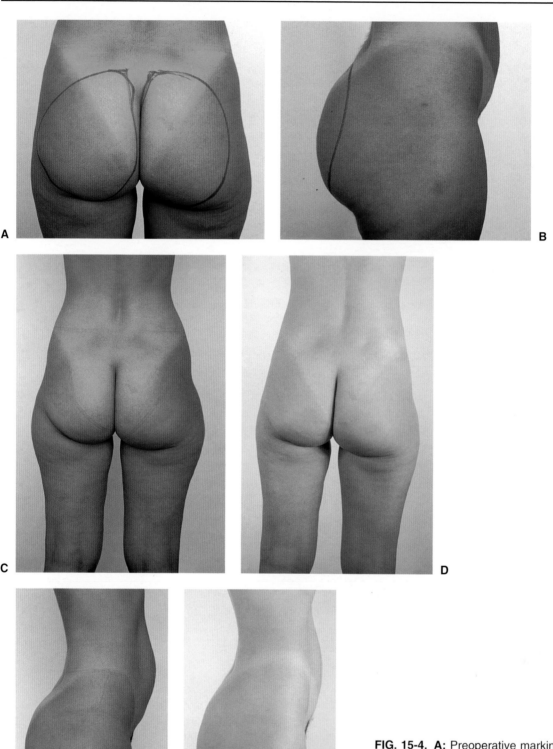

FIG. 15-4. A: Preoperative markings of a 31-year-old patient who wanted the volume of her buttocks reduced. **B:** Profile of the preoperative markings of the same patient. She wanted a reduction of the dorsal projection of the buttocks and a reduction of the lateral thighs. **C, E:** Preoperative view. Her weight was 61 kg and her measurements were 89 cm around the buttocks and 60 cm on each thigh. **D, F:** Twelve months postoperatively, with the patient weighing 58.3 kg after the removal of 1.38 liters of fat from the buttock and lateral thigh areas. Measurements were reduced by 4 cm in the buttock area and 4 cm on each thigh.

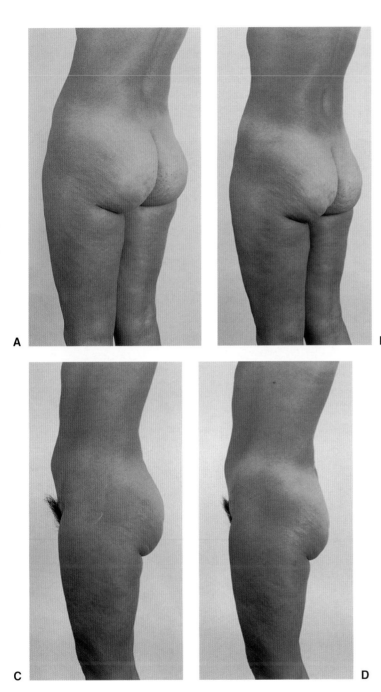

FIG. 15-5. A, C: Preoperative photos of a 49-year-old patient who complained that her buttocks had gotten bigger with age and she wanted to reduce them. We aspirated a total of 380 cc of fat from the left buttock, 360 cc from the right, plus 50 cc from the subgluteal area on each side. **B, D:** Four months postoperatively, with the patient weighing one kg more, but showing a reduction of 6 cm in the buttock area. *Figure continues on next page.*

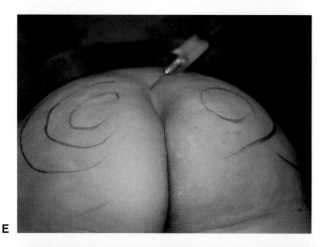

E

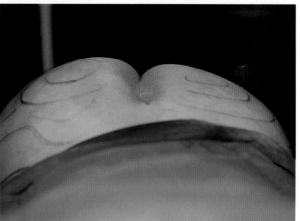

FIG. 15-5. *Continued.* **E:** Intraoperative photo of the buttock reduction procedure using the superficial liposculture method; the patient is under local tumescent anesthesia with sedation. **F, G:** Intraoperative views showing the difference in the two sides after removal of 380 cc of fat from the right side.

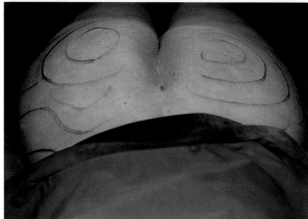

F

G

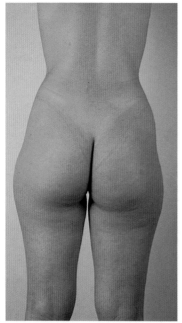

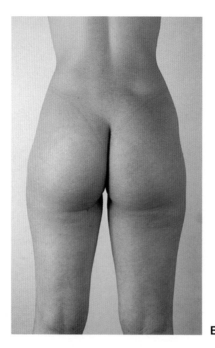

A

B

FIG. 15-6. **A:** Preoperative photo of a 28-year-old patient who had her buttocks in continuation with the thighs. **B:** Three months postoperatively, after suction of lateral thighs to give some definition to the buttocks.

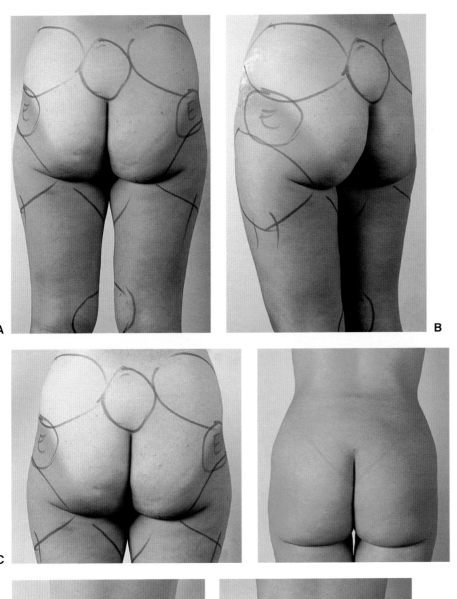

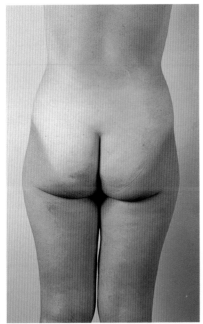

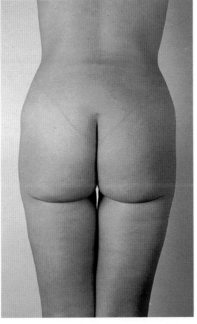

FIG. 15-7. A, B: Preoperative photos of a 36-year-old patient with very flaccid skin, showing the accumulation of fat in the flanks, medial thighs, lateral thighs, sacral region, and medial knees, and a depression in the trochanteric areas. The blue markings are the areas for suction, the red areas for injection of fat. **C, D:** Pre- and one-year postoperative photos of superficial liposculpture of the body showing an improvement in the shape of the buttocks. The flaccidity remains the same, but there were no irregularities and the fat injected into the buttock gave the impression of an elevation. **E, F:** Pre- and one-year postoperative photos of superficial liposculpture. The shape and the superficial irregularities have improved. The patient's weight remained the same.

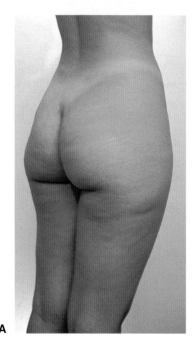
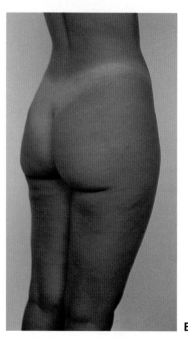

A

B

FIG. 15-8. **A:** The primary "banana fold" due to tissue flaccidity and the weight of the buttock. **B:** Correction of the "banana fold" and lateral thigh fat deposit with superficial liposculpture.

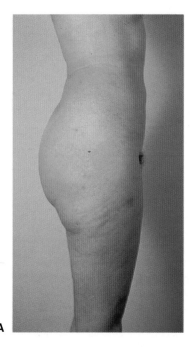
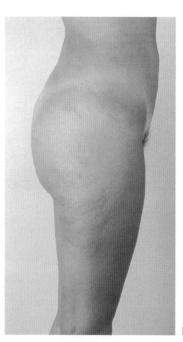

A

B

FIG. 15-9. **A:** A "banana fold" secondary to deep liposuction in the subgluteal area. **B:** Correction of the secondary "banana fold" with superficial liposculpture.

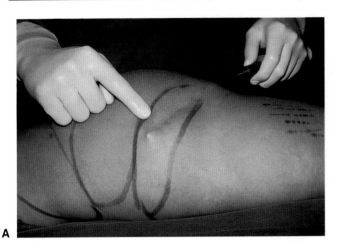

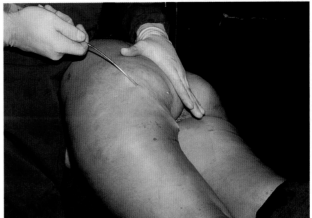

A

B

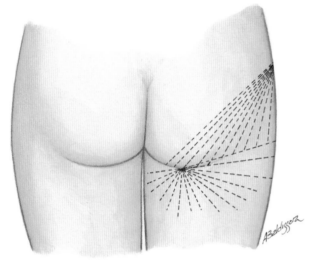

C

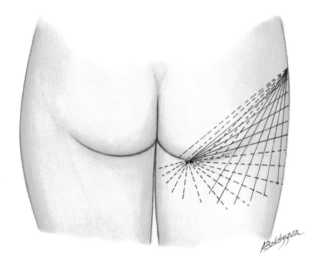

D

FIG. 15-10. A: Intraoperative photo of superficial liposculpture in the "banana fold" area to provoke skin retraction. **B:** Intraoperative photo of superficial liposculpture in the "banana fold" area. The left hand presses the buttock down to imitate the effect of gravity. **C:** Areas of superficial suction in the lower third of the buttock through a trochanteric incision and on the subgluteal ("banana fold") area through a gluteal fold incision. **D:** Crisscrossing the superficial tunnels using the trochanteric and gluteal fold incision to obtain a uniform skin retraction.

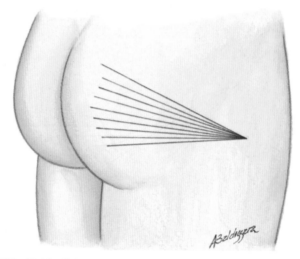

FIG. 15-11. Scheme of the area of fat injection in the upper two-thirds of the buttock. We usually inject from the trochanter incision, using a blunt 3-mm-gauge cannula. The fat is injected into the gluteus muscle and the subcutaneous area.

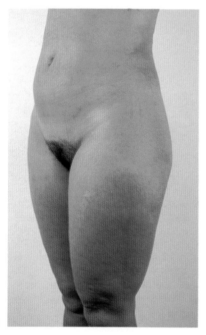
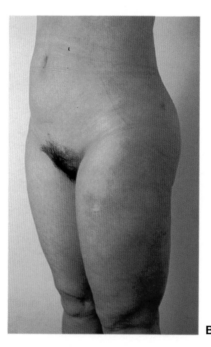

A

B

FIG. 15-12. A: Preoperative photo of a 42-year-old patient with lipodistrophy of the buttocks, lateral thighs, medial thighs, and abdomen who weighed 66 kg. **B:** One year postoperatively, with the same weight after removal of 1.86 liters of fat through superficial liposculpture. There is good retraction on the lower third of the buttock because of the superficial suction. The good projection of the upper part of the buttock is due to fat injection of 300 cc per side. Notice that the new depression on the subgluteal area enhances the curve of the buttock. The superficial irregularities were treated with the V-tip dissector cannula.

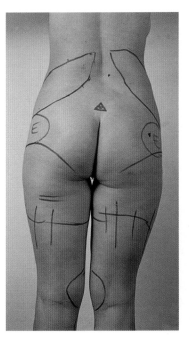
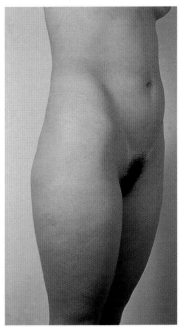
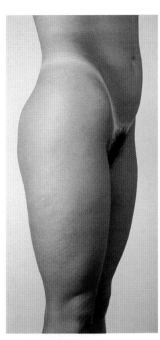

A,B

C

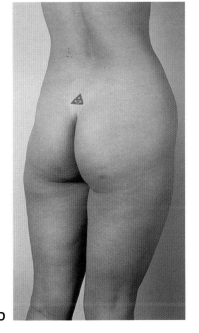
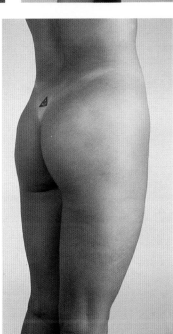

D

E

FIG. 15-13. A: Preoperative markings of a 24-year-old patient, showing an excess of fat in the flanks, thighs, and knees, marked in blue and a depression in the trochanter area marked in red, plus superficial irregularities. **B, D:** Preoperative anterior and posterior ¾ views. **C, E:** One year postoperatively, after removal of 2.5 liters of fat through superficial liposculpture from the areas marked in blue, showing a good retraction of the lower third. There is a good projection of the upper part of the buttock due to fat injection of 350 cc per side. The depression on the subgluteal area, combined with the projection of the buttock, gives the illusion of elevation. The superficial irregularities were treated with the V-tip dissector cannula. The subgluteal fold has not been lengthened.

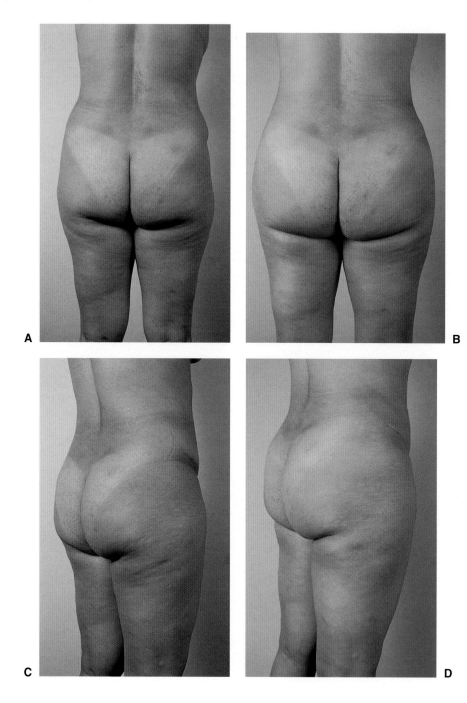

A

B

C

D

FIG. 15-14. A, C: Preoperative photo of a 45-year-old patient who had had liposuction two years before and wanted to improve the contour of her waist, buttock, and thighs. **B, D:** Two-month postoperative photos of the same patient after liposculpture of the flanks, lateral thighs, and buttocks. There was a contour improvement, but the weight of the buttocks started forming a "banana fold" deformity.

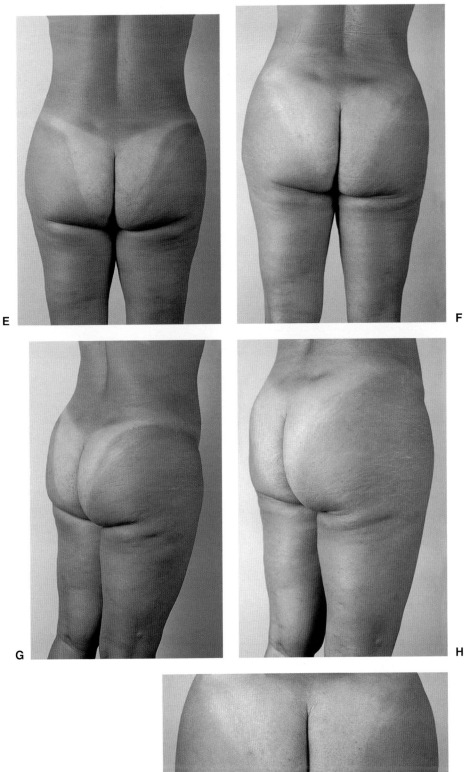

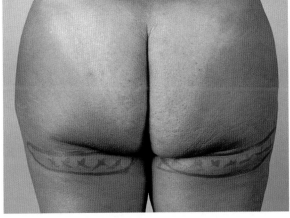

FIG. 15-14. *Continued.* **E, G:** Four months postoperatively. The "banana fold" is more evident, the subgluteal folds have been lengthened and the patient asked for aspiration of the subgluteal adiposity. We advised the patient to wait for the healing process to complete. **F, H, I:** The patient returned 21 months after the first surgery, and this is the aspect of the "banana fold." *Figure continues on next page.*

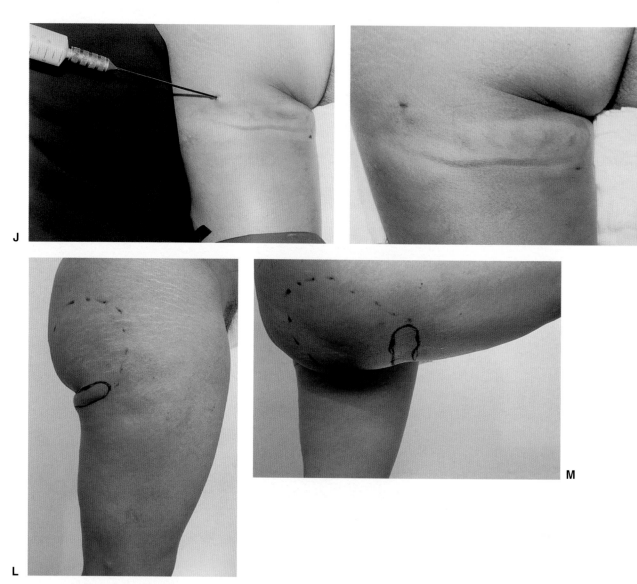

FIG. 15-14. *Continued.* **J, K:** I removed 20 cc of fat superficially from the marked area of each thigh, and injected the fat under the fold. **L, M:** Four years after the initial procedure, two years after the revision, the patient still presented a "banana fold" deformity. This was especially prominent when she was standing. She complained that when she elevated the thigh she could palpate a depression in the same area. At this point only skin resection will solve the problem.

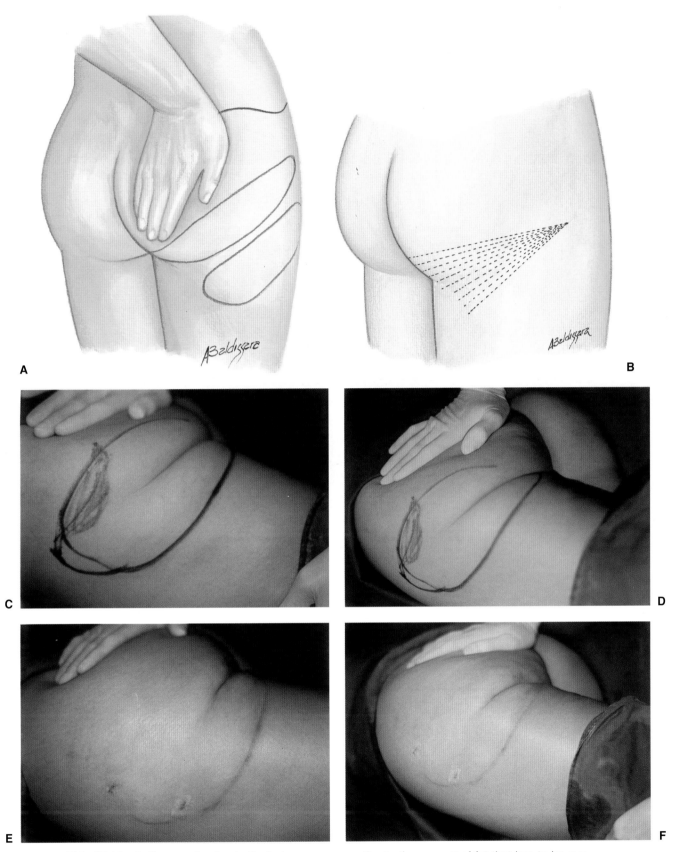

FIG. 15-15. A: By pressing the buttock down we can estimate the amount of fat that has to be suctioned from the lateral thigh, medial third of the buttock, and subgluteal area. **B:** The direction of the tunnels of superficial aspiration in the area. **C:** Intraoperative photo. Treatment of the buttock region through superficial suction using the buttock press maneuver. The area marked with black pen will be suctioned superficially. **D:** When we press the buttock using more force, we see that the subgluteal fold is extended. **E:** After superficial suction using light pressure on the buttock, the fold is almost nonexistent. We have to take into account that the area is still infiltrated with local anesthesia. **F:** After superficial suction with considerable pressure on the buttock, the fold is still shorter than before.

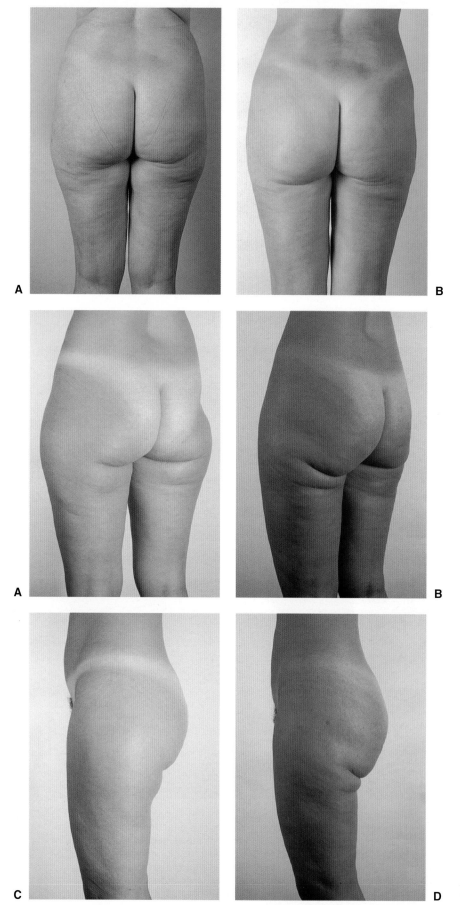

A

B

A

B

C

D

FIG. 15-16. A: A 50-year-old patient with very flaccid skin underwent two previous liposuctions, wanting to improve the waist, buttock, and thigh areas, but refused any procedure with long scars for skin removal. **B:** Six-month postoperative photo of the same patient with some improvement in the waist, buttock, and lateral thigh areas, but with a persistence of the "banana fold" deformity. We advised the patient that liposculpture was not the ideal procedure for her, and that we could improve the contour up to a certain point. The patient accepted the result; other patients might not. The problem is knowing before operating which patient will accept this result, and which patient will expect more.

FIG. 15-17. A, C: Preoperative ¾ view and profile of a 35-year-old patient with very flaccid skin, wanting liposculpture of the flanks, buttocks, and lateral thighs. The patient already had a primary "banana fold" deformity. **B, D:** One year postoperatively, with a good improvement of the flank and lateral thigh areas, but an accentuation of the "banana fold" due to too much and too deep subgluteal suction, and maintaining the same weight of the buttock.

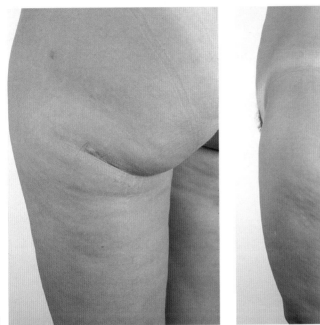

E

F

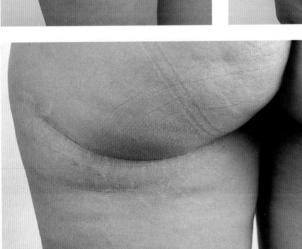

G

FIG. 15-17. *Continued.* **E, F, G:** Improvement of the "banana fold" defect three months after a fusiform dermolipectomy around the gluteal fold, removing the excess skin, but leaving the dermis and subcutaneous tissue to fill in the defect area.

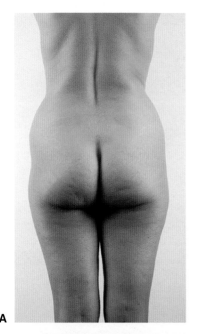
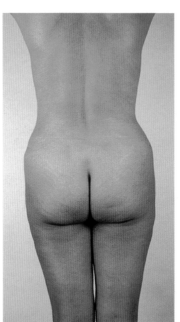

A

B

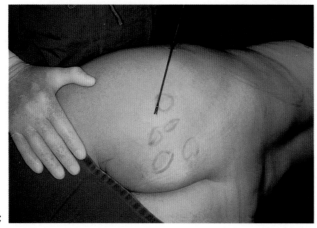

C

FIG. 15-18. A: Preoperative photo of a 42-year-old patient with excess fat on the dorsal region, flanks, buttocks, and lateral thighs, plus superficial irregularities of the buttocks. **B:** One year postoperatively, after liposculpture of dorsal region, flanks, buttocks, and lateral thighs, with good contour improvement and good treatment of the superficial irregularities of the buttocks with the Toledo V-tip dissector cannula. **C:** The use of the Toledo V-tip dissector cannula. The depression areas are marked with the patient in the standing position. The cannula is used with in-and-out movements, freeing the skin from the adhesions that pull it down. Fat is injected into the irregular area to help prevent the reattachment of the dimple.

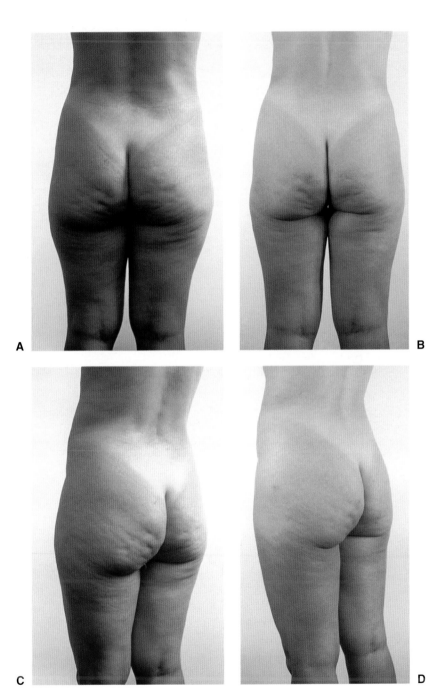

FIG. 15-19. A, C: Severe superficial irregularities in the buttocks. This patient wanted correction of the lateral thigh and gluteal area plus improvement of the "cellulite" dimples in the buttocks. **B, D:** One year postoperatively, after reduction liposculpture of the body with superficial treatment of buttock irregularities.

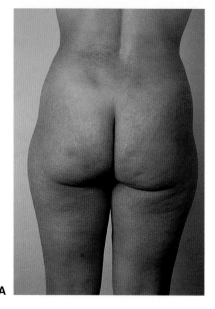

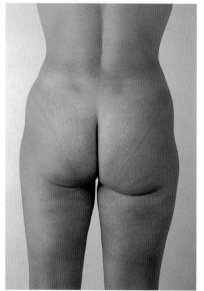

FIG. 15-20. A: Preoperative photo of a 35-year-old patient with minor defects, small adiposities in the flanks, lateral thighs, and buttocks, and some small "cellulite" buttock depressions. In my experience, patients who come for minor corrections, as in this case, are always the more demanding patients. **B:** Six-month postoperative photo of body reduction liposculpture with improvement of superficial buttock irregularities. I always advise the patient preoperatively that we should obtain a good contour improvement, but the superficial defects will improve only up to 50%, depending on their reabsorption of fat.

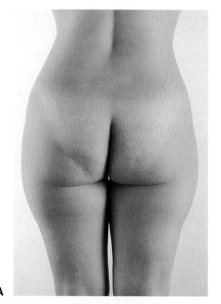

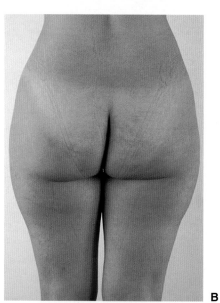

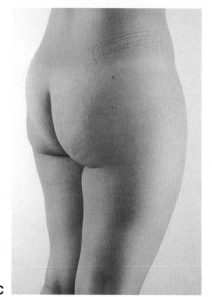

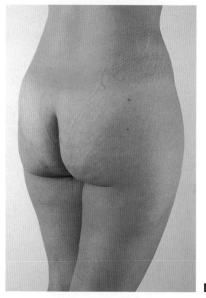

FIG. 15-21. A, C: Preoperative photos of a 38-year-old patient who had a left buttock depression from childhood, provoked by intramuscular injections. **B, D:** One year postoperatively, after two injections of 50 cc of fat under the depression, performed with a two-month interval. The result shown is 10 months after the second fat injection.

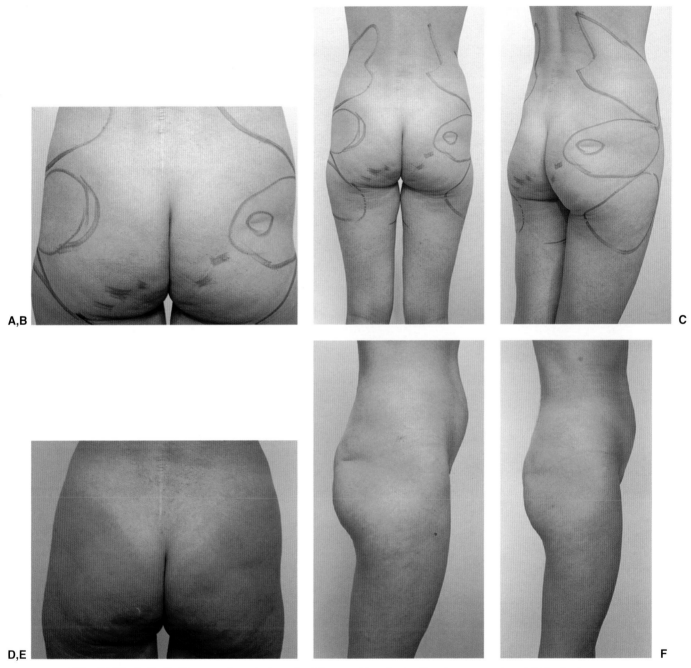

FIG. 15-22. A, B, C: Preoperative photos of a 39-year-old patient with a trauma on her right buttock, the result of a car accident. She developed a serious depression in that area. She also had excess fat in the flanks and lateral thighs that needed fat suction (marked in *blue*) and a trochanteric depression that needed fat injection, plus a few dimples and small buttock irregularities (marked in *red*). **D:** Eleven months postoperatively, after body liposculpture. Fat was aspirated with syringe liposculpture from the flanks and thighs and immediately reinjected into the depression areas. We freed and pretunneled the depression areas prior to fat injection. **E:** Preoperative profile of the right side with the trauma depression. **F:** Eleven months postoperatively, after body liposculpture. The depression was not totally corrected, but the patient was happy with the result; we estimated a 50% improvement and she believes she got more than that. *Figure continues on next page.*

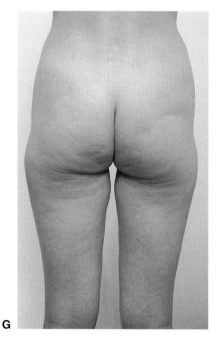

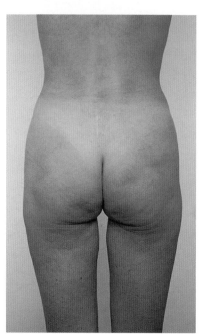

FIG. 15-22. *Continued.* **G:** Preoperative dorsal view. **H:** Dorsal view eleven months postoperatively.

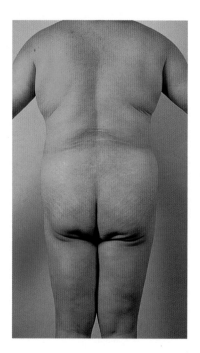

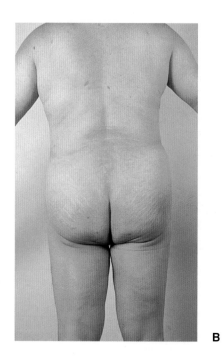

FIG. 15-23. A: A 48-year-old patient with a masculine-shaped body, fat deposits concentrated above the waistline, and flaccid flat buttocks with a painful depression on the ischium pressure areas. **B:** Eight months postoperatively, after reduction liposculpture of the arms, dorsal area, and waist, and injection of 400 cc of fat into each buttock, with a good improvement of the sitting depression. Although this initial result seems good, this is not the usual outcome for this type of problem; reabsorption in pressure areas tends to be higher than in places with no pressure.

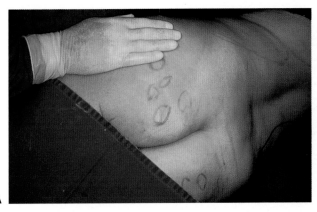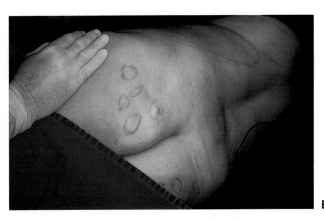

FIG. 15-24. A: We mark the depressions in red with the patient standing and use the V-tip dissector cannula with in-and-out movements to free the adhesions that pull the skin down. **B:** After the skin is freed from its attachments, we inject fat in 3-mm threads under the marked area. We overinject by about 50%.

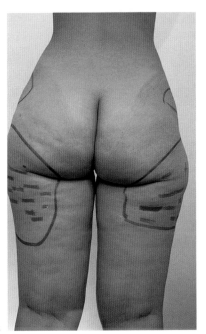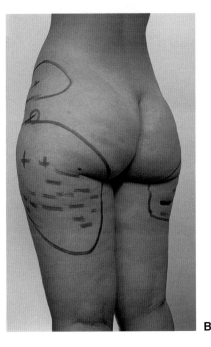

FIG. 15-25. A, B: Preoperative dorsal and ¾ views of an overweight 27-year-old patient. She has a flaccid skin tone with the fat excess concentrated below the waistline. This patient needs superficial liposculpture of the flanks, lateral thigh, and lower third of the buttock areas. The blue marks the areas of suction, the little red dots mark the areas with skin depressions for fat injection, and the two blue crosses mark the highest point on the lateral thigh. *Figure continues on next page.*

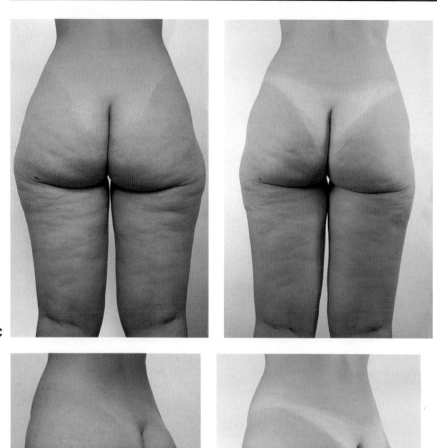

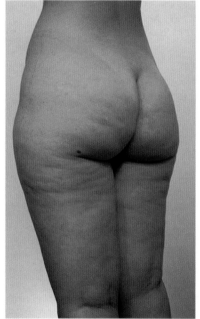

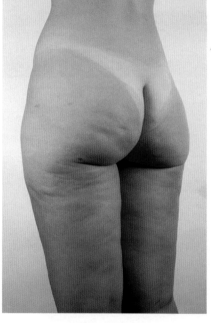

C

D

E

F

FIG. 15-25. *Continued.* **C, E:** Preoperative photos. The skin flaccidity does not allow us to improve her contour too much, but we discussed the probability of a reduction in her measurements so she would be able to wear clothes at least one size smaller, hoping this would stimulate her to exercise and lose weight. **D, F:** Ten months postoperatively. It is not a great result, but it is all we could accomplish for this patient—a reduction in the lateral thighs and some improvement in the superficial irregularities, where we overinjected by about 50%.

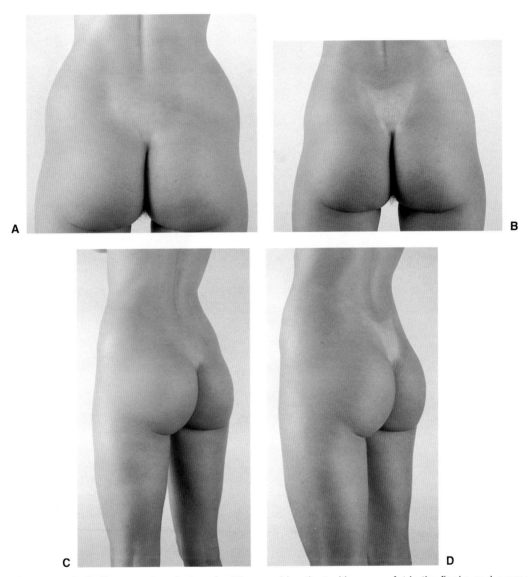

FIG. 15-26. A, C: Preoperative photos of a 23-year-old patient with excess fat in the flanks and a very bony sacral region. She referred to pain in this area when she sat in the reclined position. This is not a very common problem. **B, D:** Ten months postoperatively, after aspiration of fat from the flanks, improving her contour, and injecting into the sacral region, being careful to spread the graft in parallel 3-mm threads. We performed only one procedure on this patient, although we had planned two. She decided she did not need the second injection.

16

The Calves and Ankles

Fat aspiration of calves and ankles does not give the same satisfaction as with other areas. In one study, only 84% of patients were satisfied with the results, compared with 98% of those who underwent liposuction in other parts of the body (1). Patient selection is based on the thickness of subcutaneous fat. A minimum amount of fat should remain to avoid postoperative skin irregularity. The problems with aspiration of fat in the calves and ankles are mostly due to the anatomy of the region. It is crucial that the surgeon thinks three-dimensionally when operating on these areas, otherwise the cannula will irregularly suction the superficial fat layer and provoke defects.

There is an old belief that there are colliding zones in the dorsal region of calves and ankles, which should not be crossed to avoid irregularities. Suction should be limited to the medial and lateral parts of these areas. This idea has been challenged, and circumferential treatment has been advocated and practiced with good results (2), not limiting the correction to defined bulges. Obviously, patients who need circumferential treatment need reduction of the entire lower leg instead of just reducing the medial and lateral ankle bulges.

I rarely have to perform circumferential liposculpture. Most of my patients need only localized treatments, either in the anterior area just below the knees, or on the dorsal calves, or on the medial and lateral ankles. This procedure is rarely performed alone; it is usually part of a combined procedure.

For the last 12 years, I have been performing not only aspiration, but also injection of fat into the lower legs. In android-type patients, I usually combine aspiration of fat from the upper body with injection into the calves and ankles. In gynoid patients, I will aspirate fat from the lower legs (3).

Aspiration or injection of fat into the calves and ankles gives a very subtle result, most of the times imperceptible to other people, but many patients are very pleased with even small changes of one or two centimeters in the circumference. I always measure and photograph very precisely to show the patient postoperatively what the problem looked like before in case of dissatisfaction.

INSTRUMENTS

I use 60-cc toomey-tip syringes, 2- and 3-mm gauge, 25 to 35 cm long. Anesthesia is injected with a 2-mm-gauge multiholed-tip cannula. The cannulas I prefer are the Pyramid-tip cannulas, although I can use a 2-mm one-lateral-holed tip. For injecting fat I use a one-lateral-holed, 3-mm-gauge blunt-tip cannula.

ANESTHESIA

Anesthesia is the same as that used to treat the rest of the body, usually sedation and local tumescent. The injection is done with a fine multiholed cannula (Fig. 16-1). I infiltrate a proportion of 1:1 of my local anesthesia formula at body temperature and wait ten minutes before I begin suctioning.

POSITION

I usually treat the calves and ankles with the patient in the supine or prone position, with the leg extended or with the knee bent at 90 degrees. The assistant can hold the leg for other special positions if necessary.

INCISIONS

I will do as many incisions as necessary to have good access, but generally, I make two popliteal incisions for the dorsal calf and one or two subpatellar incisions for the pretibial area. The ankles can be treated through medial and lateral malleolus incisions. Another incision might be necessary in the midmedial part.

FAT ASPIRATION

Deep Suction

When there is a large fat deposit, I start suctioning deep, with a 3-mm-gauge long cannula in the area marked preoperatively, trying to aspirate fat uniformly following the curves of the leg to thin down the defect. Laterally and medially, when aspirating from the malleolus region, the suction can be more plane. The quantities are usually small, and the syringes allow us to measure them exactly (Figs. 16-2, 16-3).

Superficial Suction

I change to a 2-mm-gauge cannula, and aspirate fat closer to the skin. Superficial suction is rarely necessary in this area. I usually suction 4 to 5 mm deep. Skin retraction is rarely needed in the calves and ankles.

Fat Injection

I can inject fat into the muscle, in the calves, in the ankles, only subcutaneously. I prefer fat injection to silicone prostheses in the calves. Prostheses can get retracted and appear unnatural. Fat can be partially reabsorbed, but the results look natural (Figs. 16-4, 16-5).

POSTOPERATIVE CARE

I tell patients to avoid walking too much on the first postoperative days. Sleeping with the legs elevated 10 to 16 cm and the use of elastic stockings of mild compression for three weeks are also advised to avoid excessive swelling. Manual lymphatic drainage is prescribed after the second postoperative day. Exercising and sunbathing are allowed after 30 days.

REFERENCES

1. Watanabe K. Circumferential liposuction of calves and ankles. *Aesthetic Plast Surg* 1990;14: 259–269.
2. Mladick RA. Circumferential ''intermediate'' lipoplasty of the legs. *Aesthetic Plast Surg* 1994;18:165–174.
3. Matsudo PK, Toledo LS. Experience of injected fat grafting. *Aesthetic Plast Surg* 1988;12:35–38.

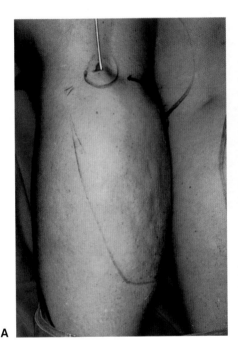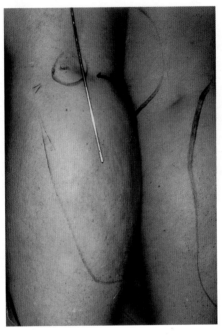

A   B

FIG. 16-1. A, B: Anesthesia is injected with a 2-mm-gauge multiholed-tip cannula.

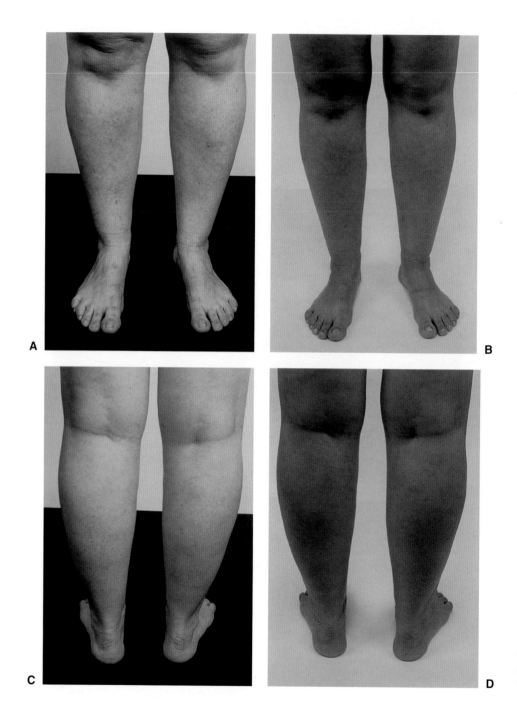

FIG. 16-2. A, C: Preoperative photos of a 39-year-old patient. **B, D:** Six months postoperatively. There was a reduction of 2 cm in the calves and 2 cm in the ankles, difficult to appreciate in the pictures.

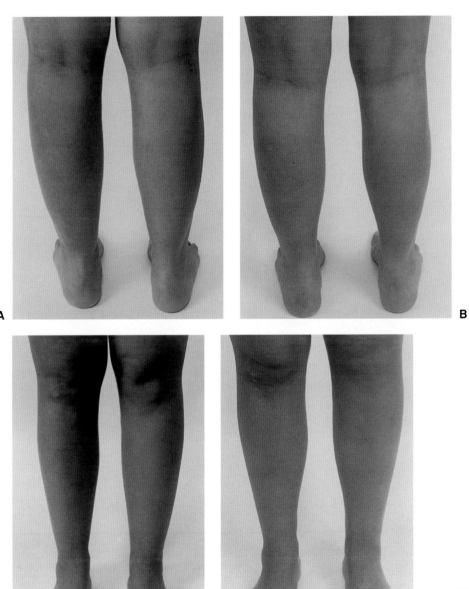

FIG. 16-3. A, C: Preoperative photos of a 25-year-old patient. She wanted a better shape to the leg and reduction of the ankles. **B, D:** One year postoperatively. Ankle reduction was 2 cm.

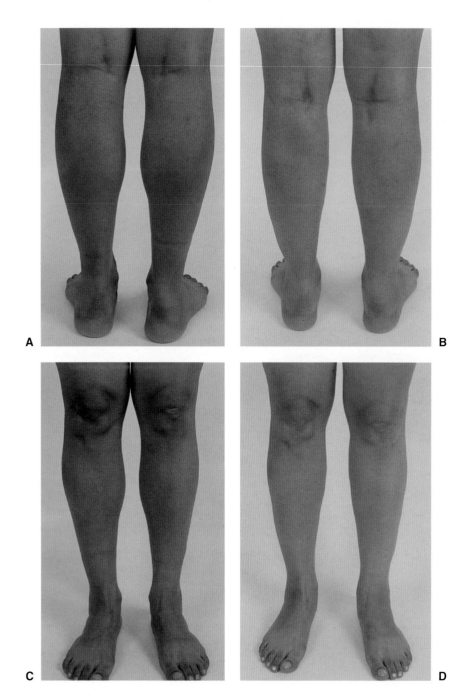

FIG. 16-4. A, C: Preoperative photos of a 45-year-old patient who wanted to smooth the shape of her thin calves and ankles. **B, D:** One year postoperatively, after injection of 60 cc on each calf, 25 cc on each medial ankle, and 30 cc on each lateral ankle.

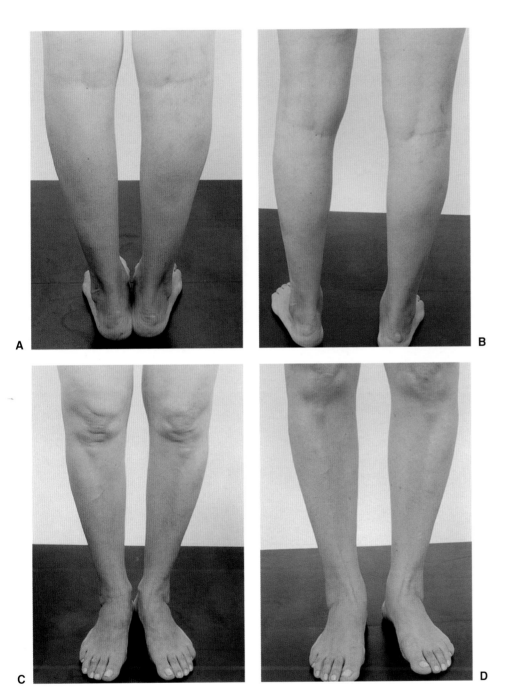

A

B

C

D

FIG. 16-5. A, C: Preoperative photos of a 52-year-old patient who wanted to improve the shape of her thin calves and ankles. **B, D:** Six months postoperatively, after injection of 50 cc on each calf, 30 cc on each medial ankle, and 30 cc on each lateral ankle.

17

The Abdomen

In 1988 (1), I stopped using the aspirator and began using syringe liposculpture (2) to treat the abdomen. In 1989, I began using superficial liposculpture (3) to treat the areas of the abdomen, such as the hypogastrium, that needed skin retraction. Because of the good retraction obtained with this technique, my practice showed a reduction in the number of patients that I would indicate for traditional abdominoplasty (4).

Due to the increased precision superficial liposculpture gives, my results with liposculpture of the abdomen improved greatly. The main reason is that with the syringe, I can see the exact amount of fat and anesthesia removed from each part of the abdomen, and do not have to rely only on the pinch test to control the final flap thickness (Fig. 17-1). Before the syringe, it was impossible to estimate the removal by looking at the 2-liter vial of the aspirator. In some borderline cases where abdominoplasty would have traditionally been advised, a satisfactory skin retraction can be obtained without the abdominoplasty (Fig. 17-2). In these cases patients will usually opt for a closed procedure with no extensive scarring, even if the final result might not be as good as the possible abdominoplasty (Fig. 17-3). This factor—the use of the superficial technique, as opposed to traditional liposuction—has greatly broadened my indication for liposuction of the abdomen. Abdominoplasty today (traditional and limited together) accounts for only 20% of my patients who are looking for improvement in the abdominal area. Before 1988 this number was 50%. One of the main concerns of the plastic surgeon and his patient is the reduction in the length of the abdominoplasty scar. After the initial enthusiasm of trying to solve too many problems with the new liposculpture technique, I am now more cautious and do not try to solve all problems through suction alone.

I do, however, constantly offer my flaccid-skin patients the opportunity to choose between an improved shape with no scars, and an optimal shape utilizing liposculpture combined with abdominoplasty, a procedure with an incision. They are also made aware that they can opt for a second suction after six months, when the healing process allows it. I can combine superficial liposculpture with suprapubic ellipse or trapezoid dermolipectomy; this usually involves just the superficial fat above the Scarpa's fascia, without having to undergo a traditional abdominoplasty with muscle-aponeurotic plication (Vasconez L., personal communication, 1993) (Figs. 17-4, 17-5). The dermolipectomy is generally performed after the suction so that there is less possibility of seromas forming, which is the most common complication when dermolipectomy and suction are performed together.

I use syringe liposculpture alone in 80% of my patients. The remaining 20% are treated either with the Callia technique (5) of classical abdominoplasty (Fig. 17-6), or with the Wilkinson technique (6) of limited or mini-abdominoplasty (Fig. 17-7).

Most of the problems related to the abdomen are caused by a lack of criteria for surgeons to classify the abdomen and choose the appropriate technique (7). Patient dissatisfaction can be minimized preoperatively by talking and explaining the possibilities and limitations of each method. Patients needing an abdominoplasty for hygiene purposes should be treated with the classical method, with extensive skin and fat resection, plus muscle-aponeurotic plication and omphaloplasty (Fig. 17-8). Not many patients need this kind of application, which was very popular in the past. When there are no diastases hernias, exercising and diet after liposculpture can solve the abdominal protrusion. The plication, in most cases, was just a simpler way of reducing the abdominal volume for the patients who did not want to exercise, at the cost of a very long horizontal and permanent scar.

INSTRUMENTS

I use 60-cc toomey-tip syringes, plunger locks, and transfers to pass fat from one 60-cc syringe to another anaerobically. For anesthesia injection I use a 2-mm or 3-mm-gauge, 35-cm-long, multiholed-tip needle. Fat is aspirated with Pyramid-tip cannulas, 2-mm to 4.6-mm-gauge, 25 cm to 35 cm long. I treat irregularities and release old scars with the 3-mm-gauge V-tip Toledo dissector cannula (8). We also utilize a balloon-tip 5-mm-gauge cannula to suction fibrotic fat areas.

ANESTHESIA

When treating only a small adiposity, or if the patient prefers, there is no need for heavy sedation, and only oral midazolam 15 mg is applied. For larger cases the anesthesiologist uses midazolam and fentanyl for sedation. Midazolam is used in doses of 0.1 mg/kg IV. The maximum dose is a total of 0.3 mg/kg, depending on the patient and the procedure. Midazolam's action is antagonized with flumazenil in doses varying from 0.2 to 1.0 mg IV. For local anesthesia I use a modification of the Klein tumescent solution (9) with 20 cc of 2% lidocaine, 5 cc 3% sodium bicarbonate, 1 cc adrenaline 1:1000, Ringer's lactate q.s.p. 500 ml (10). I inject up to 2 liters of this solution into the abdomen at body temperature. I start suctioning after 10 to 15 minutes.

POSITION

I operate with the abdomen hyperextended in the supine position to avoid perforations of the abdominal wall (Fig. 17-9).

INCISIONS

Although sometimes it is possible to operate on the abdomen through only one pubic incision (Fig. 17-10), I usually use two incisions: one pubic and one umbilical (Fig. 17-11). Sometimes, however, I need extra incisions for specific areas. For the waist I might use two iliac crest incisions (Fig. 17-12). For the epigastrium, two mammary fold incisions might be necessary (Fig. 17-13). The benefit of other incisions is the possibility of crisscrossing to obtain a regular result.

FAT ASPIRATION

Deep Suction

The abdomen can be aspirated alone or in conjunction with the flanks and waist. When I treat other areas, I use the other incisions for crisscrossing; if just the abdomen, I plan the aspiration in four stages, dividing the abdomen into four quadrants. I anesthetize the entire abdomen before I start suctioning. I start with deep suction close to the rectus muscle (Fig. 17-14). If I am treating an obese patient, I use a 4.6-mm gauge; for medium-sized patients, I start with a 3.7-mm-gauge cannula. As I get more superficial, I change the gauges, using fine cannulas, 3-mm gauge or 2-mm gauge, as I approach the dermis and need more refinement.

Preoperative photographs of the patient in the standing position are displayed in the operating room to evaluate asymmetries when the patient is lying down on the operating table (Fig. 17-15). Irregularities and asymmetries are compared and treated accordingly.

I control the regularity of the suction with either the pinch test (Fig. 17-16) or the outstretched hand (Fig. 17-17). Most abdomens will greatly improve through deep liposculpture alone and it is unnecessary to treat the superficial layer of fat (Fig. 17-18), which would augment the risk of provoking irregularities.

Superficial Suction

I perform superficial liposuction in the abdomen only in the areas where I want the skin to retract (Fig. 17-19). Usually after one or two pregnancies, the hypogastrium gets flaccid and protrudes. This area should be aspirated with great care, to avoid irregularities. The epigastrium usually needs only deep suction. We establish a sequence for aspiration of the four quadrants and follow that sequence.

After finishing one side of the abdomen, I compare both sides and check the amount of fat removed. After I finish the other side, I check both sides for evenness. Any irregularities can be corrected with a 2-mm-gauge cannula. I am always very careful with the angle of the cannula, never pointing it down to the abdominal wall. I also use a different pinching method, pulling the flap up to make sure I am working in the fat layer (Fig. 17-20). Assistants usually help me to spot uneven areas. Sometimes the assistant is at a better angle to appreciate the deformity than I am. If I agree with their comments, I will accept their input. By checking the recorded volume of aspirate and comparing with the photographs, I can tell if I need to aspirate more. Small defects can be better appreciated with the outstretched hand (Fig. 17-21). The uniformity of the suction can also be tested by changing the position of the operating room lights, by wetting the skin, or by moving the patient.

If the defect is a high point, I will perform more suction. If it is a depression, I will inject some of the two or three syringes of fat I always reserve for these occasions.

FAT INJECTION

We try to preserve the aspirated fat cells by treating them gently—slow (1,500 r/min) centrifuging, decanting, and transferring the fat with extreme care. Injection is in threads, with a blunt needle, all to avoid fat cell destruction. Fat grafts with a diameter greater than 3 mm have less possibility of survival. Fat cells obtain nutrition through plasmatic inbibition only at approximately 1.5 mm from the vascularized edge (11). I usually find that 50% of my fat grafts take.

SECONDARY PROCEDURES

Scars

I usually combine the treatment of old general surgery scars, retracted cesarean incisions, and appendectomy and old abdominoplasty scars with abdominal liposculpture. When the old abdominoplasty scar is too high, I perform an intraoperative 20-minute tissue extension and pull it down (Figs. 17-22, 17-23). If the scar is completely out of place laterally, there is nothing much that can be done, except to try to improve the scar quality and the shape of the abdomen. I do not think tissue expansion will improve this situation without extending the incisions even more (Fig. 17-24.)

When performing an abdominal liposculpture on a patient with scars, there are some techniques that can be used to avoid incisional hernias. One of them is to elevate the scar with a Backauss forceps (Fig. 17-25) and continue with our suction.

The improvement of Pfannenstiel or vertical cesarean scars can be performed in combination with aspiration and the use of the V-tip Toledo dissector cannula. I suction the excess fat above the scar and, with the patient still in the hyperextended supine position to avoid abdominal penetration, I free the scar adhesions. I inject some of the removed fat under the scar to avoid its reattachment (Figs. 17-26, 17-27).

The same technique is used to treat old retracted abdominoplasty scars (Fig. 17-28). Dog-ears of old abdominoplasty scars can be treated through superficial suction before we try a scar revision that undoubtedly lengthens the scar (Fig. 17-29).

Patients with abdominal liposuction sequelae of irregularities and depressions are treated by suctioning the excess fat, freeing the adhesions, and injecting fat into the depressed areas (Figs. 17-30, 17-31).

Pubis

The treatment of fat deposits in the pubic area was developed in the 1960s, when the horizontal incision abdominoplasty became popular. Reduction liposculpture of the suprapubic area (Fig. 17-32) is not a popular technique, but I often do it in conjunction with other body sculpture procedures. Patients with this type of fat deposit often feel discriminated against and cannot wear certain types of clothes or sports wear. Superficial liposculpture improves the results obtained with deep suction, with a better skin retraction.

POSTOPERATIVE CARE

Micropore dressings with gauze are placed on the incision points. The incisions will drain for the first 24 hours. An abdominal binder or girdle should be used for a month. Manual lymphatic drainage (Fig. 17-33) is performed by our estheticians, starting at 24 hours postoperatively, two to three times a week to diminish the swelling and provide comfort. I give my patients one gram IV of cephalosporin in the operating room and prescribe antibiotics for five days. Patients can begin walking the next day, driving on the fifth or sixth postoperative day, and start exercising and sunbathing after one month.

REFERENCES

1. Toledo LS. Syringe liposculpture for face and body. In: Toledo LS, ed. *Annals of the international symposium "recent advances in plastic surgery (RAPS) 89,"* São Paulo, Brazil, March 3–5, 1989. São Paulo: Estadão, 1989:177–192.
2. Fournier P. *Liposculpture—ma technique.* Paris: Arnette, 1989.
3. Toledo LS. Superficial syringe liposculpture. In: Toledo LS, ed. *Annals of the international symposium "recent advances in plastic surgery (RAPS) 90,"* São Paulo, Brazil, March 3–5, 1990. Rio de Janeiro: Marques Saraiva, 1990:446–453.
4. Toledo LS. Total liposculpture. In: Gasparotti M, Lewis CM, Toledo LS, eds. *Superficial liposculpture.* New York: Springer-Verlag, 1993:44.
5. Callia WEP. Contribuição para o estudo da correção cirúrgica do abdome pêndulo e globoso—técnica original. Tese de Doutoramento apresentada -a Faculdade de Medicina da Universidade de São Paulo. São Paulo:USP, 1965.
6. Wilkinson TS. Individual modifications in body contour surgery. The "limited" abdominoplasty. *Plas Reconstr Surg* 1986;77:779–784.
7. Bozola AR, Psillakis JM. Classification of abdominoplasty. *Plast Reconstr Surg* 1988;82:983–993.
8. Toledo LS. Superficial syringe liposculpture for the treatment of "cellulite" and liposuction sequelae. Lecture presented at the Recent Advances in Plastic Surgery symposium, Buenos Aires, Argentina, June 11, 1989.
9. Klein JA. Tumescent technique for regional anesthesia permits lidocaine doses of 35 mg/kg for liposuction. *J Dermatol Surg Oncol* 1990;248–263.
10. Toledo LS. Syringe liposculpture. A two year experience. *Aesthetic Plast Surg* 1991;15:321–326.
11. Carpaneda CA, Ribeiro MT. Percentage of graft viability versus injected volume in adipose autotransplants. *Aesthetic Plast Surg* 1994;18:17–19.

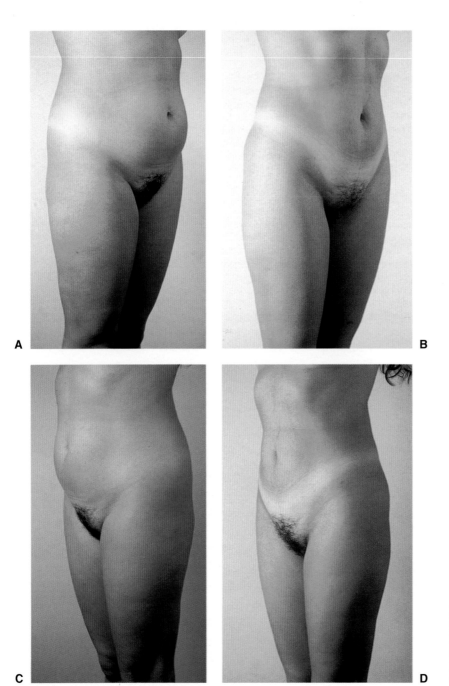

FIG. 17-1. A, C: Preoperative photos of a 32-year-old patient. A good indication for syringe liposculpture because of the precision of the method. **B, D:** One year postoperatively. The procedure motivated the patient to start dieting (lost 4 kg) and exercising.

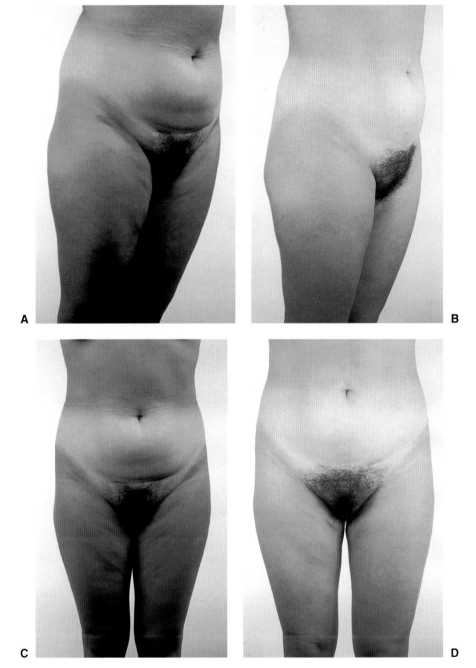

FIG. 17-2. A, C: Preoperative photos of a 36-year-old patient, with an indication for an abdominoplasty, who did not want to have the procedure but preferred abdominal liposculpture. **B, D:** One-month postoperative results of abdominal liposculpture, with a good uniform retraction although there is still a residual edema.

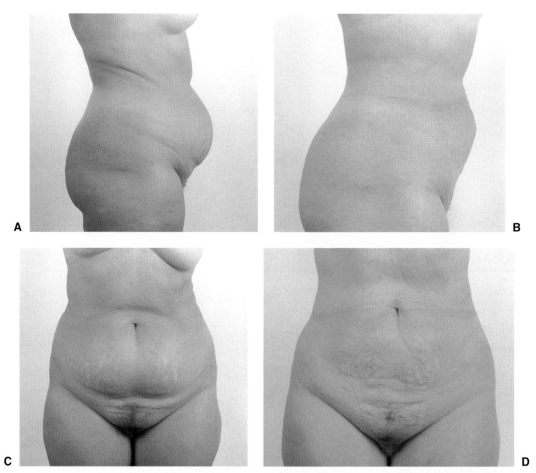

FIG. 17-3. A, C: A 51-year-old patient after three pregnancies and with excess abdominal fat plus striae. The skin was very flaccid, and our indication was for a limited abdominoplasty. **B, D:** The patient opted for an abdominal liposculpture, avoiding an abdominoplasty scar even if the final result would not be as good. She still had some fat and skin excess in the hypogastrium, but was happy with the shape of her body in clothes and did not want skin removed.

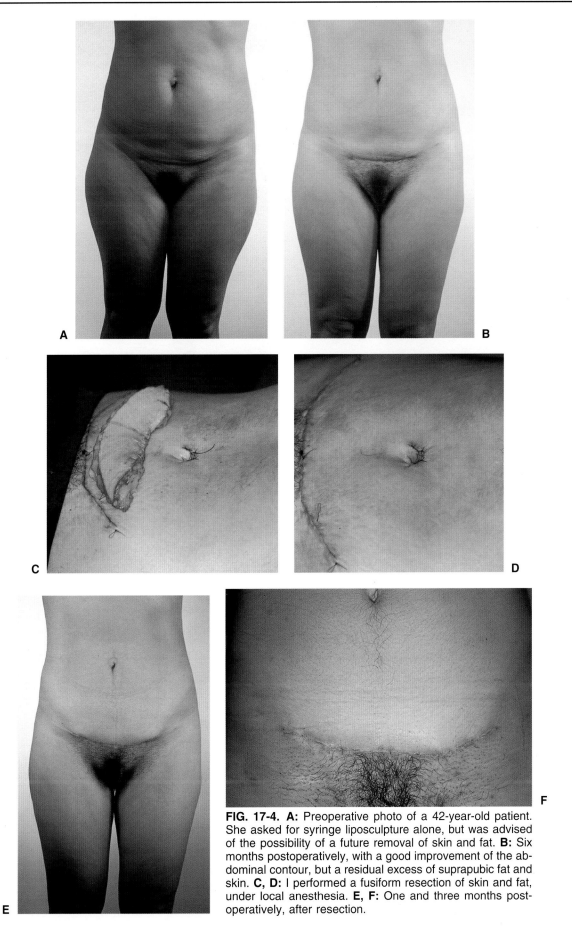

FIG. 17-4. A: Preoperative photo of a 42-year-old patient. She asked for syringe liposculpture alone, but was advised of the possibility of a future removal of skin and fat. **B:** Six months postoperatively, with a good improvement of the abdominal contour, but a residual excess of suprapubic fat and skin. **C, D:** I performed a fusiform resection of skin and fat, under local anesthesia. **E, F:** One and three months postoperatively, after resection.

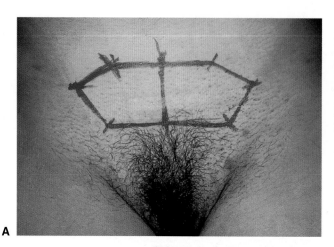
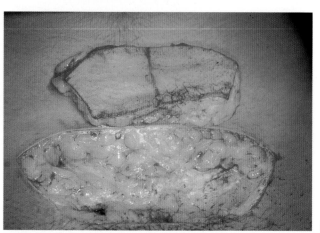

FIG. 17-5. A, B: Another shape of this resection can be a trapezoid.

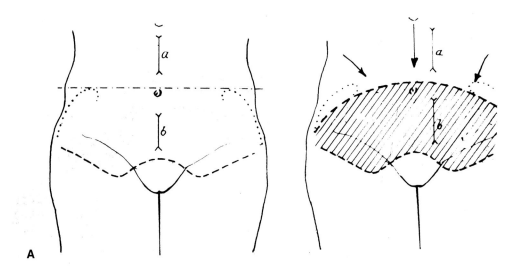

FIG. 17-6. A: The original 1961 drawings of the Callia abdominal dermolipectomy technique. (Courtesy of Prof. William E. P. Callia.)

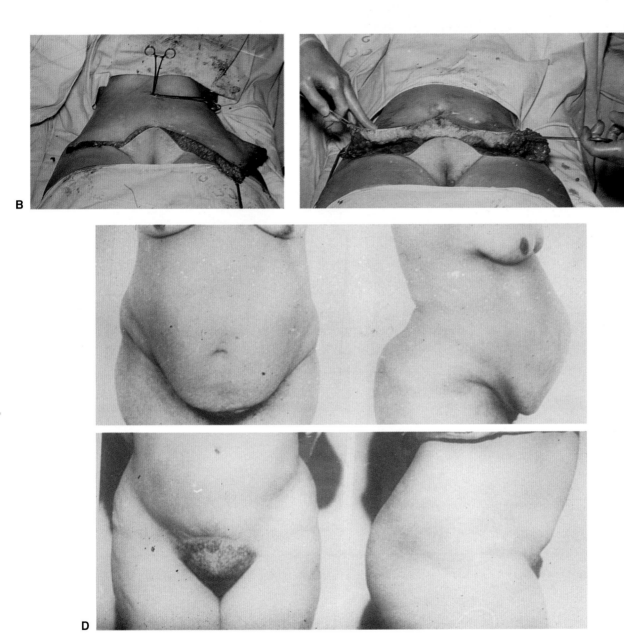

FIG. 17-6. *Continued.* **B, C:** Intraoperative photos of a Callia abdominoplasty in 1961. **D:** Pre- and postoperative photos of Callia abdominoplasty from 1961. (Courtesy of Prof. William E. P. Callia.)

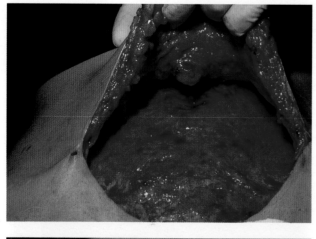

A

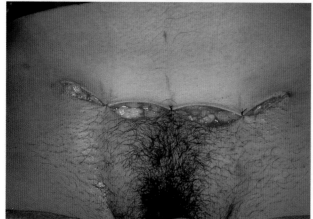

B

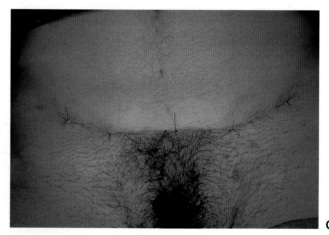

C

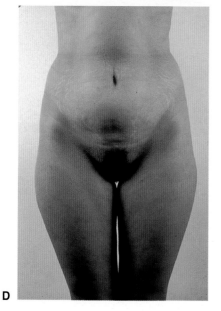

D

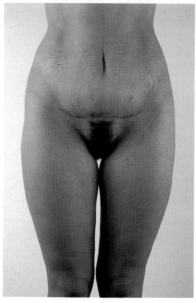

E

FIG. 17-7. A, B, C: Intraoperative photos of a limited Wilkinson abdominoplasty, with the removal of a slice of skin and fat and "floating" of the umbilicus. **D, E:** Pre- and 14-month postoperative photos of a 45-year-old patient who underwent a limited abdominoplasty.

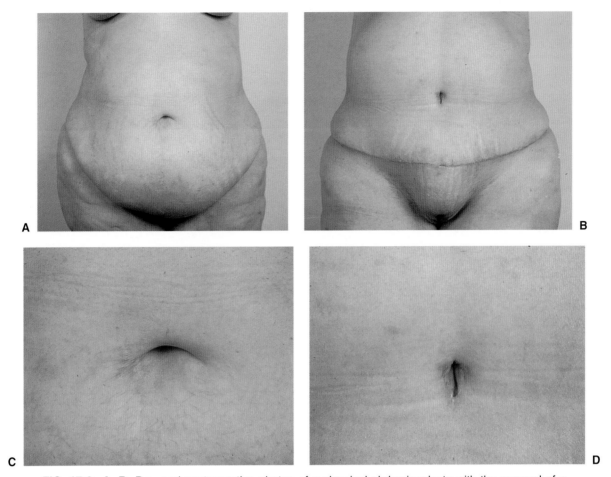

A   B

C   D

FIG. 17-8. A, B: Pre- and postoperative photos of a classical abdominoplasty with the removal of a 3.5 kg flap. **C, D:** Pre- and postoperative photos of the technique I prefer for omphaloplasty—Juri's technique.

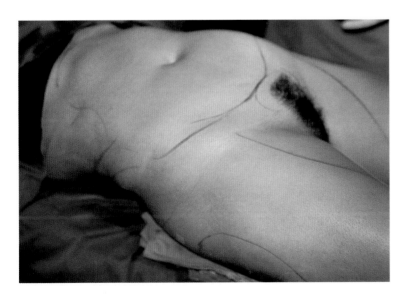

FIG. 17-9. The patient is placed on the table in the supine hyperextended position. That can be achieved either by bending the surgical table or by placing a pillow under the patient's buttocks.

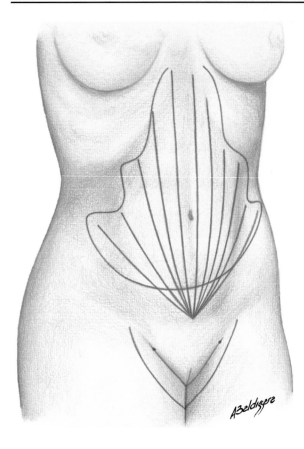

FIG. 17-10. Drawing of the pubic incision and the direction of possible tunnels. For some patients this incision alone is enough to treat the abdomen.

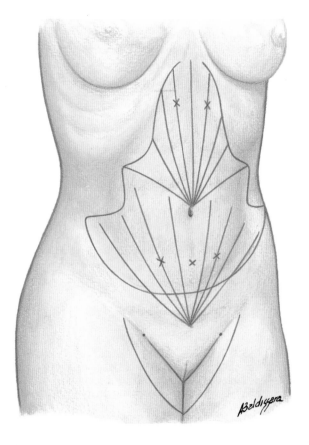

FIG. 17-11. Most patients are treated with two incisions in the abdomen, one in the pubic area and another in the umbilical scar. This will provide better access to the epigastrium as well as the possibility of crisscrossing.

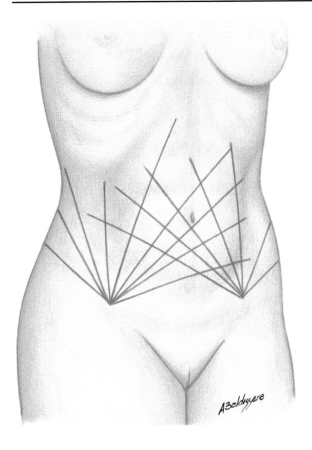

FIG. 17-12. For patients who need treatment of the waist area or who have large adiposities, we can use two iliac crest incisions, alone or combined with the pubic, the umbilical, or the trochanter incisions.

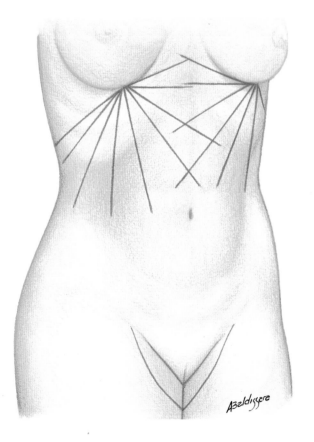

FIG. 17-13. The submammary fold incisions are used for an easier access to the epigastric area. I use them for patients with large epigastric adiposities and also to treat the epigastrium without risking penetration under the rib cage. It also helps with criss-crossing. Instead of changing hands, surgeons can change sides and continue using the syringe with the same hand.

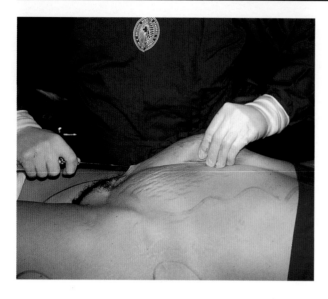

FIG. 17-14. With the abdomen hyperextended, the cannula runs parallel to the abdominal wall. Pinching the flap up high and running the cannula in the deep layer facilitates deep liposculpture. This is a modification of the pinch test where the cannula runs between the fingers.

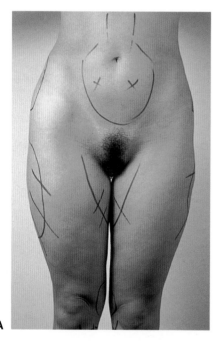
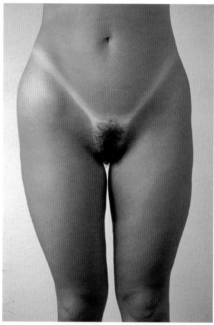

A

B

FIG. 17-15. A: The patient's preoperative photographs in the standing position are displayed in the operating room to evaluate asymmetries when the patient is lying down on the operating table. The photo with the marked irregularities serves as a guide to treat asymmetries. B: Six-month postoperative photo showing the improvement in the marked areas.

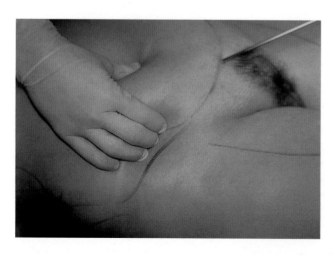

FIG. 17-16. I control the regularity of the deep suction with the pinch test.

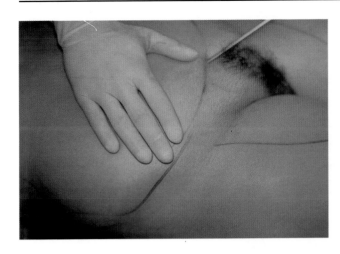

FIG. 17-17. The technique of the outstretched hand can be used to control the regularity of superficial suction.

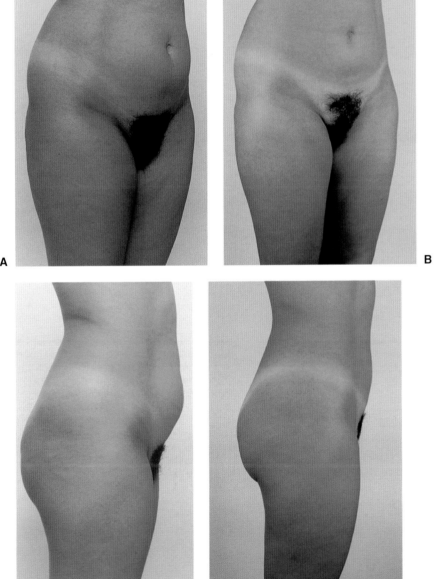

A

B

C

D

FIG. 17-18. A, C: Preoperative photos of a 27-year-old patient with good skin tone and excess fat in the abdomen, flanks, lateral thighs, and medial thighs. **B, D:** We aspirated a total of 780 cc from the abdomen through deep liposculpture alone, it being unnecessary to treat the superficial layer of fat. There was a good retraction of the tissues.

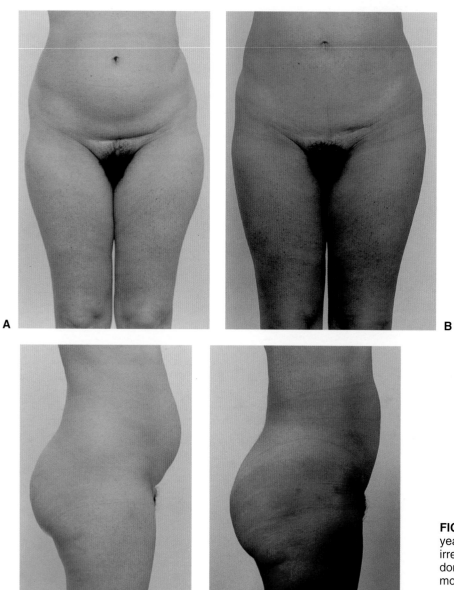

A

B

C

D

FIG. 17-19. A, C: Preoperative photos of a 38-year-old patient with flaccid skin and superficial irregularities. She needed reduction of the abdomen, flanks, and lateral thighs. **B, D:** Six months postoperatively, after superficial liposculpture. There was good retraction of the tissues. The abdominal skin excess in the suprapubic area was almost completely resolved with suction alone. I offered the patient the possibility of a cesarean scar revision, but she was satisfied with the result.

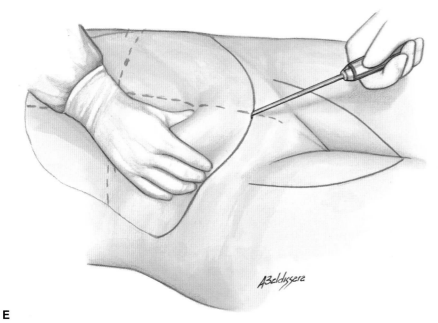

FIG. 17-19. *Continued.* **E:** Aspiration of the abdominal quadrants. By following the sequence I can be sure of a regular result. The amounts removed from each quadrant are recorded for comparison purposes.

E

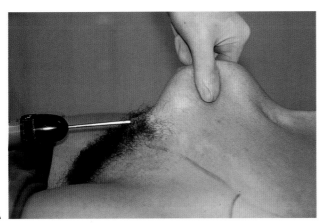

A

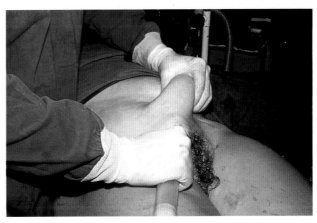

B

FIG. 17-20. A: Pulling the abdominal skin up with the left hand and aspirating with the right hand. The angle of the cannula will direct it towards the skin and not the abdominal wall. **B:** Another possibility of the traditional pinch test where the cannula runs between the fingers.

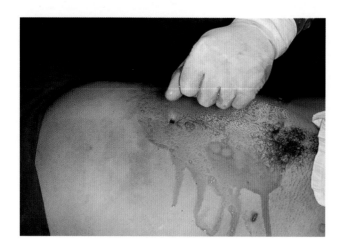

FIG. 17-21. Feeling the cannula aspirating superficially with the outstretched hand. The wet skin facilitates tactility, making it possible to evaluate the depth of the tunnels.

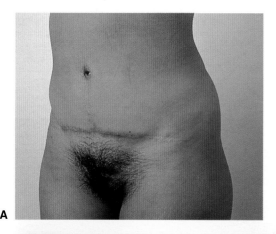

A

FIG. 17-22. A: Old high scars in the abdomen can be pulled down-through an intraoperative tissue extension. **B:** Intraoperative photo with the markings of the fusiform resection to be done. **C:** Intraoperative photo taken during the 20-minute extension of the flap, before we suture and anchor it to its new position.

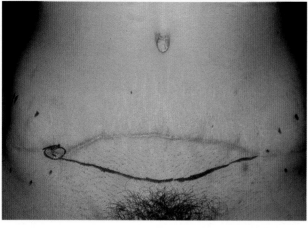

B

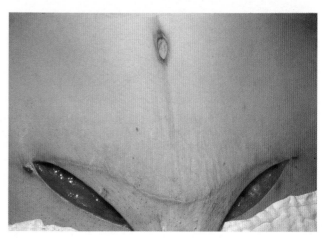

C

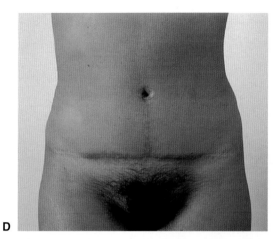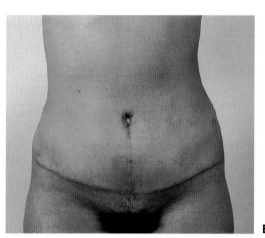

D
E

FIG. 17-22. *Continued.* **D:** Preoperative. **E:** One week postoperatively, after the removal of the stitches. The scar has descended 4 cm.

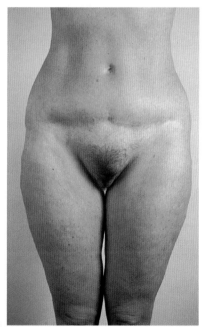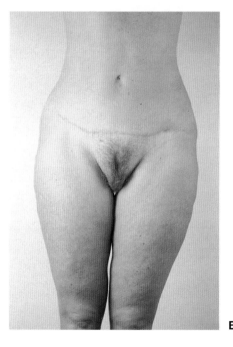

A
B

FIG. 17-23. A: Preoperative photo of a 50-year-old patient with an old, preliposuction abdominoplasty sequela. There was an excess of fat that had to be aspirated and a step deformity between the flap and the pubic region. **B:** Six months postoperatively, after syringe liposculpture of the abdomen, producing a more even result and a scar revision, and lowering the scar 4 cm.

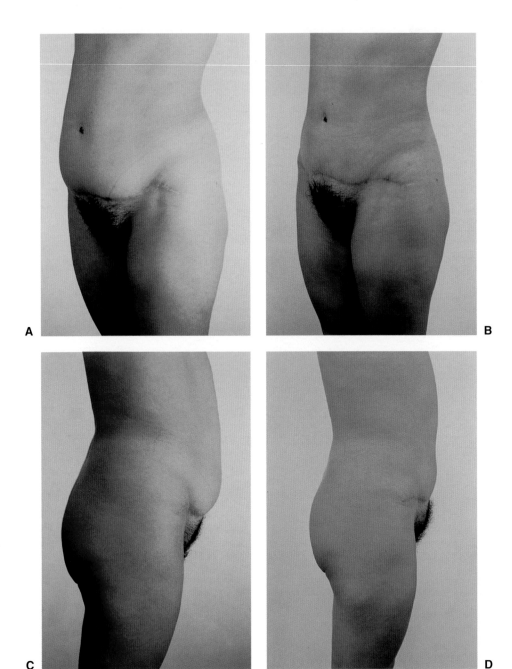

FIG. 17-24. A, C: Preoperative photos of a 43-year-old patient who underwent an old abdominoplasty, with misplaced scars on her anterior thighs and residual excess abdominal fat. **B, D:** One year postoperatively, after syringe liposculpture of the abdomen and scar revision. There was an improvement on the abdominal shape, but the scar did not improve much.

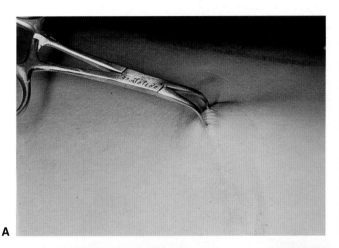

A

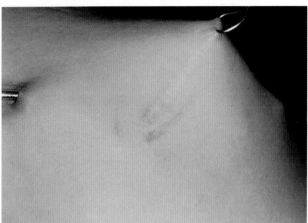

B

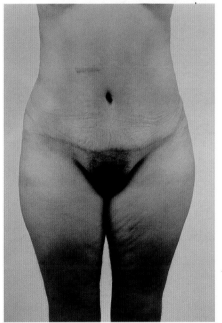

C

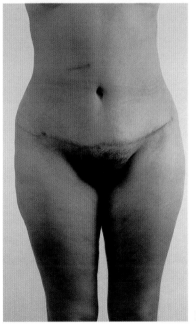

D

FIG. 17-25. A, B: If there are any clinical doubts about the presence of incisional hernias, we should ask for a magnetic resonance image (MRI) or an ultrasound preoperatively. Here I am using a Back-auss forceps to elevate the scar, and passing the cannula under it. **C, D:** Pre- and six-month postoperative photos of syringe liposculpture on a patient with abdominoplasty and cholecystotomy scars. *Figure continues on next page.*

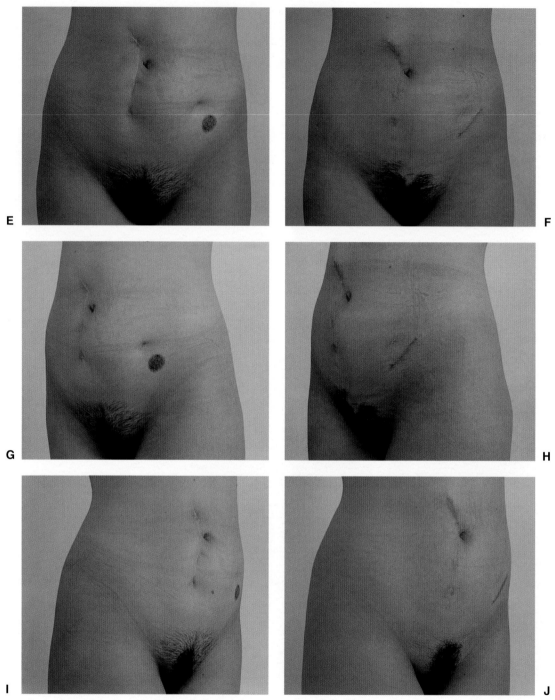

FIG. 17-25. *Continued.* **E, G, I:** Preoperative photos of a 16-year-old patient with excess abdominal fat and scars from an accident many years before. The vertical scar was not bad, but retracted. Only its upper part needed resection. There was a depression on the left hypogastrium on the drain scar and a nevus the patient wanted removed. **F, H, J:** One-month postoperative photos of syringe abdominal liposculpture, scar release, scar revision, and nevus resection. We used the Toledo V-tip dissector cannula for closed scar release. The upper part of the vertical scar and the nevus were resected and sutured.

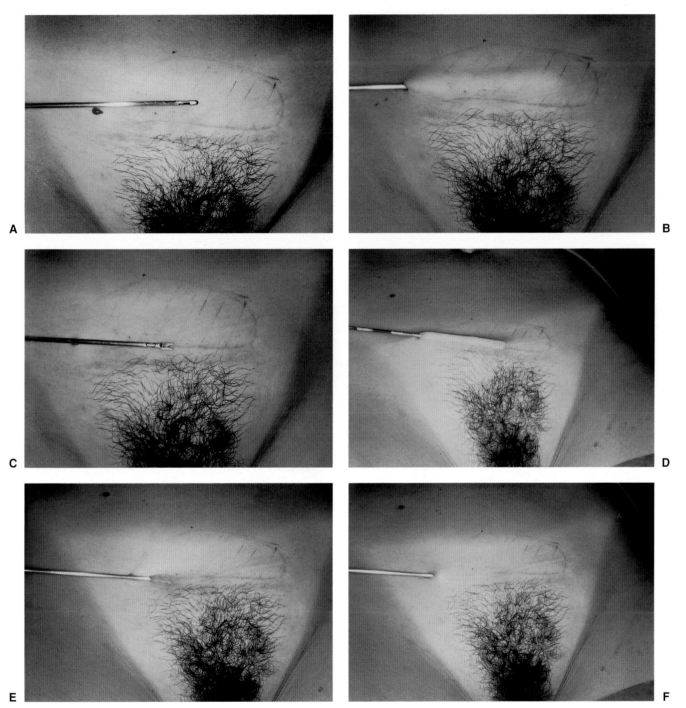

FIG. 17-26. A, B: To improve Pfannenstiel cesarean scars, I combine aspiration and the use of the V-tip Toledo dissector cannula. I suction the excess fat above the scar with a 3-mm-gauge Pyramid-tip cannula. **C, D:** With the Toledo V-tip dissector cannula I free the scar adhesions. **E, F:** With the same cannula, I inject some of the removed fat under the scar to prevent reattachment.

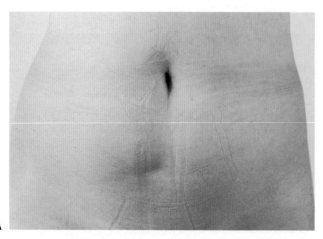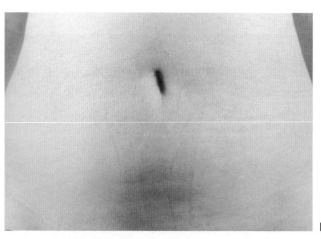

FIG. 17-27. A, B: The improvement of vertical cesarean scars can be performed in the same way. Pre- and three-month postoperative photos of abdominal liposculpture and freeing a retracted vertical scar using the V-tip Toledo dissector cannula.

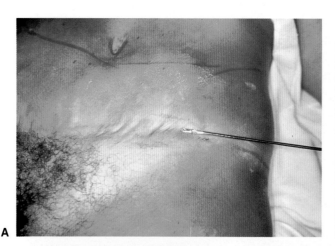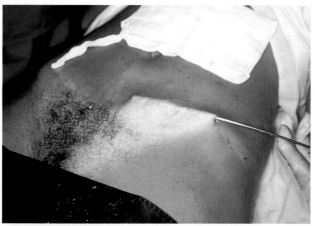

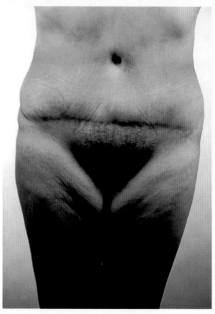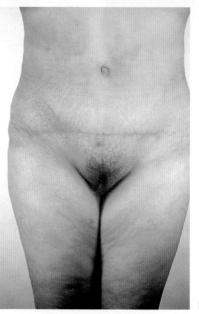

FIG. 17-28. A, B: Using the Toledo V-tip dissector cannula to free an old retracted abdominoplasty scar. Fat is injected under the scar tissue. **C, E:** Preoperative photos of a 52-year-old flaccid-skin patient with a step deformity on her old abdominoplasty scar and excess fat in the abdomen, flanks, and medial thigh areas. **D, F:** One year postoperatively, after superficial liposculpture of the flanks, abdomen, and thighs, plus scar release with the Toledo V-tip dissector cannula.

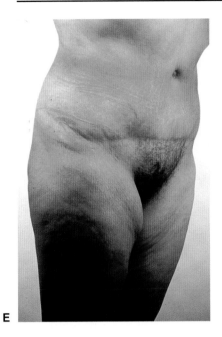
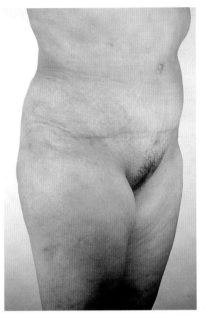

F   **FIG. 17-28.** *Continued.*

E

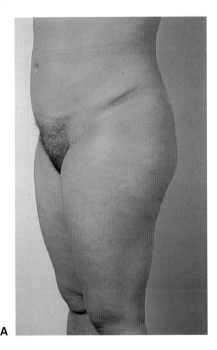
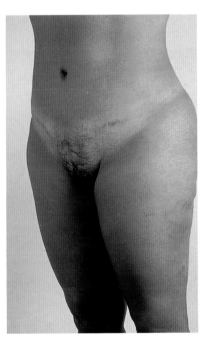

FIG. 17-29. A, B: Pre- and postoperative photos of the treatment of a "dog-ear" deformity on an abdominoplasty scar through superficial liposculpture alone.

A

B

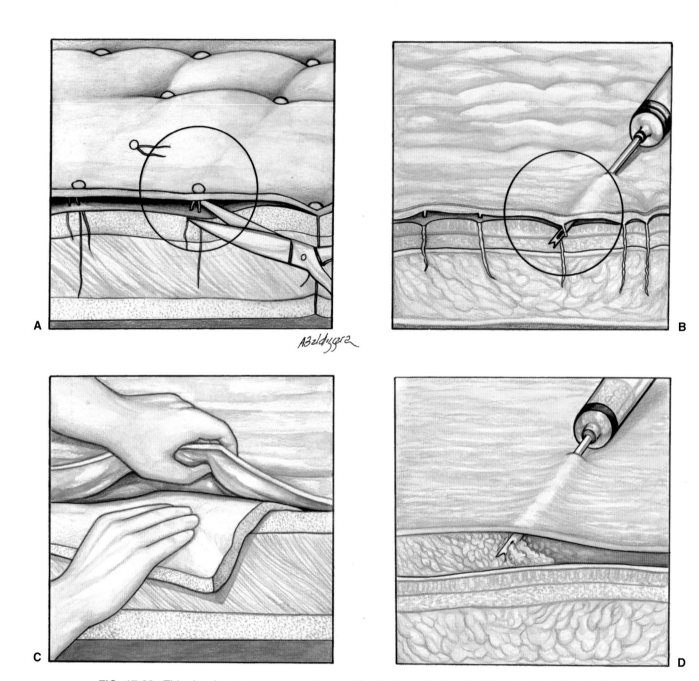

FIG. 17-30. This drawing compares a mattress with skin irregularities. **A:** The strings that retract the surface are cut with scissors. **B:** The Toledo V-tip dissector cannula severs the fibrous adhesions that pull the skin down. **C:** The mattress is stuffed. **D:** The Toledo V-tip dissector cannula injecting fat to fill the depressed areas.

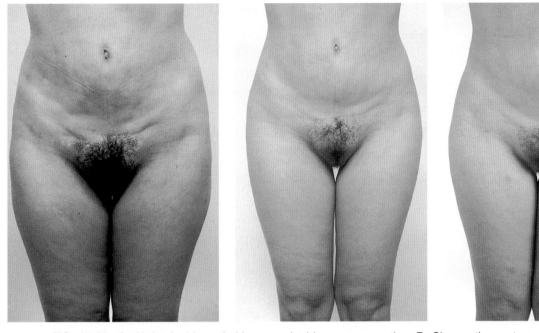

FIG. 17-31. A: Abdominal irregularities provoked by uneven suction. **B:** Six months postoperatively, after superficial liposculpture, fibrous adhesions release, and fat injection in the depressed areas. **C:** Six years postoperatively. No other treatment was performed.

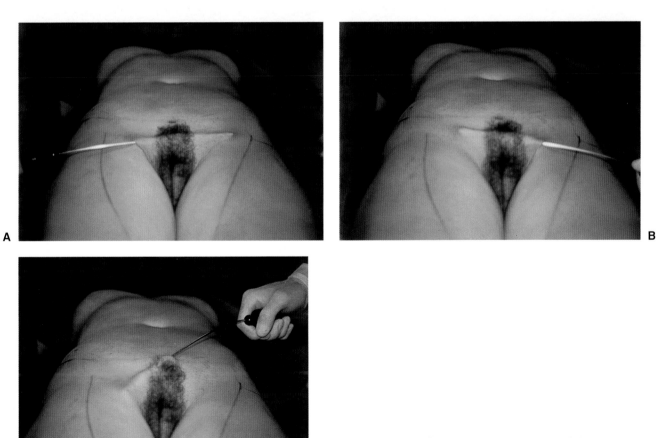

FIG. 17-32. A, B, C: Reduction liposculpture of the pubis. I crisscross the tunnels from the two inguinal incisions and the pubis incision.

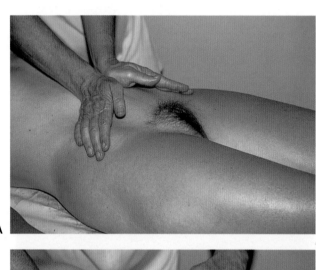

A

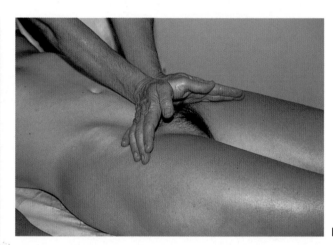

B

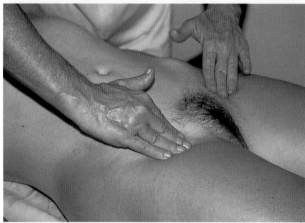

C

FIG. 17-33. A, B, C: The French technique of manual lymphatic drainage being applied to drain edema to the inguinal lymph nodes.

18

The Dorsal Region

The dorsal region is an area where fat deposits will change the contour of the body. This is one of the areas that could not be treated before liposuction, except through dermolipectomy. People who accumulate more fat above the waistline will develop rolls of fat in the dorsal region, starting in the axillary region, the middorsal area, the waist, and the flanks. The divisions between these rolls will present folds where the skin connects to the muscle through fibrous adhesions. The usual complaints about the dorsal area are the lack of a marked waistline and the fat excess that shows when the patient wears a bra or a bikini top, compressing the region. This can happen in young patients (Fig. 18-1) but it is more common with age (Fig. 18-2). Back rolls can be one of the signs of aging, and superficial liposculpture in this area has a rejuvenating effect.

INSTRUMENTS

The 60-cc toomey-tip syringe and cannulas varying from 3-mm to 5-mm gauge are used. I start with thicker cannulas and change to finer gauges as I get closer to the skin. The Pyramid is the most used tip. Sometimes it is necessary to use a two-holed flat tip or even the Toledo V-tip dissector cannula.

ANESTHESIA

Small areas can be treated with local anesthesia alone or in combination with oral midazolam sedation. For larger areas I will use local anesthesia combined with IV sedation. Patients who undergo this procedure often need contouring of other parts of the body as well. The local anesthesia is injected slowly at body temperature. I use the same formula and inject all the adiposities on that side before I start suctioning (Fig. 18-3).

POSITION

I can operate the dorsal area with the patient in the prone, supine, or lateral position, depending on what I have to treat. Some patients need treatment combined in different positions (Fig. 18-4).

INCISIONS

I usually treat the area through a posterior axillary incision, a lateral or dorsal midthoracic incision, and the trochanteric incision (Fig. 18-5), depending on the position of the patient on the operating table. Other incisions might be necessary depending on the problem. The important thing is not to make symmetrical incisions that will always indicate aesthetic surgery. If the incisions are asymmetrical and they are apparent postoperatively, they will look like scars from the removal of a wart or mole. I connect the incisions through the anesthesia infiltration and also through suction.

FAT ASPIRATION

Deep Suction

I always start suctioning deep. The whole dorsal region can be treated through deep suction. Some patients have more fibrotic fat in this area, which is difficult to aspirate. The difficulty is related more to the type of cannula used for aspiration than to the vacuum source. Whenever I find it hard to suction with the Pyramid tip, I change to the two-holed flat tip, and that cannula can always aspirate the excess fat. When I obtain a good contour with deep suction alone I will not aspirate superficially.

Superficial Suction

The dorsum is a very forgiving area for superficial liposculpture, much more so than the abdomen, where any little irregularity will show. This would be the area of choice for surgeons starting to practice superficial liposculpture as there is less possibility of leaving sequelae. Even patients with flaccid skin can obtain a good retraction in the dorsal region.

I usually start with deep suction and after I have obtained the desired shape, I pass to the superficial layer to improve skin retraction (Fig. 18-6). It is always wise to save some syringes of aspirated fat in case there is the need for immediate reinjection. The dorsum is one of the areas that surgeons sometimes find difficult to treat because they use the wrong cannula. This has been one of the areas that advocates of internal ultrasound say are ''impossible'' to treat properly without ultrasound. I believe, however, that if one has the right cannulas there are no areas of the body that cannot be treated effectively with syringe liposculpture. The more aggressive cannulas, like the V-tip or 2-hole flat tip, are especially useful to aspirate areas where the fat is more fibrotic, usually in men but also in female patients (Fig. 18-7).

Results obtained with liposculpture of the dorsal region are usually very gratifying to patients of all ages. The improvements show when patients are not only in bathing suits but also in clothes, with significant reductions in the sizes worn. The recontouring of the upper body can lead to significant changes in body proportions and in patients' attitudes (Figs. 18-8–18-16). Patients often ask me if they should diet first and have the operation after weight loss. My answer is that the reduction in measurements produced by the surgery often stimulates the need to continue the improvement in body contour with dieting. I prefer to operate first, and if, after weight reduction, there are still some fat deposits, I can treat them separately under local anesthesia. Another possibility is to perform ''serial'' treatments to achieve the desired result, giving the tissues time to retract.

POSTOPERATIVE CARE

It is difficult to prescribe girdles that do not mark the dorsal region. Patients can provoke permanent depressions and irregularities if they wear tight bras immediately after superficial liposculpture. Postoperative treatment with manual or machine lymphatic drainage, combined with the use of loose clothes with no elastics in the area, will allow for good healing.

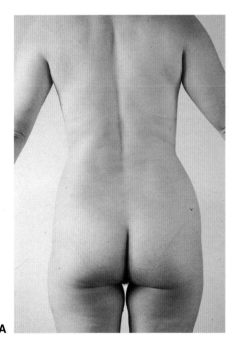
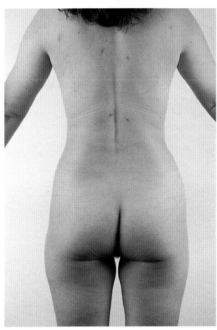

A

B

FIG. 18-1. A: Preoperative photo of a 26-year-old patient with excess fat in the dorsal axillary, middorsal, and flank regions. Excess fat forms a bulge when the patient wears a bra or a bikini top, compressing the region. **B:** Two months postoperatively, with a good contour of the dorsal area and improvement of the waistline and flanks.

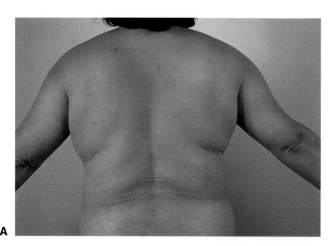
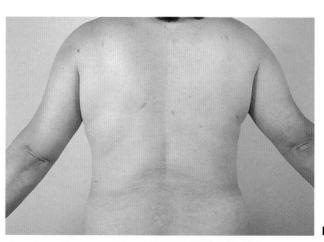

A   B

FIG. 18-2. A: The same problem is more common with age. Here a 53-year-old patient with back rolls and a thick waistline. **B:** One year postoperatively. The improvement provided by superficial liposculpture contouring procedure has reduced the signs of aging in this area and had a rejuvenating effect.

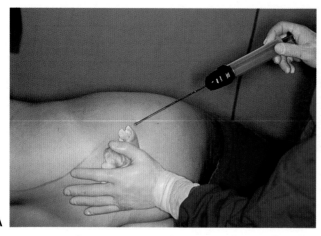
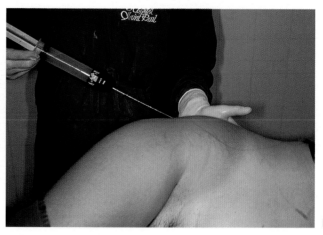

A   B

FIG. 18-3. A, B: Local anesthesia is injected into the dorsal region slowly at body temperature.

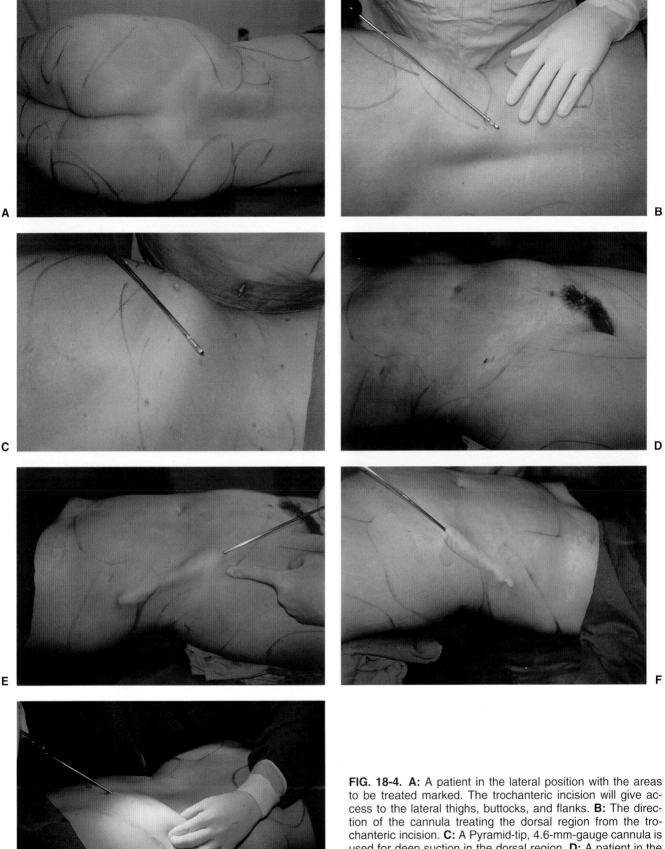

FIG. 18-4. A: A patient in the lateral position with the areas to be treated marked. The trochanteric incision will give access to the lateral thighs, buttocks, and flanks. **B:** The direction of the cannula treating the dorsal region from the trochanteric incision. **C:** A Pyramid-tip, 4.6-mm-gauge cannula is used for deep suction in the dorsal region. **D:** A patient in the supine position for treatment of the abdomen, waist, and medial thighs. **E, F:** A patient in the supine position being treated in the waist region through lateral thoracic incisions. **G:** A patient in the prone position during treatment of the dorsal region fat deposits.

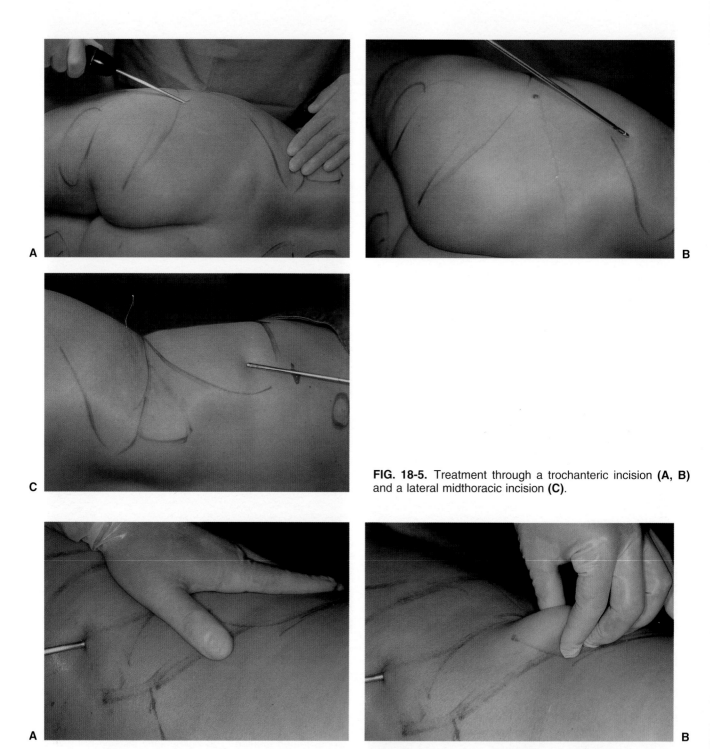

FIG. 18-5. Treatment through a trochanteric incision **(A, B)** and a lateral midthoracic incision **(C)**.

FIG. 18-6. **A:** The depth of the cannula during deep liposculpture in the dorsal region and waist can be controlled with the outstretched hand. **B:** The depth of the cannula during superficial liposculpture in the dorsal region and waist can be controlled with the pinch test.

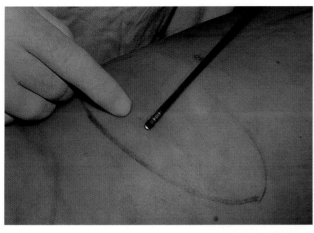

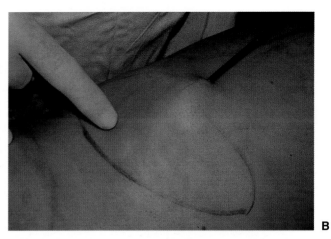

A

B

FIG. 18-7. A: Using the two-holed flat-tip 5-mm-gauge cannula to aspirate fibrous fat tissue from the dorsal region. **B:** To obtain skin retraction in the dorsal region, I can aspirate superficially with the two-holed flat-tip cannula with the holes towards the dermis. It has to be a uniform suction to avoid superficial tunnel depressions.

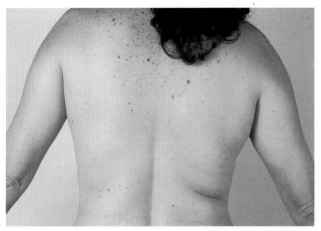

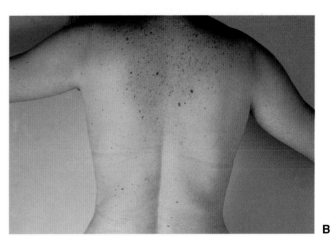

A

B

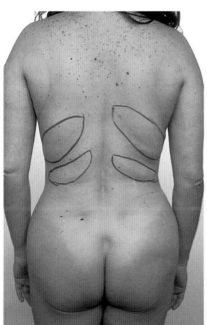

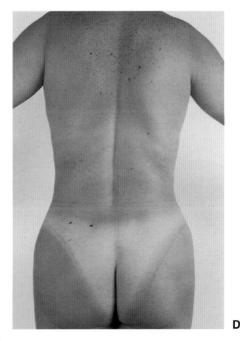

C

D

FIG. 18-8. A, B: Pre- and one-year postoperative photos of a 39-year-old patient after superficial liposculpture for fat deposits in the axillary and dorsal regions. **C, D:** Pre- and six-year postoperative photos. The patient is now 45 years old and her dorsal region looks younger than when she was 39.

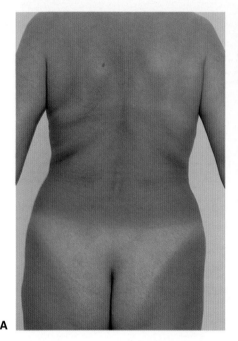

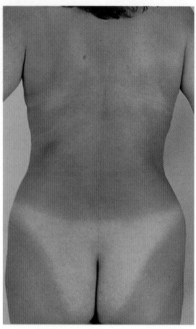

FIG. 18-9. A, B: Pre- and four-month postoperative photos of a 29-year-old patient after superficial liposculpture for fat deposits in the axillary and dorsal regions. This patient's main complaint was that bulges formed above and below her bra.

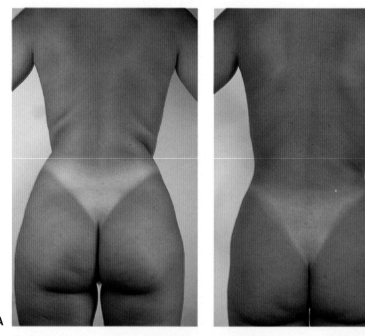

FIG. 18-10. A, C: Preoperative photos of a 29-year-old patient with fat deposits in the dorsal region in the waist area. Her main complaint was that rolls formed above and below her belt. B, D: Six months postoperatively, after superficial liposculpture of the waist and dorsal region. The folds between the rolls were freed with the Toledo V-tip dissector cannula.

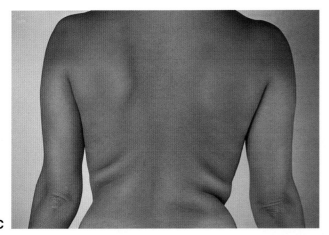
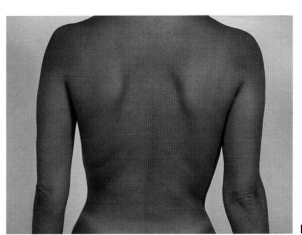

C   D

FIG. 18-10. *Continued.*

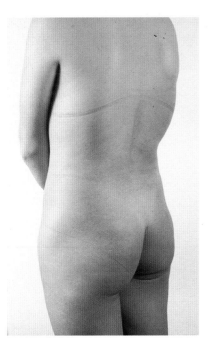
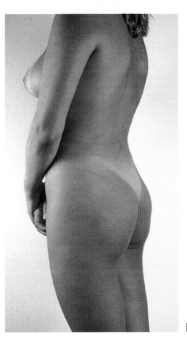

A   B

FIG. 18-11. A: A 22-year-old patient with a very masculine upper body. **B:** One year postoperatively, after suction of the dorsal region, arms, and flanks. I also injected 500 cc of fat per buttock. After one year, the reduction in the dorsal region was 5 cm and in the flanks, 4 cm. There was an increase of 10 cm in the buttock measurements. The procedure changed this patient's attitude towards life, and she became much more confident and happier with herself.

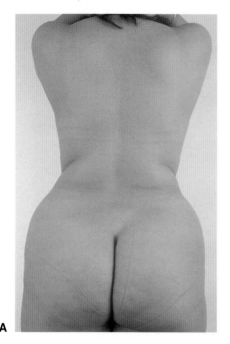

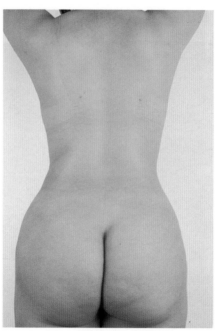

A

B

FIG. 18-12. A: This 22-year-old patient needed a big reduction in her adiposities. I indicated body liposculpture. One of her complaints was that even with her arms up she would still present some rolls in her waist. **B:** One month postoperatively. There was an improvement in the flanks and waist. The rolls disappeared. Notice the two small incisions in the dorsal region and the two incisions in the axilla.

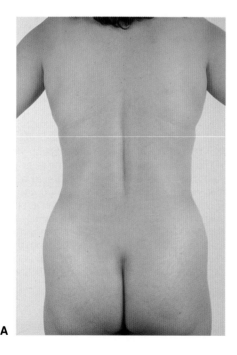

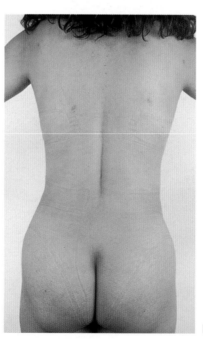

A

B

FIG. 18-13. A: Preoperative photo of a 34-year-old patient who wanted to improve the axillary and dorsal region, plus the waistline and the flanks. **B:** One month postoperatively, after superficial liposculpture. Notice the two small incisions in the dorsal region and the two incisions in the axilla. The flanks were treated through the trochanter incisions.

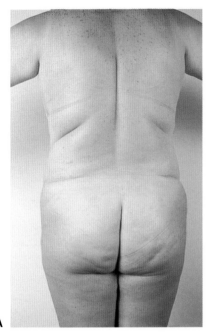
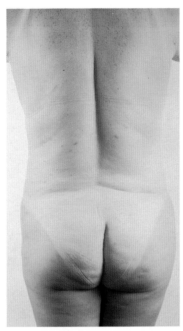

A   **B**

FIG. 18-14. A: Preoperative photo of a 55-year-old patient who wanted to improve her waistline and dorsal region. **B:** Three months postoperatively. Although the improvement was limited, it gave this patient the motivation she needed to start dieting and exercising.

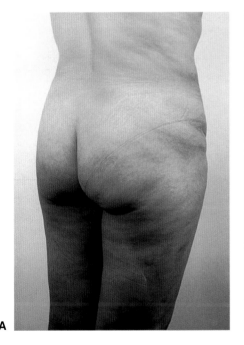
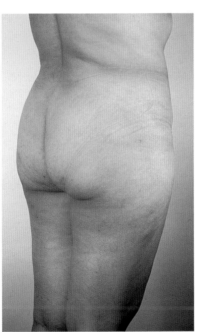

A   **B**

FIG. 18-15. A, B: Pre- and one-month postoperative photos of a 54-year-old patient with flaccid skin and fat deposits in the dorsal region, waist, and flanks. I performed superficial liposculpture. There was an improvement in the contour and in the superficial irregularities.

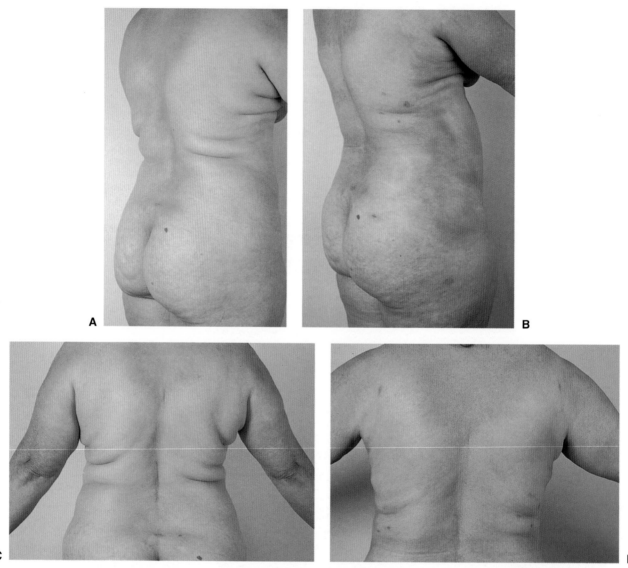

FIG. 18-16. A, C: Preoperative photos of a 59-year-old overweight patient who wanted to improve her dorsal region, waist, and flanks. **B, D:** Six months postoperatively, after superficial liposculpture, with a good reduction in the adiposities and the patient's measurements.

19

The Arms

Reduction liposculpture of the arms is a procedure that is usually combined with other body contour treatments, although it can be performed in isolation. I combine arm reduction liposculpture with the treatment of the dorsal and anterior part of the axilla.

Younger patients with good skin tone can be treated by suction alone. Superficial liposculpture will help retract the skin of the arms, although the dermis should not be scraped with the cannula, especially in the ventral part, at the risk of provoking irregularities. Older patients with flaccid skin and subcutaneous tissue will benefit from a combination of reduction liposculpture and dermolipectomy. I prefer this combination because superficial liposculpture reduces the thickness of the arm uniformly, and the excess skin is removed through an axillary fusiform incision. There are patients who need dermolipectomy along the ventral part of the arm from the axilla to the elbow. I seldom get these patients in my practice. Some surgeons have established wonderful operative techniques to treat this type of patient (1).

INSTRUMENTS

I use 60-cc 2- and 3-mm-gauge, 25- to 35-cm toomey-tip syringes. Anesthesia is injected with a 2-mm-gauge multiholed-tip cannula. The cannulas I prefer are the Pyramid-tip cannulas, although I can use a 2-mm one-lateral-holed tip. For injecting fat, I use a one-lateral-holed 3-mm-gauge blunt-tip cannula.

ANESTHESIA

Anesthesia is the same as is used to treat the rest of the body, usually sedation and local tumescent. The injection is done with a fine multiholed cannula. I infiltrate a proportion of 1:1 of my local anesthesia formula at body temperature and wait ten minutes before I start suctioning.

POSITION

I treat the arms and anterior axilla with the patient in the supine position or in the prone position when I have to treat the dorsal axilla. The assistant can hold the arm if necessary.

INCISIONS

I will do as many incisions as necessary to have good access, but generally two axillary one anterior and one dorsal, to treat the axilla and the arms, and probably a third one at the elbow for crisscrossing. The axillary dermolipectomy surgical sequence is shown in Appendix 1, Example Case 1.

FAT ASPIRATION

Deep Suction

I start suctioning deep in the lateral bulge of the arm and change to superficial suctioning when I treat the dorsal area. I do not suction the ventral fine skin area, where the fat layer is too fine to aspirate. I use a 3-mm-gauge long cannula in the area marked preoperatively, aspirating fat uniformly following the curves of the arm, to thin down the defect.

Superficial Suction

I change to a 2-mm-gauge cannula and aspirate fat closer to the skin. Superficial suction is performed with a 2-mm-gauge cannula, with care taken not to provoke skin depressions (Figs. 19-1–19-3).

POSTOPERATIVE CARE

There are no good girdles for the arms. Most of my liposculpture patients have only a small Micropore dressing at the incision. A mild compression bandage can stay on for the first 24 hours. The dermolipectomy incision is also covered with a Micropore and gauze dressing for the first 24 hours and after that only with Micropore until the stitches are removed. Manual lymphatic drainage can be started after 24 hours to reduce swelling. The patient should avoid keeping the arms down for long periods of time in the early postoperative period and should not exercise for the first 30 days.

REFERENCES

1. Vogt P, Baroudi R. Brachioplasty and brachial suction-assisted lipectomy. In: Cohen M, ed. *Mastery of plastic and reconstructive surgery,* vol. 3. Boston: Little Brown and Company, 1994; 2219–2236.

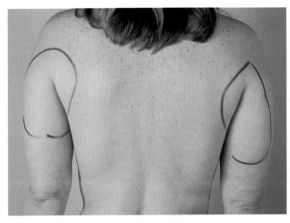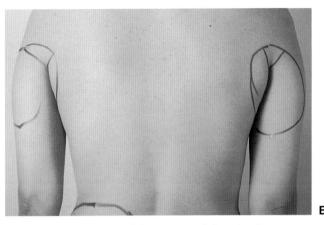

FIG. 19-1. A, B: Patients marked in the standing position for treatment of the arms and dorsal axilla. From one incision in the dorsal axilla I can reach the dorsal region and the lateral and dorsal part of the arms.

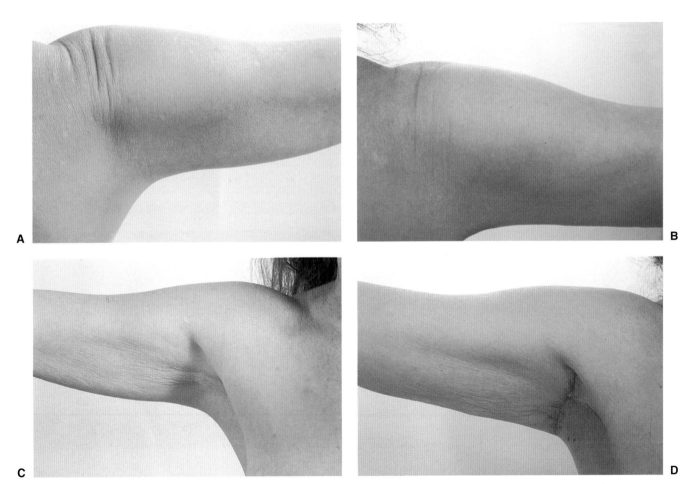

FIG. 19-2. A, C: Preoperative photos of a 65-year-old patient with fat deposits on her arms and skin flaccidity. **B, D:** Two months postoperatively, following superficial liposculpture and axillary dermolipectomy of the arms. There was an improvement in shape and in flaccidity without using a vertical incision.

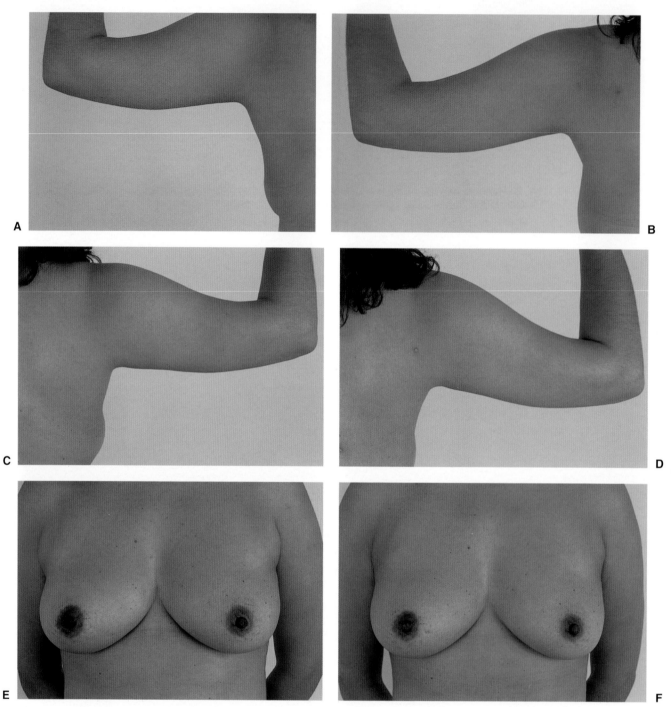

FIG. 19-3. A, C: Preoperative photos of a 37-year-old patient with excess fat in the axilla and arms. **B, D:** Two-month postoperative photos of superficial liposculpture of the arms and axilla. The area was treated through one axillary incision. **E, F:** Pre- and two-month postoperative photos of superficial liposculpture of the anterior axillary region. This solved the patient's problem. When she wore a bra it would press the area, showing fat deposits.

20

The Hands

Hand rejuvenation is an important aspect of my practice. People usually have no idea that something can be done to improve the appearance of their hands.

I use a combination of fat grafting and chemical peels which improves the look of older patients' hands (1). This is important when patients undergo facial rejuvenation and the aging hands are in contrast with the face's youthful look.

The dorsal skin of the hands gets thin with age, and the veins and tendons start showing by transparency. This aspect can be extended to the fingers, and I also inject a few cc of fat in the dorsal part of the fingers. The skin can also get wrinkled and show photo age spots. I treat these two problems simultaneously. I increase skin thickness with subcutaneous fat injection and I treat the superficial problems with chemical peels. I have tried trichloroacetic acid (TCA), but I was frightened by its strength. I prefer to repeat two or three 70% glycolic acid peels and prescribe a home treatment with 8% glycolic with either kojic acid to bleach the age spots or 3% hydroquinone.

INSTRUMENTS

I use 10-cc syringes, a carpule, my tumescent formula, a 2-mm cannula for aspiration of fat, and a blunt 2-mm-gauge needle for injection. I also use a no. 16 needle to perforate the skin before I introduce the blunt needle. Peels are preprepared and are done after the fat injection.

FAT INJECTION

Under local anesthesia (Fig. 20-1), I harvest 20 to 30 cc of fat from the flanks or lateral thighs, centrifuge it at 1,500 r/min, separate the anesthetic fluid, and transfer the fat to a 10-cc syringe connected to a pistol (Fig. 20-2). This is the same process that is used for fat injection on the face. After I put a dressing on the donor area, I inject a dermal button of anesthesia with the carpule on the wrist area, perforate the skin with the no. 16 needle, introduce the blunt needle under the skin, and inject a fine layer of fat (Figs. 20-3–20-10). The possibility of vascularization of this graft is very good. If a 2-mm-thick layer is injected, there will be a good chance of survival because the neovascularization process comes from both sides. The layer of fat thickens the skin and improves elasticity. I usually inject between 8 and 10 cc in the dorsal part of the hands and between 1 and 2 cc in the dorsal part of each finger, if necessary. The process should be repeated after six months to compensate for any excessive fat reabsorption.

POSTOPERATIVE CARE

Dressings worn for the first one or two days will remind patients they should be careful not to change the position of the fat graft. Gloves can be worn to avoid sun exposure, although it is not absolutely necessary.

REFERENCES

1. Aboudib Junior JH, de Castro CC, Gradel J. Hand rejuvenescence by fat filling. *Ann Plast Surg* 1992;28:559–564.

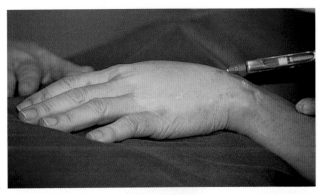

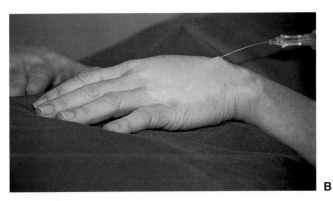

FIG. 20-1. A, B: Anesthesia of the dorsal part of the hand.

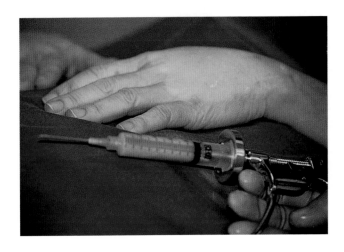

FIG. 20-2. The syringe with pure fat is adapted to a pistol for injection with precision.

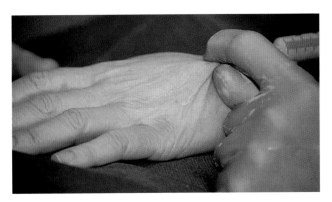

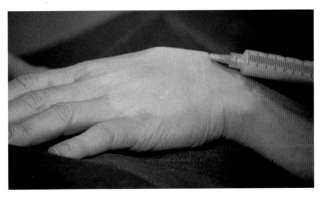

FIG. 20-3. The blunt needle is inserted under the skin. I inject between 8 and 10 cc into the dorsal part of the hand.

FIG. 20-4. By elevating the needle parallel to the skin, I avoid provoking unnecessary ecchymosis.

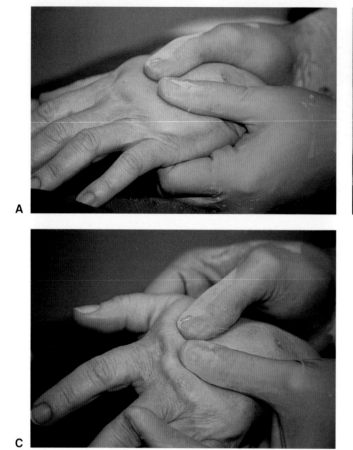

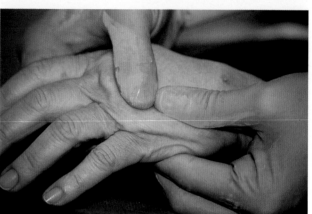

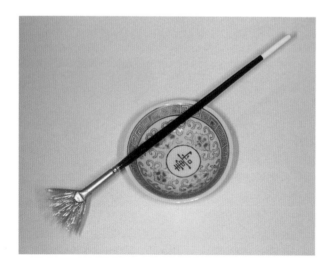

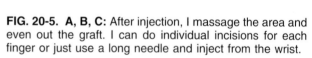

FIG. 20-5. A, B, C: After injection, I massage the area and even out the graft. I can do individual incisions for each finger or just use a long needle and inject from the wrist.

FIG. 20-6. The 70% glycolic acid peel utensils.

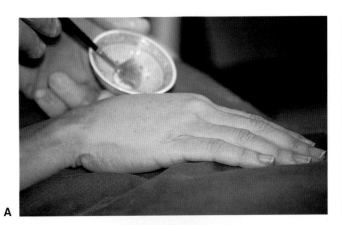

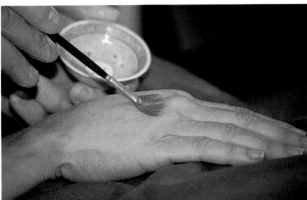

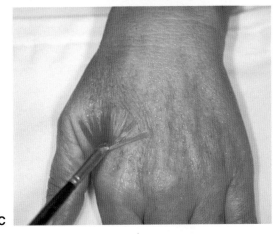

FIG. 20-7. A, B, C: Applying the 70% glycolic acid peel.

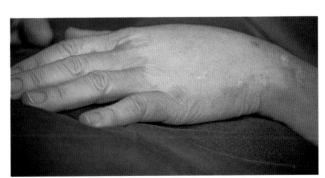

FIG. 20-8. Immediately postoperatively.

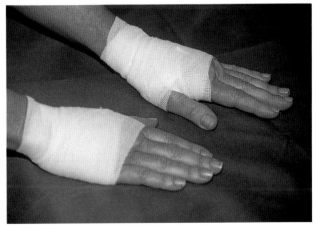

FIG. 20-9. Dressings are important for the first one or two days to remind patients and friends to avoid firm handshakes that can change the position of the fat graft.

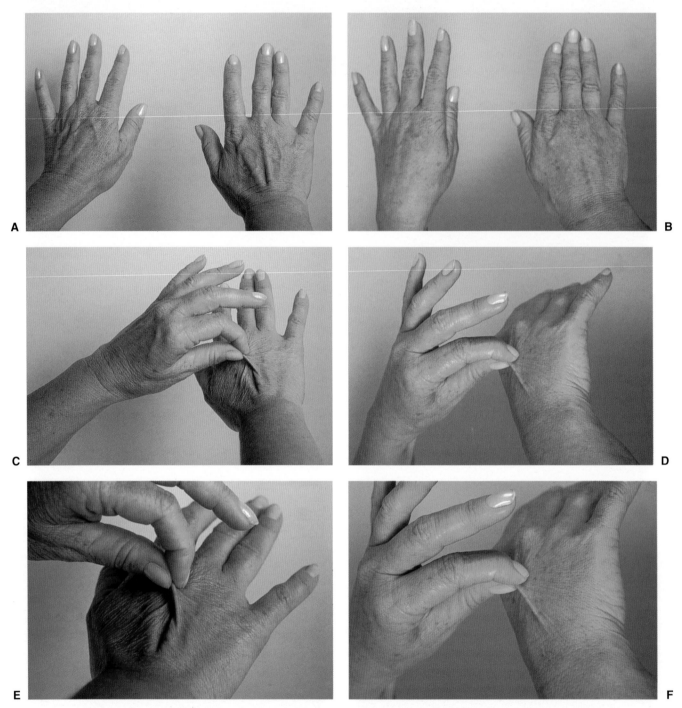

FIG. 20-10. A, C, E: Preoperative photo of a 55-year-old patient. **B, D, F:** Six months postoperatively. There is a visual improvement and also an improvement in the skin texture.

21

The Breasts

The introduction of liposuction (1) and later syringe liposculpture (2) made it possible to improve the shape of the breasts with shorter scars. With liposuction it is possible to change form without long incisions. Most breast hypertrophies are caused by excess fat. Reduction liposculpture can be used as an adjunct to mammoplasty. It is a simple way of reducing excess fat from the breasts and surrounding areas without extending incisions. Fat can be aspirated from the breast itself or from the lateral part of the thorax. One of the main problems with aspirating fat from the breasts was the general belief that the possible calcifications provoked by suction could be confused with a tumor and provoke unnecessary biopsies. Today, with ultrasound, computed tomography (CT), and magnetic resonance imaging (MRI), a diagnosis can be established distinguishing between a simple fibrosis and a tumor.

Today, it is possible to considerably reduce fatty breasts through liposuction alone, without the need for any other incisions.

Brazilian mammoplasty patients usually undergo reduction through the Pitanguy breast reduction technique, with its inverted T scar (3). In 1985, I performed liposuction of the breast with an aspirator and combined the procedure with a periareolar skin and gland resection. The results were presented in 1987 (4,5), with a one-year follow-up. By 1988 (6), I was using syringes esclusively for all my facial and body work, for more precision. I started gland resection in the upper pole as well, to elevate the areola after the lower pole resection. In 1989 (7), I started resecting an oval of skin before gland resection and using an areolar purse-string stitch to help prevent areolar enlargement.

I often indicate reduction liposculpture alone for breast reduction, especially for young patients (Fig. 21-1). When there is skin excess or for older patients it can be combined with mastopexy (Figs. 21-2–21-4). A mammography is recommended preoperatively and six months postoperatively. After this period of time the exam should follow the usual timetable, according to the patient's age. 2.9% of patients undergoing cosmetic surgery of the breast found breast cancer through routine preoperative mammography. Their prognosis was better due to the early detection of the disease (8).

INSTRUMENTS

The cannulas used are the same as those used for the dorsal region. I use 60-cc toomey-tip syringes and cannulas varying from 3-mm to 5-mm gauge. I start with thicker cannulas and change to finer gauges as I get closer to the skin. If I cannot suction easily with a Pyramid tip I change to a two-holed flat tip or even the Toledo V-tip dissector cannula.

ANESTHESIA

If I am planning only a reduction through liposculpture I use local anesthesia. When aspiration is combined with breast reduction or mastopexy, I use general anesthesia.

POSITION

I operate on the breasts with the patient in the supine position, with the dorsal region elevated 30 degrees. The arms should be held horizontally, perpendicular to the body.

INCISIONS

Through a submammary fold incision I introduce a 20- to 35-cm-long 3- to 5-mm-gauge Pyramid-tip cannula connected to a 60-cc toomey-tip disposable syringe filled with 5 cc of Ringer's solution. Through this incision the cannula can reach all the areas of the breast. I also aspirate from another axillary incision for crisscrossing. If after aspiration I still need to remove the gland, I can opt for a periareolar incision or an inverted T.

FAT ASPIRATION

The thickest cannula I use for the breast is a 5-mm gauge. As in other areas, I start suctioning deep with the thicker cannulas and as I get closer to the skin I change to smaller gauges.

Deep Suction

The aspiration of fatty breasts starts closer to the pectoral muscle, and I build tunnels as in any other area of the body, respecting the conic shape of the breast. When the breast has fibrous tissue, I change the Pyramid tip for a two-holed flat tip. I avoid aspiration closer to the skin with thick cannulas. The skin is fine and it is easy to provoke irregularities and depressions. I aspirate the axillary and medial parts of the breast. This treatment reduces the size of the breast. If I am performing a gland reduction or mastopexy together with the suction, I start with liposuction, the breast gets smaller, and I can use a shorter incision to remove the gland.

Superficial Suction

After the reduction in size, I can improve shape and provoke skin retraction by aspirating fat superficially. Superficial suction on the breast varies according to skin thickness, but can vary from 2 to 5 mm below the dermis. I use very fine cannulas for that—2- to 3-mm gauge, because small gauge cannulas allow for more delicate work. By aspirating from two incisions and crossing the tunnels I can obtain an even retraction of the breast. I usually avoid aspirating under the areola.

INDICATION FOR COMBINED GLAND RESECTION

Today, I indicate the periareolar technique in very specific cases: for patients who will not benefit from aspiration alone, patients who prefer a round-shaped breast, young patients who are still subject to a change of breast size and shape, young patients with posture problems, and patients who will not accept the inverted T incision even if told it is the best option for them. All these patients have to be aware that they might need to undergo a revision procedure.

In the periareolar resection I will resect a slice of gland from the inferior pole. If the areola is too low or is pointing down after the suture, I will resect the gland in the shape of a pyramid or a prism from the upper pole. I resect from the area between the lateral and medial mammary artery branches so as not to affect the pedicle of the breast. The skin is sutured first with a dermal purse-string stitch, then with separate 5–0 nylon stitches.

When I use the inverted T incision, I try to keep the horizontal scar as short as possible and within the breast area. Excessive concern over the final scar size should not interfere with the final results of the mammaplasty, as far as shape, volume, and lasting results are concerned (9). I indicate the inverted T incision for patients who prefer a pear-shaped breast (with the periareolar technique I will not produce this shape), patients with posture problems who are not concerned with the length of the incision, for older patients who need a good shape in clothes, and for out-of-town patients because of the faster recovery period.

These combined techniques have given me a good experience with breast aspiration and I have coauthored a book about these techniques (10).

POSTOPERATIVE CARE

I prescribe manual lymphatic drainage every other day postoperatively for the first ten days to help accelerate the recovery time by reducing fluid retention and eliminating discomfort. Patients wear a medical bra for a month and must avoid physical exertion and exercising for that period of time.

TREATMENT OF GYNECOMASTIA WITH AREOLA AND NIPPLE REDUCTION

Gynecomastia, the benign enlargement of the male breast (11), can be due to proliferation of ducts and periductal tissues. When there is deposition of adipose tissue along with excess skin, it is called pseudogynecomastia. The cause can be endocrine, and drug factors can also be involved, but half of the cases are idiopathic (12). Treatment can involve mastectomy alone (13), mastectomy plus skin resection (14,15), mastectomy plus liposuction, (16–20), or liposuction alone (21–24). To treat gynecomastia I can combine the syringe liposculpture technique (5,25) to reduce the fatty portion of the breast, a surgical removal of the breast gland, a periareolar reduction of the size of the areola, and a ring resection of the nipple to reduce projection, all in a single surgical stage without compromising the vascularization of the nipple–areolar complex.

A 33-year-old male presented with a steroid-induced gynecomastia with moderate breast augmentation and areola and nipple enlargement. One year after the interruption of the steroid treatment, the breast size was reduced, but there remained a residual fatty breast with a palpable gland. The areola and nipple size were still too large and unacceptable to the patient.

Technique

With the patient under midazolam IV sedation, I injected each breast (Fig. 21-5) with 100 ml of my modified tumescent anesthesia formula—500 ml Ringer's lactate, 20 ml 2% lidocaine, 1 ml 1:1000 epinephrine, 5 ml 3% Na CO_3 (26). Fifteen minutes after the infiltration, when there was good control of bleeding (27), I started the liposculpture with a 35-cc syringe connected to a 3-mm Pyramid-tip cannula inserted at the inframammary fold. I aspirated 25 cc of fat from each breast, out of 60 cc of total aspirate per breast, feathering the suction to the sides to avoid any ridges and irregularities (Fig. 21-6).

I anesthetized the skin and gland using 10 ml of 2% lidocaine with 1:100.000 epinephrine. Without damaging the dermis, I excised a ring of periareolar epithelium (Fig. 21-7) to reduce the areola to the desired size and also a ring of the epithelium at the base of the nipple to reduce its projection (Fig. 21-8). Through a 1-cm dermis incision, I dissected and removed the breast gland (Fig. 21-9). Hemostasis was performed. A 3–0 Vicryl purse-string suture was passed subdermally along the outer areolar incision to reduce the areola to its desired size (28) (Fig. 21-10). Skin was sutured with 5–0 nylon stitches; the knots were left in the areola size (Fig. 21-11). A Penrose drain was inserted through the cannula incision and left for 24 hours. To avoid marking the skin portion of the suture, I placed it subdermally on that side. The nipples were sutured with a 6-0 nylon (Fig. 21-12).

I believe this is an ideal treatment for moderate gynecomastia. It recontours the fatty part of the chest, resects the breast gland, and reduces areolar size and nipple projection in one stage. When there is no need for areolar reduction, I do not remove any skin (Fig. 21-13).

REFERENCES

1. Illouz YG. Une nouvelle technique por les lipodistrophies localizes. *Rev Chir Est Lang Franç* 1980;6:19.
2. Fournier P. *Liposculpture—ma technique.* Paris: Arnette, 1989.
3. Pitanguy I. Mamaplastias. Estudo de 234 casos consecutivos e apresentação de técnica pessoal. *Rev Bras Cir* 1961;42:201–1961.
4. Toledo LS, Matsudo PKR. Mammoplasty using liposuction and the periareolar incision [abstract]. In: *Abstract book of the 9th international congress of ISAPS.* New York, 1987:35.
5. Toledo LS, Matsudo PKR. Mammoplasty using liposuction and the periareolar incision. *Aesthetic Plast Surg* 1989;13:9–13.
6. Toledo LS. Periareolar mammoplasty with syringe liposuction. In: Toledo LS, ed. *Annals of the international symposium "Recent advances in plastic surgery (RAPS) 89."* São Paulo, Brazil, March 3–5, 1989. São Paulo: Estadão, 1989:256–265.
7. Toledo LS. Mammoplasty using syringe liposuction and periareolar incision—a four year experience. In: Riventer, ed. *Annals of the second international symposium "Recent advances in plastic surgery (RAPS) 90,"* São Paulo, Brazil, March 28–30, 1990. Rio de Janeiro: Marques-Saraiva, 1990:127–133.
8. Perras C. Fifteen years of mammography in cosmetic surgery of the breast. *Aesthetic Plast Surg,* 1990;14:81–84.
9. de Pina DP. Mammaplasty: shape, volume, and scar size. *Aesthetic Plast Surg* 1990;14:27–33.
10. Wilkinson TS, Aiache A, Toledo LS. *Circumareolar techniques for breast surgery.* New York: Springer-Verlag, 1995.
11. Letterman G, Schurter M. Suggested nomenclature for aesthetic and reconstructive surgery of the breast. Part III: gynecomastia. *Aesthetic Plast Surg* 1986;10:55–57.
12. Abbes M, Bourgeon Y, De Graeve B. Apropos of 72 gynecomastias. *J Chir (Paris)* 1988;125:327–331.

13. Aiache AE. Surgical treatment of gynecomastia in the body builder. *Plast Reconstr Surg* 1989;83:61–66.

14. Schrudde J, Petrovici V, Steffens K. Surgical therapy of pronounced gynecomastia. *Chirurg* 1986;57:88–91.

15. Ward CM, Khalid K. Surgical treatment of grade III gynaecomastia. *Ann R Coll Surg Engl* 1989;71:226–228.

16. Xuan QY. Suction lipectomy for male gynecomastia. *Chung Hua Cheng Hsing Shao Shang Wai Ko Tsa Chih* 1993;9:243–244, 317.

17. Samdal F, Kleppe G, Amland PF, Abyholm F. Surgical treatment of gynaecomastia. Five years' experience with liposuction. *Scand J Plast Reconstr Surg Hand Surg* 1994;28:123–130.

18. Pitanguy I, Muller P, Davalo P, Barzi A, Persichetti P. Treatment of gynecomastia using a trans-areolar incision. *Minerva Chir* 1989;44:1941–1948.

19. Mladick RA. Gynecomastia. Liposuction and excision. *Clin Plast Surg* 1991;18:815–822.

20. Courtiss EH. Gynecomastia: analysis of 159 patients and current recommendations for treatment. *Plast Reconstr Surg* 1987;79:740–753.

21. Stark GB, Grandel S, Spilker G. Tissue suction of the male and female breast. *Aesthetic Plast Surg* 1992;16:317–324.

22. Lewis CM. Lipoplasty: treatment for gynecomastia. *Aesthetic Plast Surg* 1985;9:287–292.

23. Rosenberg GJ. A new cannula for suction removal of parenchymal tissue of gynecomastia. *Plast Reconstr Surg* 1994;94:548–551.

24. Becker H. The treatment of gynecomastia without sharp excision. *Ann Plast Surg* 1990;24:380–383.

25. Toledo LS. Periareolar mammoplasty with syringe liposuction. In: Toledo LS, ed. *Annals of the international symposium "Recent advances in plastic surgery (RAPS) 89."* São Paulo, Brazil, March 3–5, 1989. São Paulo: Estadão, 1989:256–265.

26. Toledo LS. Superficial syringe liposculpture. In: Toledo LS, ed. *Annals of the international symposium "Recent advances in Plastic Surgery (RAPS) 90."* São Paulo, Brazil, March 3–5, 1990. Rio de Janeiro: Marques-Saraiva, 1990:446–453.

27. Varma SK, Henderson HP. A prospective trial of adrenaline infiltration for controlling bleeding during surgery for gynaecomastia. *Br J Plast Surg* 1990;43:590–593.

28. Peled IJ, Zagher U, Wexler MR. Purse-string suture for reduction and closure of skin defects. *Ann Plast Surg* 1985;14:465–469.

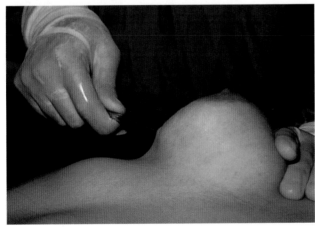

FIG. 21-1. Syringe aspiration of the breast.

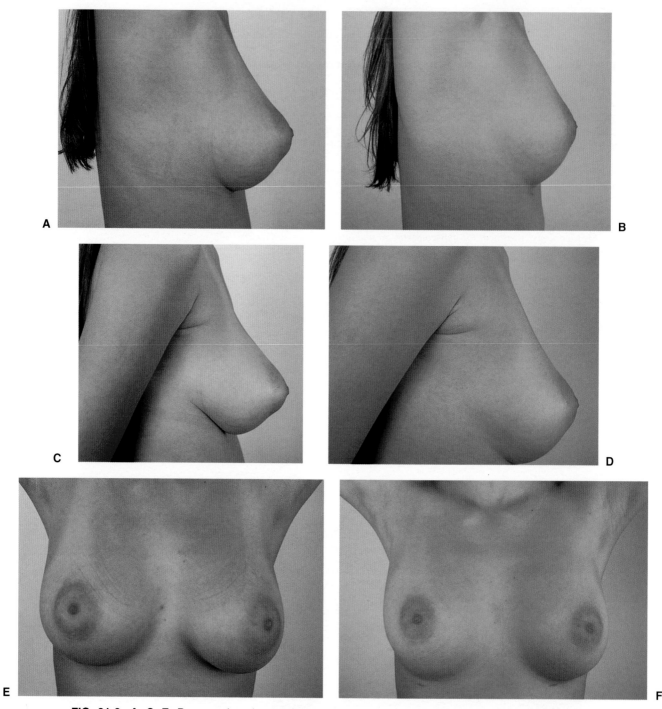

FIG. 21-2. A, C, E: Preoperative photos of reduction liposculpture on a 16-year-old patient. **B, D, F:** Six months postoperatively, with a good reduction in size and improvement of the shape without any visible scars.

FIG. 21-3. A, C, E, G: Preoperative photo of a 36-year-old patient who underwent reduction liposculpture and periareolar mastopexy. **B, D, F, H:** One year postoperatively, with a good reduction, elevation of the areola, and only a periareolar scar.

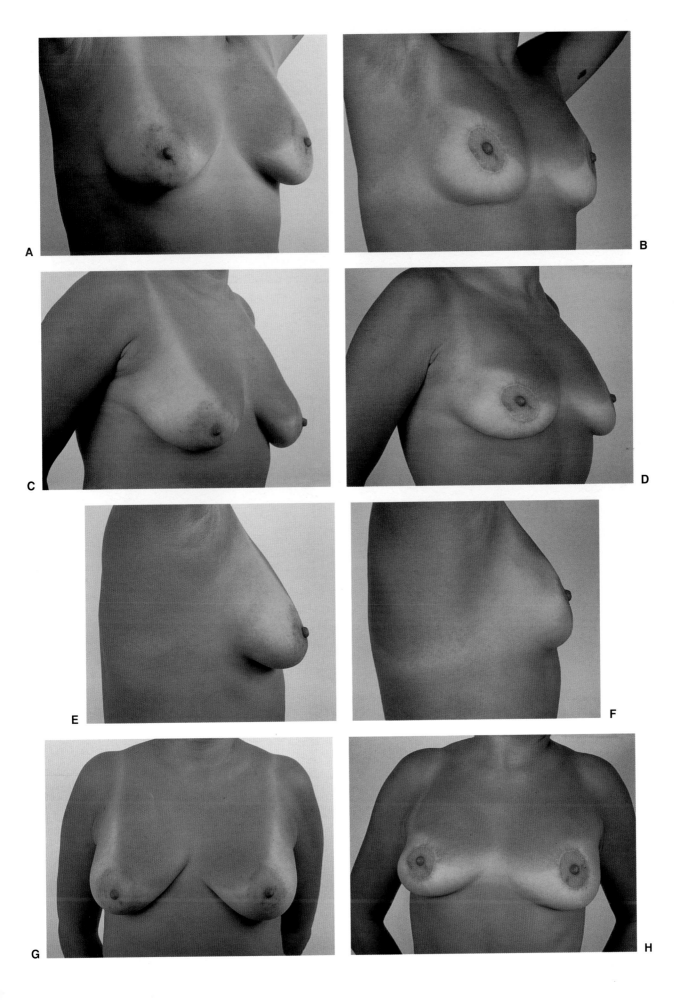

A

B

C

D

E

F

G

H

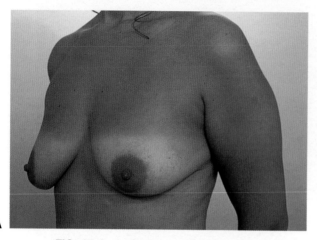 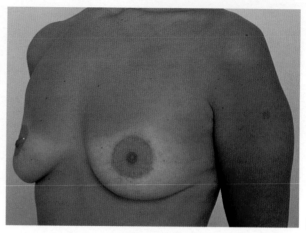

A   **B**

FIG. 21-4. A, B: Pre- and postoperative photos of a 32-year-old patient after periareolar mastopexy and reduction liposculpture.

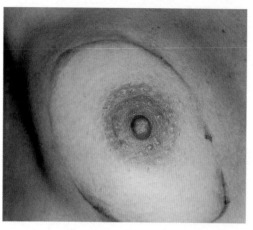

FIG. 21-5. The breast of a 33-year-old male patient with a steroid-induced moderate gynecomastia, with areola and nipple enlargement, after infiltration of 100 ml of my modified tumescent anesthesia formula.

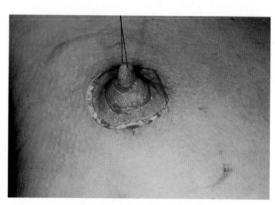

FIG. 21-7. We excised a ring of periareolar epithelium to reduce the areola to the desired size.

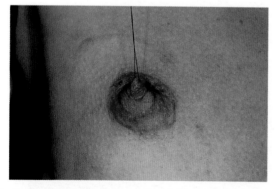

FIG. 21-6. The breast after we aspirated 60 cc of total aspirate, 25 cc of fat, feathering the suction to the sides to avoid any ridges and irregularities.

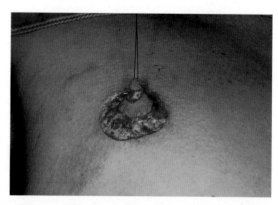

FIG. 21-8. A ring of the epithelium at the base of the nipple is excised to reduce its projection.

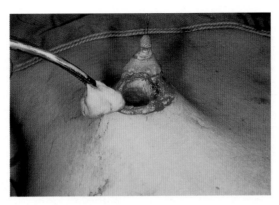

FIG. 21-9. Through a 1-cm dermis incision, we dissected and removed the breast gland.

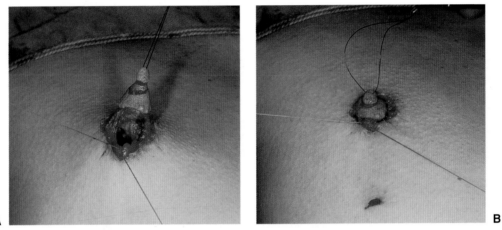

A   B

FIG. 21-10. A, B: A 3-0 Vicryl purse-string suture is passed subdermally along the outer areolar incision to reduce the areola to its desired size.

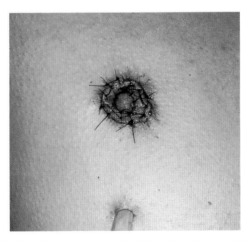

FIG. 21-11. Skin is sutured with 5-0 nylon stitches; the knots were left in the areola side.

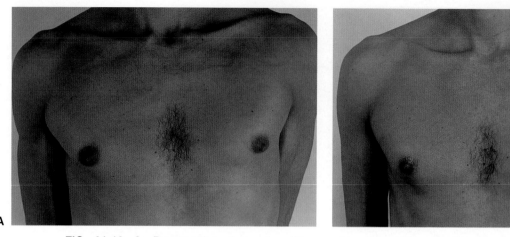

FIG. 21-12. A: Preoperative photo of a 33-year-old patient with steroid-induced gynecomastia. **B:** Three months postoperatively, with a good contour of the fatty part of the breast, breast gland resection, areolar size, and nipple projection reduction, in one stage.

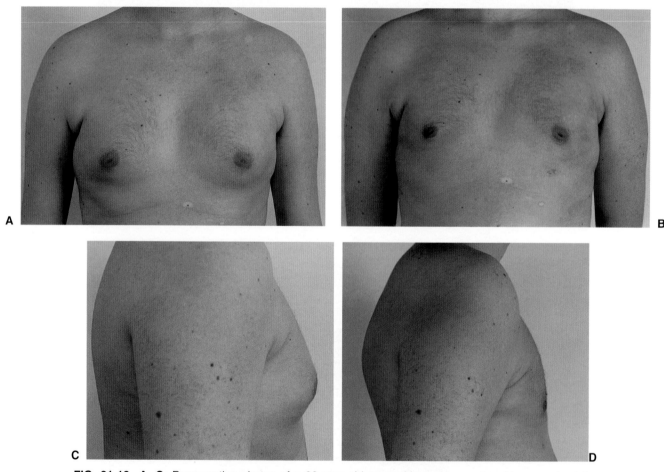

FIG. 21-13. A, C: Preoperative photos of a 23-year-old man with gynecomastia of hormonal origin. **B, D:** One month postoperatively, after reduction liposculpture of the fatty part of the breast and gland removal through a periareolar incision. The areola was not reduced.

APPENDIX 1

Combined Body Liposculpture Procedures

EXAMPLE CASE 1

A 22-year-old patient weighing 70 kg preoperatively wanted to improve her body contour. I indicated syringe liposculpture of the dorsal region, flanks, lateral and medial thighs, and abdomen (Fig. A1-1).

I removed a total aspirate of 5,290 cc, being 4,535 cc of pure fat, representing 6.4% of her body weight. After one month her weight was down to 63 kg. She started exercising, and three months after the surgery her weight was down to 55 kg. Her pre- and postoperative measurements are outlined in Table A1-1. The main objectives of this procedure were: to get a good retraction of the dorsal region, to reduce the lateral thighs and lower buttock, without dropping the buttocks, and to reduce the abdomen evenly, getting a good skin retraction.

After IV sedation with midazolam and fentanyl, the patient was placed in the lateral position and the anesthetic formula was infiltrated on the first side to be treated. The amounts were 180 cc on the axilla, 30 cc on the dorsal area, 860 cc on the flank, and 720 cc on the lateral thigh, including the lower third of the buttock.

The dorsal region was treated through three incisions: one in the dorsal part of the axilla, one in the dorsal area, and another in the flank. I started suctioning deep with a 4.6-mm-gauge Pyramid-tip cannula. After I reduced the volume in the axillary area, I changed to a flat-tip two-holed 4.6-mm-gauge cannula and suctioned superficially, with the holes towards the dermis. The total aspirate was 60 cc, 30 cc of which was pure fat.

I changed to a 3-mm-gauge Toledo V-tip dissector cannula to break the adhesions between this adiposity and the dorsal midroll of fat. This roll was suctioned with the same sequence of cannulas, and the areas were crisscrossed at the end from the axillary and the dorsal incisions. We removed 120 cc, 60 cc of which was pure fat. Through the trochanteric incision, I suctioned 555 cc, 405

Table A1-1. *Measurements and weight for Example Case 1*

	October 4	November 4	December 12	January 27
Thorax (submammary) (cm)	85	76	75	74
Thorax (axilla) (cm)	92	84	84	83
Waist (umbilicus) (cm)	84	78	72	70
Abdomen (iliac crest) (cm)	105	101	96	91
Hips (trochanter) (cm)	111	105	102	98
Right thigh (groin) (cm)	68	60	59	54
Left thigh (groin) (cm)	68	60	59	54
Weight (kg)	70.3	63	61.2	55

cc of pure fat, from the flank. After suction, I crisscrossed these dorsal and axillary areas from the three incisions with the flat-tip cannula to provoke a uniform skin retraction. Almost no fat came out on this last passage of the cannula in the dorsal region, but I tried to stimulate the dermis by rasping it gently. It is not necessary to do this on the flank, because there is no need to retract that area.

I treated the lateral thigh and the lower buttock through two incisions, one in the trochanter area and another in the infragluteal fold. After the infiltration of the anesthetic solution, the area becomes very tumescent. I started suctioning deep with a 4.6-mm-gauge Pyramid-tip cannula to reduce the volume. After the removal of 500 cc, I changed to a 3-mm gauge and started suctioning more superficially in the subgluteal area and on the lower third of the buttock. To reduce these areas without dropping the buttocks, I suctioned the subgluteal area and the lower third of the buttock superficially. The total fat aspirated was 900 cc.

To help understand what the deformity looks like in the standing position, I pressed the buttock, elevating the lateral thigh. I aspirated the excess fat and created a curve between the buttock and the thigh, defining the contour. Aspiration of the deep structures in the dorsal area of the thigh can affect the position and shape of the buttock.

After I treated the other side, I put the patient in supine position to treat the abdomen and the medial thighs. To prevent perforation of the abdominal wall, I bent the table and placed a support under the patient's buttocks, elevating them. This forced the cannula that entered the pubic area to have a trajectory outward in the epigastrium, avoiding perforation of the abdominal wall. I injected 1,500 cc of anesthetic solution into the abdomen and 180 cc into each medial thigh. To reduce the abdomen evenly, I started suctioning deep with a 4.6-mm-gauge pyramid-tip cannula. I prefer 35-cm-long cannulas to treat the abdomen, because they allow long, more uniform passes to treat the upper and lower abdomen simultaneously. I treated the left side first for comparison, and then the right side. The abdomen rarely needs superficial suction unless a great retraction is required. This patient needed no superficial suction in the abdomen. I changed to a 3.7-mm-gauge cannula for refinement at the end, but I did not have to treat the areolar layer of fat in this case. Sometimes I may suction the lower abdomen to get a good skin retraction, but it is very rarely necessary to suction the whole abdomen superficially. The total aspirate here was 1,730 cc, 1,400 cc of which was pure fat.

The medial thighs are a difficult area to treat because it is easy to get a depression there if suction is too superficial. I aspirated only 155 cc from each side. I usually tell my patients the percentage of improvement they can expect on their medial thighs, depending on their skin flaccidity. If I tell them it will improve only 50% and they want more improvement, I will reevaluate the skin retraction after six months to assess whether they need a second suction or whether only a dermolipectomy can solve the problem.

This procedure enhanced this patient's self-esteem, and she began dieting and exercising on a regular basis after the first postoperative month. So her good result is not only due to surgical technique but also is a consequence of the better lifestyle she adopted after the procedure.

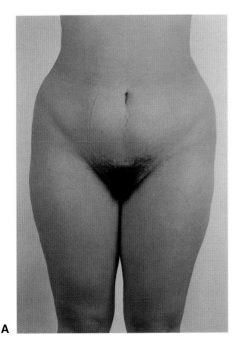

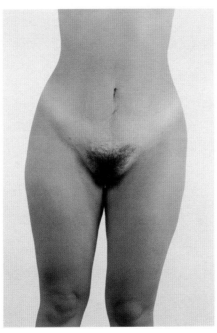

A   B

FIG. A1-1. A, C, E: Preoperative photos. **B, D, F:** Three-month postoperative photos of syringe liposculpture of the dorsal region, flanks, lateral and medial thighs, and abdomen. *Figure continues on next page.*

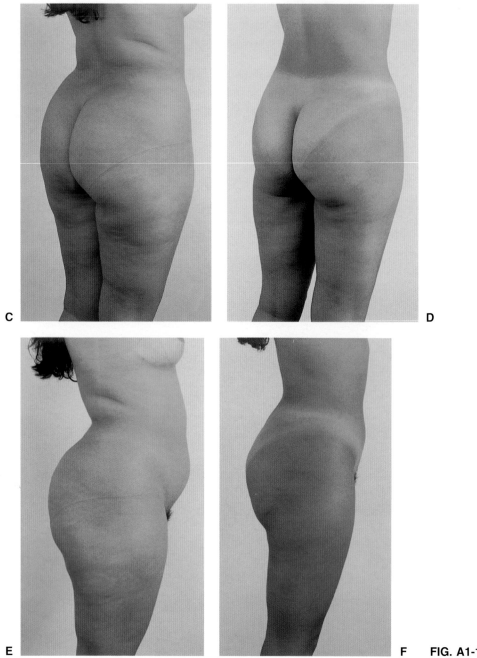

C

D

E

F   **FIG. A1-1.** *Continued.*

EXAMPLE CASE 2

A 28-year-old patient, 1.59 m high and weighing 63 kg, thought she looked fat and wanted to improve her body contour. She went to an endocrinologist who referred her for body sculpture. The areas she was not pleased with were the dorsal region, flanks, lateral, dorsal and medial thighs, buttocks, knees, and abdomen. I indicated syringe liposculpture of these areas (Fig. A1-2). I removed a total aspirate of 1,640 cc of pure fat and injected only 30 cc on a left buttock depression. Her pre- and postoperative measurements are outlined in Table A1-2. The main objectives of this procedure were to reduce the rolls around the waist, and to improve overall body contour.

After IV sedation with midazolam and fentanyl, the patient was placed in the lateral position and the anesthetic formula was infiltrated on the first side to be treated. The dorsal region was treated through three incisions, two in the dorsal area and another in the flank. I began suctioning deep with a 4.6-mm-gauge Pyramid-tip cannula. I changed to a flat-tip two-holed 4.6-mm-gauge cannula and suctioned superficially, with the holes towards the dermis. With the 3-mm-gauge Toledo V-tip dissector cannula, I severed the adhesions between the back rolls and the flank. The total aspirate was 160 cc of pure fat. Through the trochanteric incision, I suctioned 160 cc of pure fat from the flank. After suction, I crisscrossed these dorsal flank areas from the three incisions to make sure there were no retractions or adhesions.

I treated the lateral and dorsal thigh and the lower buttock through two incisions, one in the trochanter area and another in the infragluteal fold. After the infiltration of the anesthetic solution, the area becomes very tumescent. I prefer to start suctioning deeply in the lateral thigh with a 4.6-mm-gauge Pyramid-tip cannula to reduce the volume. After this, I changed to a 3-mm gauge and began suctioning more superficially in the subgluteal area and on the lower third of the buttock to reduce these areas without dropping the buttocks. The total fat aspirated here was 300 cc. I also injected 30 cc of fat into the depression in the left buttock. After I treated the other side, I put the patient in a supine hyperextended position to treat the abdomen and the medial thighs. To reduce the abdomen evenly, I suctioned deep with a 3.7-mm-gauge Pyramid-tip 35-cm-long cannula. This abdomen did not need superficial suction. The total aspirate here was 240 cc of pure fat. The medial thighs were aspirated (only 90 cc), as well as the knees (20 cc from each side). The stitches were removed on the fifth postoperative day and the patient was sent to the aesthetic clinic for manual lymphatic drainage. She had two sessions a week for four weeks. After this period she was weighed and measured. There was only 1 kg difference in her weight and she was feeling very swollen. She was also still unusually bruised. But as the measurements in Table A1-2 show, she continued to lose weight in the months that

Table A1-2. *Measurements and weight for Example Case 2*

	November 3 1993	December 7 1993	January 19 1994	May 25 1994
Waist (umbilicus) (cm)	74	70	68	66
Abdomen (iliac crest) (cm)	90	87	86	83
Hips (trochanter) (cm)	103	98	97	93
Right thigh (groin) (cm)	60	54	53	53
Left thigh (groin) (cm)	60	54	53	53
Right knee (cm)	41	34	34	34
Left knee (cm)	41	34	34	34
Weight (kg)	63	62	56.5	56.5

followed, and by the sixth postoperative month, she had a reduction of 6½ kg, a 10% reduction from her preoperative weight. Her measurements showed a good improvement, and she was happy with her new figure. The patient then mentioned that she had undergone the procedure to try to keep her boyfriend, who was dating a younger, leaner girl. After she acquired the body she wanted, she realized she did not want that boyfriend anymore. They split up, and she was much happier in another relationship.

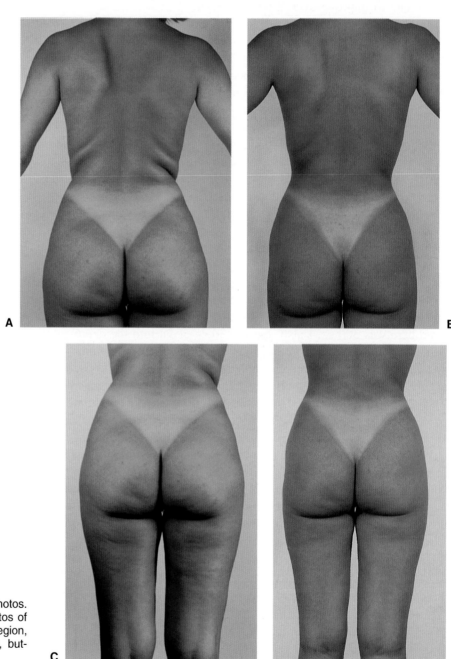

FIG. A1-2. A, C, E, G: Preoperative photos. **B, D, F, H:** Six-month postoperative photos of syringe liposculpture of the dorsal region, flanks, lateral, dorsal and medial thighs, buttocks, knees, and abdomen.

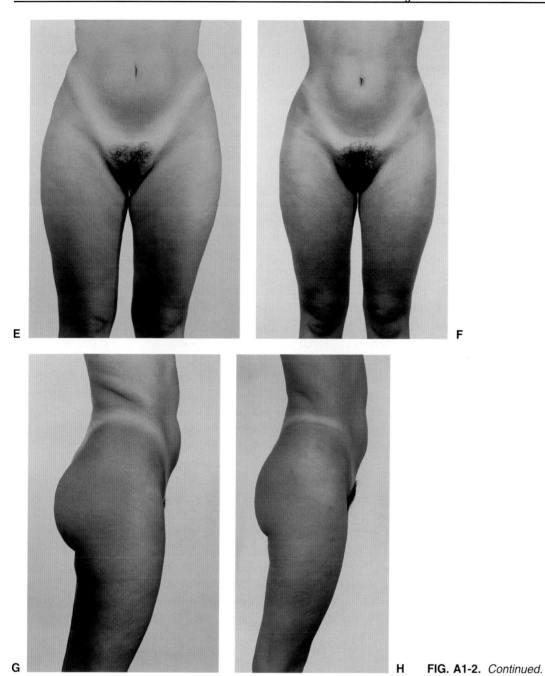

E

F

G

H   **FIG. A1-2.** *Continued.*

EXAMPLE CASE 3

A 33-year-old patient weighing 70 kg, 1.72 m tall with very flaccid skin, complained that she had to have her clothes made to order because her right thigh was 4 cm thicker than the left. She wanted more even thighs and to improve the body contour below the waist.

I indicated syringe liposculpture of the lateral and medial thighs and knees (Fig. A1-3). I told her the contour would improve, but not the skin tone, and through superficial liposculpture we could avoid an increase of the flaccidity. Postoperative exercise was also prescribed. I removed a total aspirate of 1,430 cc of pure fat—2% of her body weight. After one month, her weight was down to 65.3 kg. Her pre- and postoperative measurements are outlined in Table A1-3. The main objectives of this procedure were to reduce the lateral thighs, more the right thigh than the left, and the lower buttocks, without dropping the buttocks, and to reduce the medial thighs and knees, without increasing skin flaccidity.

After IV sedation with midazolam and fentanyl, the patient was placed in the lateral position, and the anesthetic formula was infiltrated on the first side to be treated. We treated the right side first, and then the left. After both sides were treated, the patient was placed in the supine position, and we treated the medial thighs and knees.

Through the trochanteric incision, I suctioned fat from the lateral thigh superficially using first a 3.7-mm-gauge Pyramid-tip cannula and later subdermally, a 3-mm gauge. The lower buttock was suctioned through the two incisions, with a 3-mm gauge only. The amounts aspirated were 500 cc of pure fat from the right lateral thigh, and 360 cc from the left.

The medial thighs were suctioned in the supine position through inguinal incisions using a 3.7-mm-gauge cannula. We checked the regularity of the suction by bending the knees and spreading the legs laterally. By pulling the skin down with the outstretched hand, it is possible to feel the skin texture and avoid aspirating too much fat, which would cause the need for skin resection at the groin level. The medial knees were treated with a 3-mm-gauge cannula through a popliteal incision. A total of 305 cc of pure fat was removed from the left medial thigh and 205 cc from the right, plus 30 cc from each medial knee. This procedure was a small one, but was important to the patient, who was very pleased with the result—not a dramatic change, not a great result, but just what she wanted.

Table A1-3. *Measurements and weight for Example Case 3*

	January 13	March 5
Hips (trochanter) (cm)	106	102
Right thigh (groin) (cm)	67	60
Left thigh (groin) (cm)	63	58
Right knee (cm)	41	40
Left knee (cm)	41	40
Weight (kg)	70	65.3

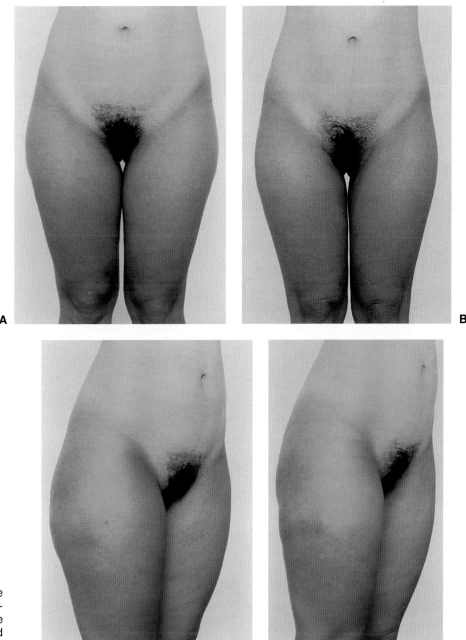

FIG. A1-3. A, C, E, G: Preoperative photos. **B, D, F, H:** Two-month postoperative photos of syringe liposculpture of the lateral and medial thighs and knees. *Figure continues on next page.*

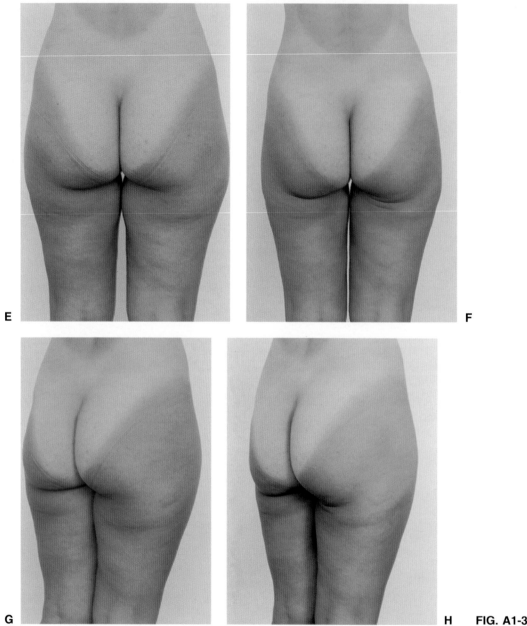

E

F

G

H   **FIG. A1-3.** *Continued.*

EXAMPLE CASE 4

A 54-year-old patient weighing 65.2 kg preoperatively wanted to improve her abdomen. She mentioned that she did not want a dermolipectomy but wanted to reduce the volume of her abdomen to look good in clothes. I indicated syringe liposculpture of the dorsal region, flanks, and abdomen. I mentioned to her that she might need a second procedure on the abdomen after six months, depending on the skin retraction (Fig. A1-4).

I removed a total aspirate of 2,705 cc, being 2,330 cc of pure fat, which was 3.5% of her body weight. After two months her weight was down to 61.5 kg.

Her pre- and postoperative measurements are outlined in Table A1-4. The main objectives of this procedure were to reduce the abdomen evenly, getting a good skin retraction, and to reduce the flanks and the dorsal region. This patient was an obvious candidate for an abdominoplasty, but she did not want that procedure because she was afraid of feeling postoperative pain, she did not have time for recovery, she wanted to look good in clothes and not in swimwear, she preferred a cheaper procedure, and she did not mind her stretch marks.

After IV sedation with midazolam and fentanyl, the patient was placed in the lateral position, and the anesthetic formula was infiltrated on the first side to be treated. The amounts per side were 360 cc on the dorsal area and 480 cc on the flank.

The dorsal region was treated through two incisions, one in the dorsal area and another in the flank. I started suctioning deep with a 4.6-mm-gauge Pyramid-tip cannula. After reducing the volume in the dorsal area, I changed to a flat-tip two-holed 4.6-mm-gauge cannula and suctioned superficially, with the holes towards the dermis. The total aspirate on this side was 130 cc, 110 cc of which was pure fat. I changed to a 3-mm-gauge Toledo V-tip dissector cannula to break the adhesions between this adiposity and the flank. A total of 390 cc, 355 cc of pure fat, was removed from the flank. After suction, I crisscrossed the dorsal and flank areas from the two incisions with the flat-tip cannula to provoke a uniform skin retraction.

After I had treated the other side, I put the patient in the supine position to treat the abdomen. The table was bent and a support placed under the buttocks, elevating the hips, to prevent abdominal wall perforation. I injected a total of 2,180 cc of anesthetic solution into the abdomen. Four incisions were used: pubic, umbilical, and one on each iliac crest. To reduce the abdomen evenly, I started suctioning deep with a 4.6-mm-gauge pyramid-tip cannula. This abdomen needed superficial suction to improve skin retraction. I changed to a 3-mm-gauge cannula to treat the areolar layer of fat of the epigastrium and hypogastrium. The total aspirate from the abdomen was 1,730 cc, 1,420 cc of which was pure fat.

This patient's result was far from the beauty contest category, but it was exactly what she wanted—a cheap, noninvasive procedure, with a short recovery time, less postoperative morbidity, and a great improvement in her clothes measurements. Two months after the operation, she came for facial liposculpture and has returned for ''maintenance'' procedures on her face.

Table A1-4. *Measurements and weight for Example Case 4*

	September 4	November 22
Thorax (axilla) (cm)	83	78
Waist (umbilicus) (cm)	82	77
Abdomen (iliac crest) (cm)	102	95
Hips (trochanter) (cm)	104	98

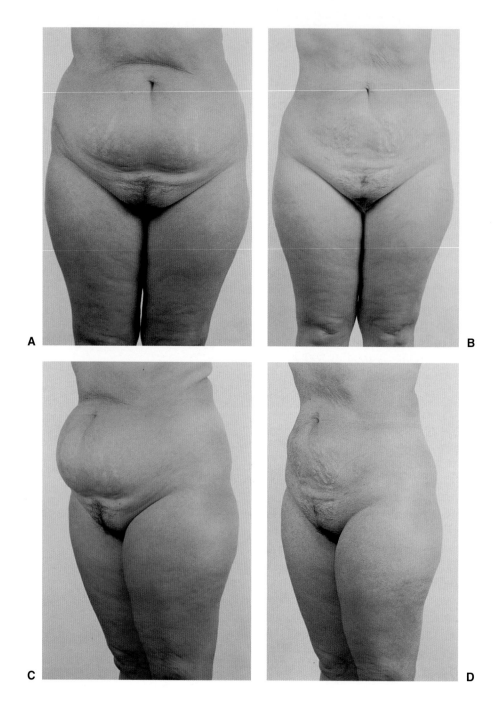

FIG. A1-4. A, C, E, G, I: Preoperative photos. **B, D, F, H, J:** Two-month post-operative photos of syringe liposculpture of the dorsal region, flanks, and abdomen.

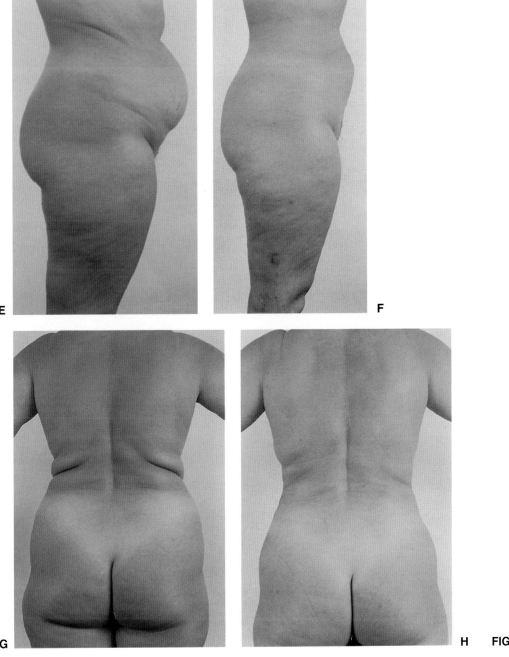

E

F

G

H FIG. A1-4. *Continued.*

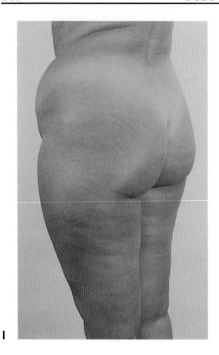

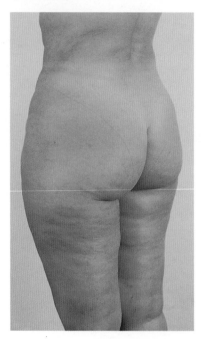

I   J   **FIG. A1-4.** *Continued.*

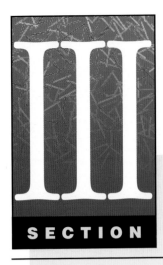

SECTION III

*F*acial Contouring

22

Facial Rejuvenation

An Overview

In the last decade, I have improved my techniques for facial rejuvenation. I have developed a different way to treat my patients, without the rigid confines taught in my early years of plastic surgery. I have learned to appreciate the desires of the patients, looking to improve their appearance with simpler, faster procedures other than rhytidoplasty. I can now offer smaller procedures under local anesthesia with no need for hospitalization, which is often a major consideration for patients.

THE EARLY SIGNS OF AGING

Patients can start showing signs of aging at different ages. I have performed blepharoplasty on a 23-year-old patient, yet sometimes a 50-year-old does not show any wrinkle or fat deposits around the eyes. Generally, between 30 and 40 years of age, people start showing one or several of the following signs (Figs. 22-1, 22-2): nasolabial, jowl, and submental fat deposits, and nasolabial, malar, and glabella depression. Between 40 and 50 years of age, there are other signs: an accentuation of the periorbital depression, thinning of the lips, and perioral and periorbital wrinkles.

After 50 years of age, skin flaccidity can provoke a general formation of wrinkles and folds on the face and neck (Fig. 22-3). The degree of aging of the skin depends on several factors, such as genetics, exposure to sun, diet, etc.

INDICATIONS

I have been performing what I call "refreshing" techniques, offering an alternative to the classical face-lift. I can start treating my patients at an earlier age, maintaining a younger look, or I can improve the aspect of older faces of patients who do not want to undergo or whose faces have been overstretched by rhytidoplasties.

Some patients complain that their face-lift, performed 10 years earlier, has "expired," and they want to improve their looks but refuse to undergo the same procedure again (Fig. 22-4). Using simple techniques, I can enhance the facial appearance of patients of all ages. I treat problems as they occur. The folds and fat deposits are aspirated and the depressions are filled. Skin flaccidity is either resurfaced or removed.

I like to tell my patients they should get into a maintenance program. Instead of letting everything "fall down" before thinking of plastic surgery, and then changing to a totally different look, they should take care of themselves as the small problems appear. Small problems need small procedures. Small changes are less noticeable, and the younger look can be kept for a longer period of time. I advise my patients to come for maintenance consultations at least every two years.

For superficial liposculpture (1), I use disposable syringes and the finest cannulas to aspirate fat from the neck, recontour the jawline, inject fat into the nasolabial, malar, orbital, and glabellar regions, and thus postpone the first face-lift or complement an older patient's face-lift. "Refreshing" does not give the same results as rhytidoplasty; I do not advocate that rhytidoplasty be abandoned. Instead, "refreshing" is a more gentle facial recontouring procedure—a temporary substitute, or a complement to other techniques.

A STATE OF MIND

Feeling young is intimately connected with the state of mind, but improving the appearance helps to improve the state of mind. "It is much better to look young and have no wrinkles than to carry the burden of an old face," said one patient. Changes need not be drastic to provoke a more youthful appearance and elevate the spirit and the "tired" face. The human appearance is the sum of a number of components (2). It has been studied for centuries by artists and more recently by psychologists (3) and plastic surgeons. The face can have some features that immediately classify people into stereotypes, such as a round faced, a crooked faced, etc. Small changes can alter our perceptions of these features and change the entire personality of an individual (Fig. 22-5). The extreme sensibility we have to the perception of small changes in facial features has been demonstrated (Figs. 22-6–22-8) (4). If makeup artists can (5) use simple tricks of color and light to change our perception of someone's face, plastic surgeons can produce amazing alterations with small procedures. Most of my patients, when asked about the alterations they would like on their faces, are very adamant about not wanting to change their expression. Their usual request is, "I just want to look good for my age," and that is the reason we should perform small changes. The comments they like to hear from their friends are: "You look rested," or "You look good today, have you been to a spa?"

Of course, in rare cases a patient will say, "I want to look ridiculously younger," but that is the exception, not the rule. A patient like this will not be satisfied with small changes, and is looking for radical changes, and I consider this a bad indication for surgery.

I like to have one point very clear in my mind so I can advise my patients. At some stage, facial rejuvenation can be achieved only by removing excess skin and repositioning the facial structures. The question is, when is that stage reached? It varies from person to person, but I will give you a few examples from my experience.

Some older patients do not want a rhytidoplasty and will agree if they are told that a smaller procedure can be done, but the result will not be the same as with rhytidoplasty (Fig. 22-9). Other patients in the postoperative period forget what they have been told about the result. They will complain about the result, saying the improvement was not enough. This is why it is necessary to have in writing that the patient knows this smaller procedure is not the ideal indication for their case. It is just an improvement, a temporary procedure to postpone the ideal surgery until a better time.

AVOIDING STIGMAS

I had to alter my concept of facial rejuvenation. I was never happy performing face-lifts on young patients of 35 to 45 years of age. First, I hesitate to put an extensive and permanent scar on a "borderline age" case, and I felt there should be an approach other than stretching the skin to accomplish a younger look. A stretched face with that "what's happening?" look, alters the facial proportions and the outward personality of the patient (Fig. 22-10). This can be avoided by a good surgeon.

RHYTIDOPLASTY

Even a good rhytidoplasty result will leave permanent scars. Of course I perform the procedure when indicated, but I find that this is not often and only in select cases. There are patients who will not want a face-lift and will probably opt for a substitute technique instead of having no surgery at all. Several patients in the 25 to 45 age group, when asking for rejuvenation, say they want to "have something done" to improve their appearance. Before liposuction, there were few options. The so-called "minilift," either forehead or cervical, is still a rhytidoplasty and should be indicated as one.

BLEPHAROPLASTY

Blepharoplasty is a wonderful procedure that solves the problems of excess skin, muscle, and fat within the orbital region. Blepharoplasty, is quick and safe with the use of the CO_2 Ultrapulse laser, giving a fast recovery time for the busy patient of 3 to 7 days. There is no substitute for it. It solves eyelid problems thoroughly and leaves inconspicuous scars. Using the transconjunctival incision, we can avoid the lower eyelid skin incision. After the removal of fat, skin retracts in 90% of these young patients, with no need for skin resection. I often combine CO_2 laser blepharoplasty with facial liposculpture, improving the eyelids and the facial contour at the same time.

PEELS

Fine wrinkles that do not disappear with a procedure can be treated with either the light alpha-hydroxy acid (AHA) peels (6), especially with 70% glycolic acid if the patient does not want postoperative redness. AHA peels are done fortnightly and also prescribed as daily creams. The peels improve fine wrinkles and old age spots, giving the skin a more youthful and healthy appearance. I have been using fewer phenol and trichloroacetic acid (TCA) peels. Laser resurfacing will be prescribed for patients who want a more predictable result but who do not mind having a longer recovery period. I have been prescribing laser peels for rejuvenation and for acne scars. I have been preparing patients' skin before and after laser resurfacing, improving surgical results. We prescribe retinoic acid treatment in low doses, controlled by weekly visits to the office for a period of at least six weeks preresurfacing. Dark-skinned patients will also use hydroquinone preoperatively and after the third postoperative week of laser resurfacing.

FACIAL LIPOSCULPTURE

By 1988, I was using only syringes for our facial liposculpture. In younger patients, I generally inject fat into the nasolabial folds, the malar region, and the glabellar region. In patients in their late 30s, I suction the jowls and submandibular area to redefine the jawline. Suction is usually performed once and fat injection three times. Injection is performed in 3-mm threads and repeated after 35 days (7,8). This means that a facial liposculpture patient is ready to return to normal activities the following day after only fat injection, or two to three days after suction, depending on the amount of fat removed and on the patient's predisposition to bruising. Corrective makeup is useful when clients have a busy schedule.

REFERENCES

1. Toledo LS. Superficial syringe liposculpture. In: Toledo LS, ed. *Annals of the international symposium "Recent advances in plastic surgery (RAPS) 90,"* São Paulo, Brazil, March 3–5, 1990. Rio de Janeiro: Marques-Saraiva, 1990:446–453.
2. Toepffer R. *Essai de physiognomonie,* Geneva, 1845.
3. Gombrich EH, Hochberg J, Black M. *Arte, percepción y realidad,* ed. Paidós. Barcelona: Mandelbaum, 1973:42.
4. Brunwick E, Reiter L. Eindrucks charaktere schematisierter Gesichter, *Z Psychol Z Angew Psychol* 1937:67–134.
5. Gombrich EH, Hochberg J, Black M. *Arte, percepción y realidad.* Paidós, ed. Barcelona: Mandelbaum, 1973:59.
6. Rubin M. Non-phenol chemical peels. In: Toledo LS, ed. *Annals of the international symposium "Recent advances in plastic surgery (RAPS) 90,"* São Paulo, Brazil, March 3–5, 1990. Rio de Janeiro: Marques-Saraiva, 1990:614–617.
7. Carpaneda CA, Ribeiro MT. Study of the histologic alterations and viability of the adipose graft in humans. *Aesthetic Plast Surg* 1993;17:43–47.
8. Toledo LS. Syringe liposculpture. A two-year experience. *Aesthetic Plast Surg* 1991;15:321–326.

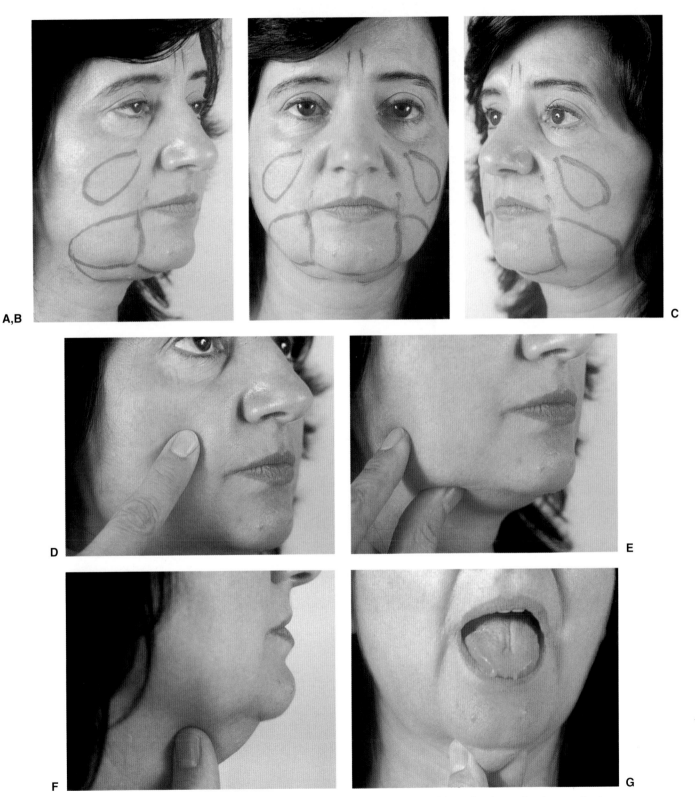

FIG. 22-1. A, B, C: Preoperative photos of a 39-year-old patient with early signs of aging marked: malar, glabellar and nasolabial depressions, jowl and submental fat deposits. **D:** The malar depression will accentuate the nasolabial fold. **E:** The jowl fat deposit blurs the definition of the jawline. **F:** The submental fat deposit. **G:** The test to find if the deposit consists of pre- or retroplatysmal fat. When the tongue is poked out easily, this must be preplatysmal fat, pinched between the fingers. *Figure continues on next page.*

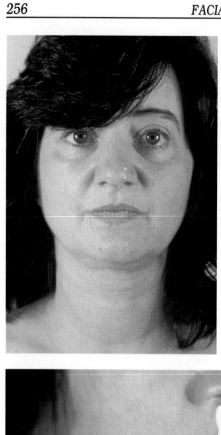

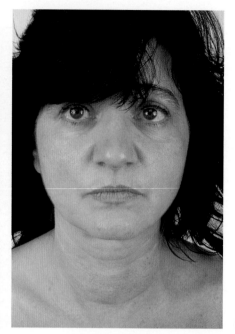

H

I

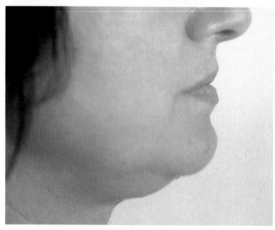

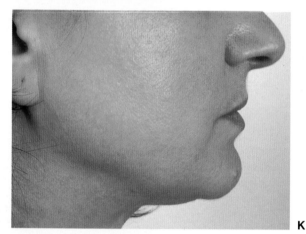

J

K

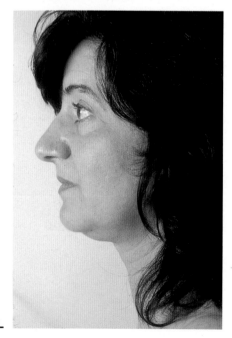

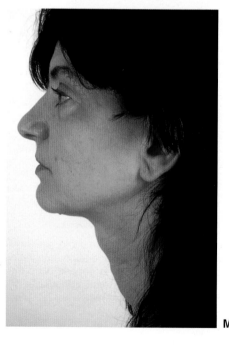

L

M

FIG. 22-1. *Continued.* **H, I:** Pre- and two-year postoperative photos of facial liposculpture, after one aspiration of fat from the jowls and submental region plus three fat injections into the depressed areas. The last fat injection was 18 months earlier. **J, K:** Pre- and two-year postoperative photos. No rhytidoplasty. **L, M:** Pre- and four-year postoperative photos. The patient is now 43 years old and looks better than when she was 39. The last procedure was 3 ½ years ago when she came back for another small procedure. She is thinking about having a neck-lift in the near future.

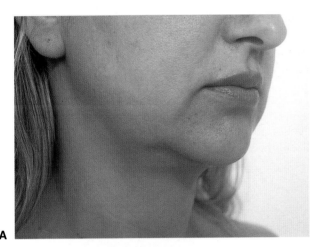

A

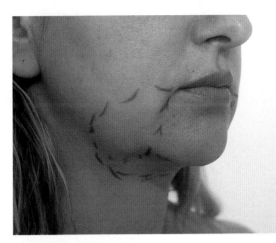

B

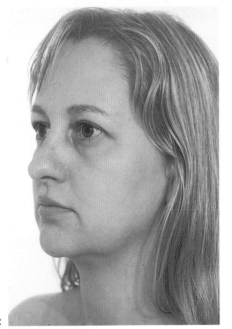

C

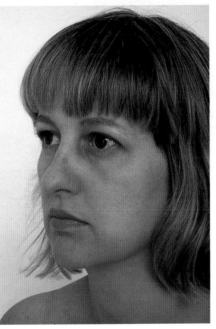

D

FIG. 22-2. A, B: Preoperative photos of a 42-year-old patient with jowls and submental fat deposits. **C, D:** Pre- and one-year postoperative photos following facial liposculpture. This patient had only fat aspiration from the jowls and submental fat deposits.

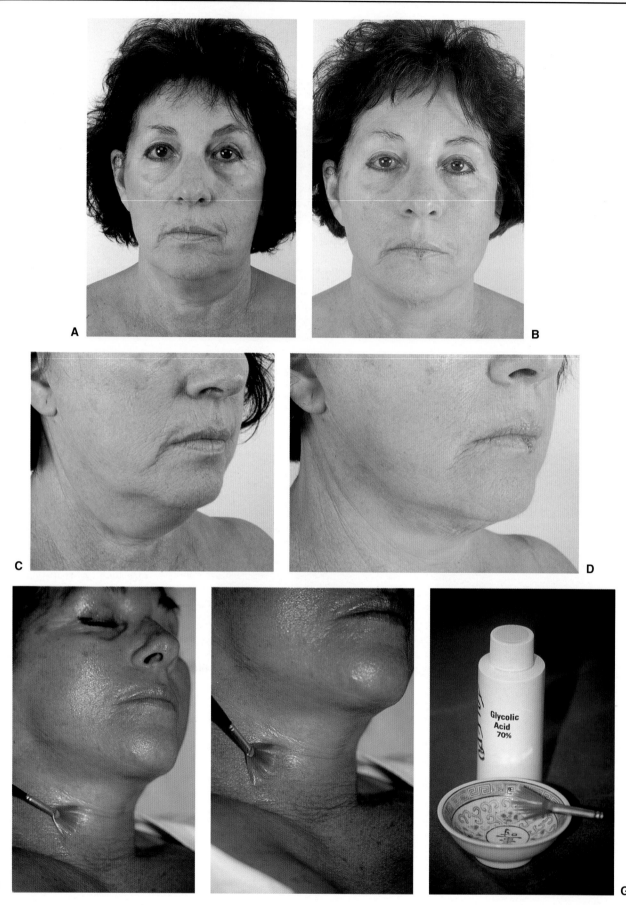

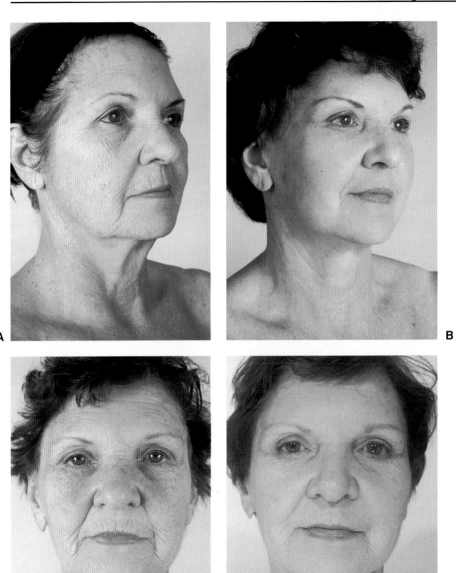

FIG. 22-4. A: Preoperative photo of a 71-year-old patient who wanted a rhytidoplasty. **B:** One-year postoperative photo of rhytidoplasty and blepharoplasty. **C:** Ten years postoperatively. The patient said that, at 81, she wanted to have some rejuvenation done but did not want a face-lift again. **D:** Three months postoperatively, after facial liposculpture. I aspirated fat from the neck, reducing the "platysmal bands," injected fat on her malar and nasolabial folds, and put her into a skin care alpha-hydroxy acid program.

FIG. 22-3. A, C: Preoperative photos of a 55-year-old patient with sun-damaged skin and fat deposits in the jowls and submental regions plus nasolabial, malar, and periorbital depressions. **B, D:** Two-month postoperative photos of facial liposculpture with fat aspiration of the jowls and neck plus fat injection in the nasolabial folds, malar, and periorbital regions. **E, F:** This patient also started on the alpha-hydroxy-acid program and had a good skin improvement in this short period of time. Her face and neck were peeled. She had four 70% glycolic acid six-minute peels and used 12% glycolic acid cream at night. **G:** The 70% glycolic acid with the soft brush used for the peel.

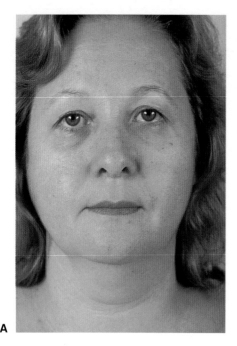

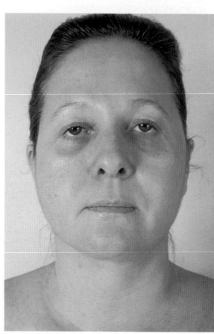

A

B

FIG. 22-5. A, B: Pre- and two-month postoperative photos of a 45-year-old patient with a round face. There was a refinement of her features just by aspirating fat from her cheeks and neck.

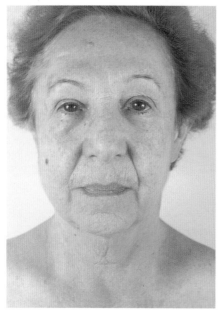

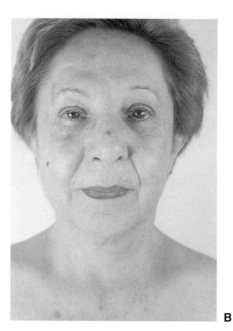

A

B

FIG. 22-6. A, B: Pre- and two-month postoperative photos of a 71-year-old patient with a crooked face. Through facial liposculpture we managed to change these features and give her face a more balanced and younger look.

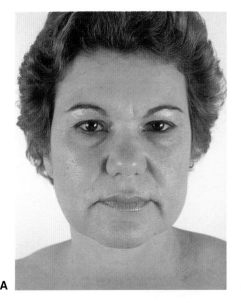

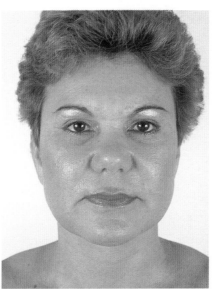

FIG. 22-7. A, B: Pre- and three-month postoperative photos of a 43-year-old patient with a "mountain" or "pear" face. The reshaping of the lower part of her face through liposculpture produced a more graceful, balanced, and younger look.

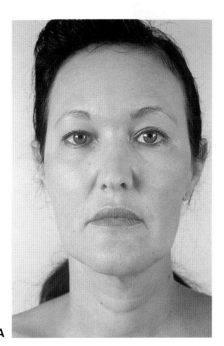

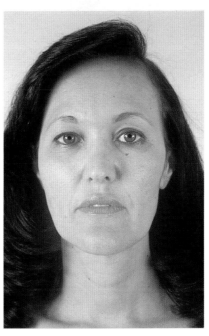

FIG. 22-8. A, B: Pre- and two-month postoperative photos of a 44-year-old patient with a "jade" or "lozenge" face. The blending of the features was performed through liposculpture, by enhancing the malar area and reducing the mandibular area.

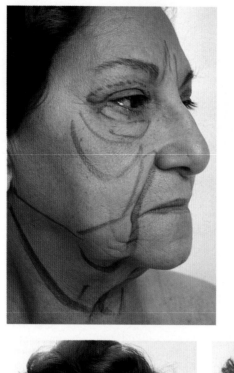

A

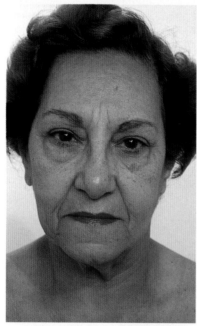

B

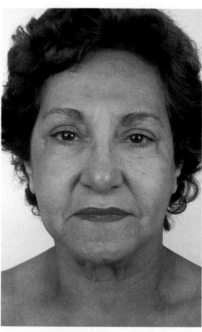

C

FIG. 22-9. A: Preoperative markings of a 72-year-old patient who wanted to rejuvenate without rhy-tidoplasty. The areas in *blue* on the neck and jowls represent the areas of superficial liposculpture; the area in *red* in the malars represents fat injection. The *purple* markings on the eyelids are for a CO_2 laser blepharoplasty. **B, D, F:** Preoperative photos of a 72-year-old patient. **C, E, G:** One year postoperatively. There was good retraction in the neck region, although no skin was removed. There was an improvement in the jowl area and mandibular line. I have also aspirated some fat from the nasolabial deposit to flatten the area, and injected fat into the nasolabial depression. The skin tone has improved with skin care and AHA peels. **H, I:** Pre- and one-year postoperative photos of CO_2 laser blepharoplasty with removal of skin, muscle, and fat from the upper eyelids and a transconjunctival removal of the lower eyelids' fat pockets. There was no skin resection. One month after the operation I performed a 35% trichloroacetic acid peel of the lower eyelids. This was before laser resurfacing, which I would prefer today.

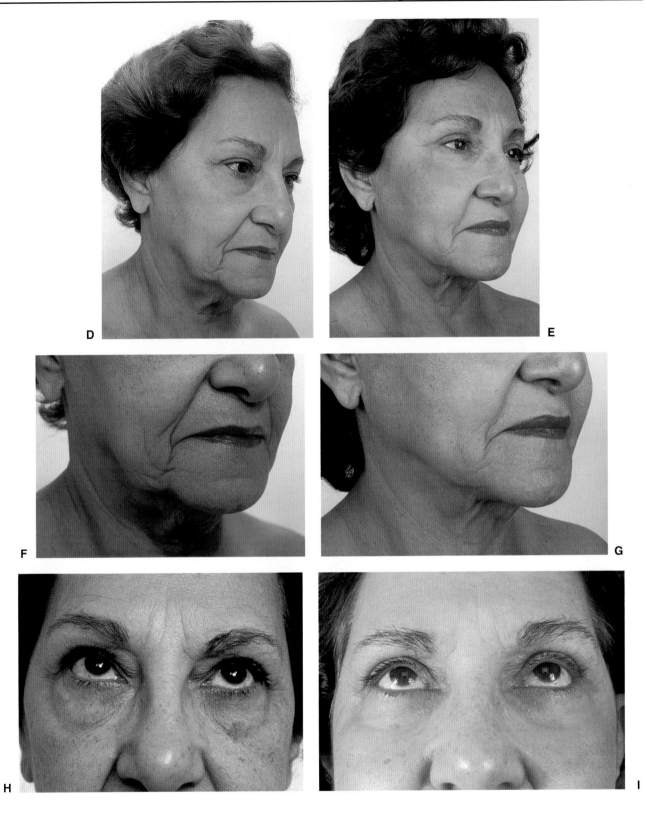

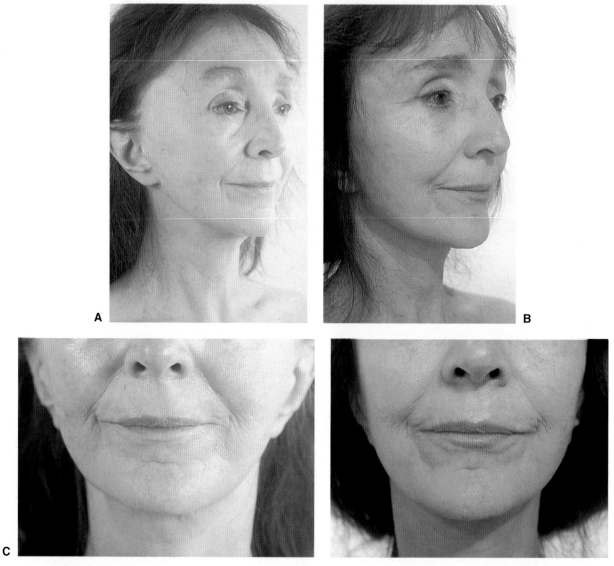

FIG. 22-10. A, C: Preoperative photos of a 63-year-old patient who had had three rhytidoplasty procedures performed by different surgeons in the past. Her face was flat, the skin was too stretched, and she lacked definition and contour to her face. **B, D:** Although this is a very subtle result, there is a difference in the projection of the malars and in the depth of her wrinkles and folds. Six months after facial liposculpture, the appearance is more natural. Fat was injected in her periorbital, malar, and nasolabial areas, and lips.

23

Facial Liposculpture

Syringe Aspiration

In the early 1980s, I started using liposuction to improve facial contours. Cannulas were thick in those days—4 mm to 6 mm—and the results then, as in all cases of liposuction, were limited by the patient's skin quality and the depth of suction. Patients were considered candidates for liposuction if they were young with good skin tone.

By 1985, I had started injecting aspirated fat into the face and body, and by 1986 I was using 10-cc disposable syringes for my facial liposculpture work. This procedure became extremely delicate with the introduction of much finer cannulas—1.5-mm to 3-mm gauge—and the injection gun that allowed minute quantities of fat to be injected at a time.

Liposuction is usually considered as an adjunct to rhytidoplasty (1,2). In my mind it is the opposite. Small procedures are very common in my practice, mostly for those who seek rejuvenation when they start noticing the signs of aging on the face. The face-lift (rhytidectomy, rhytidoplasty) became an adjunctive procedure to the smaller interventions such as blepharoplasty, fat aspiration, fat injection, laser peel, etc. This means that when a patient was ready for a rhytidoplasty, he or she had already undergone several smaller procedures to postpone the face-lift. Even when there is a clear indication for a face-lift, I will perform the rhytidoplasty combined with syringe liposculpture. It can be difficult to obtain ideal results with cervicofacial rhytidoplasty alone, especially when removing local excesses of adipose tissue in the parotid, nasolabial, submental and submandibular areas to improve definition of the facial, mandibular, and cervical contours (3). I offer facial liposculpture as an outpatient contouring procedure under local anesthesia. Small procedures can be performed with oral or intravenous sedation in an ambulatory surgical facility. Anesthesia has greatly improved with the tumescent technique. Outpatient surgery has become 90% of my work; the ease and safety of the procedure has drastically reduced the number of hospital surgeries.

SKIN RETRACTION

Perhaps the greatest change I have noticed in our results over the past years is related to the role of skin retraction. The skin of the neck, treated with lipo-superficial fat aspiration, seems to be more retractable than in other sites (Fig. 23-1). The considerable elasticity of the skin of the neck contrasts with the poor ability of facial skin to retract (4).

In 1987 I was using 3-mm-gauge cannulas to treat the face and the neck area. My results were good at the time, but in 1989 I felt I could improve them by aspirating even more superficially, closer to the skin, using the same principle I was using to provoke skin retraction in the abdominal and femoral regions with superficial syringe liposculpture.

I started performing superficial liposculpture in March 1989, to improve the facial and body contour of flaccid skin patients. The liposuction rule that we should stay at least 1 to 2 mm below the skin level can never be applied in facial suction. Rarely can we stay as deep as 2 mm, or even 1 mm, when treating the face and neck.

INDICATIONS

Facial harmony depends on a combination of prominent zygomas, a subtle cheek hollow, flat nasolabial folds, and a well-defined jawline. To reach this goal I can use several aesthetic contouring procedures, such as facial liposculpture (suction and injection of fat), blepharoplasty, and rhytidoplasty.

The indication for each procedure varies according to the problems of each individual. Some will have submental fat excess only, and this is what will be treated. I do not operate on areas about which the patient does not complain. I will, however, tell the patient that the final result will be enhanced by a chin augmentation, for example, if facial harmony will be achieved that way, even if that was not the initial complaint. This is one of the few examples in my practice of directing the patient to something that has not been addressed in the consultation (Fig. 23-2).

For patients with fat deposits on the jowls and neck, subcutaneous suction of the jowls and submandibular area is performed, redefining the "lost" jawline. Older patients who do not want a rhytidoplasty will still have excess skin after this procedure; this is their choice and I respect it, but some degree of improvement in the patient's looks can still be obtained (Fig. 23-3). I avoid suctioning fat from the face above (cephalad) the mandibular line, but sometimes it is necessary (Fig. 23-4). The jowl area, the area above the nasolabial fold, and, in heavier patients, the preauricular area are some exceptions to this rule as well as the overweight patient who lacks definition between the face and neck and needs reduction of the thickness of the fat layer to redefine the features (Fig. 23-5).

ANESTHESIA

I use oral sedation with midazolam, plus local tumescent anesthesia. IV sedation with midazolam and fentanyl is administered by an anesthesiologist.

The numerous advantages of the tumescent technique are readily applied to the cervicofacial area (5), including a better and safer method to perform a rhytidoplasty. The technique creates an essentially bloodless field and a decreased surgical morbidity (Fig. 23-6). I use my own local anesthesia formula (see Chapter 5).

Once the patient is sedated, the prepared anesthesia solution is injected into the areas of the face and neck that were marked with the patient in the standing position. The formula is injected at body temperature, with a 2-mm-gauge 15-cm-long multiholed-tip blunt cannula and a 10-ml disposable syringe, using one submental and two retroauricular 2-mm incisions. The amount of injection should be sufficient to expand the area and cause good compression of the capillaries, anesthetizing the area and reducing bleeding. Suctioning begins 10 minutes after the injection.

FAT ASPIRATION

Deep Suction

Using the submental incision, I insert a 3-mm-gauge Pyramid-tip 15-cm-long cannula connected to a 10-cc syringe and begin aspiration of the neck in this area. After a few strokes for pretunneling, I pull the plunger and start suctioning the deep layer of fat close to the platysma muscle (Figs. 23-7, 23-8). A pinch test with the other hand helps to regulate the depth of the tunnels and reveals any irregularities that need treatment. After completing the aspiration from the submental incision, I repeat the process through the other two retroauricular incisions, crisscrossing the tunnels and trying to obtain a uniform thickness in the fat layer connected to the skin. At this point it is important to leave a fine (2-mm) layer of fat connected to the platysma. This will avoid future retraction of the skin when we perform superficial suction.

Superficial Suction

After removing the neck adiposity, it is time for the more refined and meticulous work of thinning the cervical flap to allow for its retraction and adaptation to the new neck angle, and treating the jowl deformities. With the help of a 1.5-mm two-holed-flat-tipped 15-cm-long cannula adapted to a 10-cc syringe, I treat the jowls and submental area (Fig. 23-9). After fat suction, the cannula is turned with the holes facing the dermis to scrape the skin gently, provoking an even, controlled retraction of the area (Fig. 23-10).

Suction of the Jowls

When suctioning the jowls, special care must be taken with the mental nerves. We have had cases of temporary weakness of one half of the lower lip caused by traumatizing these branches, and it usually takes two months to return to normal. Again, the jowls should be treated using all the incisions to obtain an uniform retraction of the area. Usually only 1 to 2 ml of fat is aspirated from each jowl; this should be enough to obtain a good improvement. This is one of the great advantages of the syringe over the aspirator—you can measure extremely precise small amounts of aspirated or injected fat.

I have seen sequelae of superficial suction of the face and neck with unacceptable retracted skin areas that are difficult to correct. To avoid defects, it is necessary to obtain an even, uniform, and controlled suction (Fig. 23-11). Retraction should occur only when and where it is intended (Fig. 23-12). If suction is irregular in depth, it can leave depressions and subcutaneous adhesions that often show the passage of the cannula too superficially. Skin sloughs can also result if the cannula is too superficial. Suction is usually performed once but can be repeated after six months for a better skin retraction if necessary.

"Turkey Neck"

Some cases will still show excess skin after suction, and this is often diagnosed as a case for resection (6). Instead of the resection, I have performed more suction (Fig. 23-13), even though it may appear that there is no more fat left and that the excess is formed by either excess skin or platysmal flaccidity. After the local anesthetic infiltration and after suction, fat would still appear in the syringe to my surprise. In many cases we have managed to recontour the neck without having to resect skin or correct the platysma muscle, especially on patients who will not accept an auricular face-lift scar. Men are good candidates for this procedure. Most men want to look younger but do not want the scars of a face-lift. This is a good option for a natural result (Fig. 23-14). It is explained to the patient that at some stage skin resection will be necessary to maintain a good contour and eliminate flaccidity (Fig. 23-15). With this technique, a very fine line separates the optimal result from the skeletonized neck.

Neck Tightening

There is one more procedure that can be utilized to recontour the cervical mental angle before skin is removed. This is for the patient who does not mind some degree of skin redundancy and does not want to undergo a face-lift.

With the help of an endoscope (7), the skin is dissected, the fat flap of the neck dissected from the platysma, and a suture is placed that runs from mastoid to mastoid. This enhances the neck angle and helps to highlight the mandibular border. Instead of interlocking sutures (8), I prefer a simple suture that runs easily and can be removed if necessary without complications (Figs. 23-16–23-18). We also perform endoscopic cervical elevation with endoscopic malar elevation plus facial liposculpture (9) (Fig. 23-19).

The Bichat Fat Pad

I do not remove this fat pad. The removal of the Bichat fat pad, the corpus adiposum buccae (CAB) has been utilized as a way to achieve a subtle cheek hollow (10). Anatomically, the CAB stretches from the temporal region to the cheek, under the superficial musculoaponeurotic system (SMAS), passing through the zygomatic-malar tunnel and the pterygomandibular fossa (11). This buccal fat pad has ten extensions that differ in size, volume, and aspect from one person to another and from one side of the face to the other. Although its cheek extensions disappear with age, its outline remains characteristic. Intraoral approaches for buccal fat resection have been described, and the procedure has been indicated for select groups of patients to reduce the fullness of the cheek (12). I have not, however, found a patient requiring that type of surgery.

Disfiguring Lipomatosis

One other exception of fat aspiration of the face is the presence of Launois-Bensaude (13) or Madelung's disease (14) (Fig. 23-20), a rare disfiguring lipomatosis of unknown etiology, usually associated with alcohol abuse. The treatment is usually difficult and associated with a number of complications. Other types of benign multiple symmetric lipomatosis and giant lipomas have been treated by liposuction to reduce the size of the skin incision (15–17). Although long-term follow-ups show a high percentage of recurrences, liposuction, with the simplicity of the procedure and the absence of long scars is the procedure of choice over open resection, especially on the face and neck.

Various surgical techniques have been used, including conventional surgery and liposuction, to help restore a normal life to patients deformed by disease. Despite the high rate of complications and the tendency to recur, the therapy may be palliative and both techniques might be very useful. We have seen patients obtain good results with conventional surgery, and other cases where liposuction provides a good result following an unsuccessful open resection.

Freeing Adhesions and Scars

I use the Toledo V-tip dissector cannula to treat depressed scars on the face as a closed method. After anesthesia, I introduce the tip of the cannula under the fibrotic tissue and, with in-and-out movements, free the adhesions. A small amount of fat is injected into the depressed area to avoid reattachment (Fig. 23-21).

DISCUSSION

Suction is only a part of our ''refreshing'' procedure. Subtle changes can radically alter our perception of a person's face. When suction, fat injection, and light peels are used in combination, the results can be comparable to the results obtained through a more extensive, more complicated surgery that frequently involves hospitalization and a higher risk and cost.

The possible complications of syringe liposculpture for cervical rejuvenation are slight skin laxity, temporary hypoesthesia, and subcutaneous nodules. In a study (18) over a five-year period, 71 patients evaluated the result of their procedure according to a four-grade scale: very satisfied (n=41), satisfied (n=21), less satisfied (n=4), and dissatisfied (n=1). All patients except for one would have recommended the procedure to other patients with similar problems. I agree with the study's conclusion that syringe liposculpture of the neck is a simple, safe, and rewarding procedure, even for some older patients. Remodeling of the facial fat through fine aspiration is an indispensable element to be incorporated into the current concept of facial rejuvenation surgery (19). The traditional procedures have not been abandoned, but their indications have been revised. Facial liposculpture patients are ready to return to normal activities in two to three days if they had suction, depending on the amount of fat removed and on the patient's predisposition to bruising. Manual lymphatic drainage in the early postoperative days helps in reducing edema and bruising (Fig. 23-22). Corrective makeup is useful for those patients with a busy schedule who cannot stay away from work (or fun) for too long.

REFERENCES

1. Mladick RA. Lipoplasty: an ideal adjunctive procedure for the face lift. *Clin Plast Surg* 1989;16:333–341.
2. Davis PT, Cunningham CD. Adjunctive procedures in surgery of the aging face. *J S C Med Assoc* 1989;85:429–433.
3. Adamson PA, Cormier R, Tropper GJ, McGraw BL. Cervicofacial liposuction: results and controversies. *J Otolaryngol* 1990;19:267–273.
4. Goddio AS. Cutaneous retraction. Data from liposuction and other clinical procedures. *Ann Chir Plast Esthet* 1992;37:194–201.
5. Schoen SA, Taylor CO, Owsley TG. Tumescent technique in cervicofacial rhytidectomy. *J Oral Maxillofac Surg* 1994;52:344–347.
6. Kamer FM, Minoli JJ. Postoperative platysmal band deformity. A pitfall of submental liposuction. *Arch Otolaryngol Head Neck Surg* 1993;119:193–196.
7. Toledo LS. Video-endoscopic facelift. *Aesthetic Plast Surg* 1994;18:149–152.

8. Giampapa VC, Di Bernardo BE. Neck recontouring with suture suspension and liposuction: an alternative for the early rhytidectomy candidate. *Aesthetic Plast Surg* 1995;19:217–223.

9. Toledo LS. Facial Rejuvenation—technique and rationale. In: Fodor PB, Isse NG, eds. *Endoscopically assisted aesthetic plastic surgery.* St. Louis: Mosby, 1996;91–101.

10. Matarasso A. Buccal fat pad excision: aesthetic improvement of the midface. *Ann Plast Surg* 1991;26:413–418.

11. Le Pesteur J. "CAB" (corpus adiposum buccae). Anatomical description and surgical reflexions apropos of buccal fat pads. *Ann Chir Plast Esthet* 1994;38:289–301.

12. Stuzin JM, Wagstrom L, Kawamoto HK, Baker TJ, Wolfe SA. The anatomy and clinical applications of the buccal fat pad. *Plast Reconstr Surg* 1990;85:29–37.

13. Grolleau JL, Rouge D, Collin JF, et al. Launois Bensaude disease. Focus apropos of 16 cases. *Ann Chir Plast Esthet* 1994;38:302–306.

14. Horl C, Biemer E. Benign symmetrical lipomatosis. Lipectomy and liposuction in the treatment of Madelung disease. *Handchir Mikrochir Plast Chir* 1992;24:93–96.

15. Basse P, Lohmann M, Hovgard C, Alsbjorn B. Multiple symmetric lipomatosis: combined surgical treatment and liposuction. Case report. *Scand J Plast Reconstr Surg Hand Surg* 1992;26:111–112.

16. Samdal F, Kleppe G, Tonvang G. Benign symmetric lipomatosis of the neck treated by liposuction. Case report. *Scand J Plast Reconstr Surg Hand Surg* 1991;25:281–284.

17. Raemdonck D, De Mey A, Goldschmidt D. The treatment of giant lipomas. *Acta Chir Belg* 1992;92:213–216.

18. Samdal F, Amland PF, Abyholm F. Syringe-assisted microliposuction for cervical rejuvenation. A five year experience. *Scand J Plast Reconstr Surg Hand Surg* 1995;29:1–8.

19. Daher JC, Cosac OM, Domingues S. Face-lift: the importance of redefining facial contours through facial liposuction. *Ann Plast Surg* 1988;21:1–10.

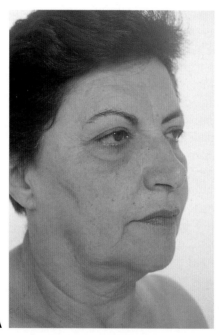 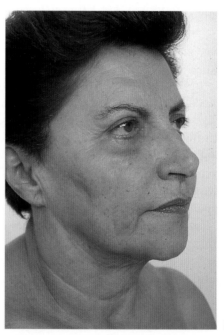

A   B

FIG. 23-1. A, C: Skin retraction is one of the fields of plastic surgery where great advances are expected in the future. The skin of the neck treated with superficial aspiration seems considerably more retractable than in other sites. Preoperative photos of a 60-year-old patient who wanted to improve her face and neck contour without rhytidoplasty. **B, D:** Three months postoperatively, after facial liposculpture of the neck and jowls plus upper and lower blepharoplasty.

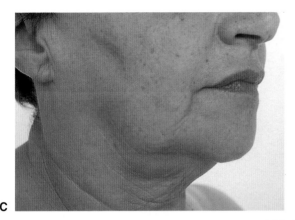
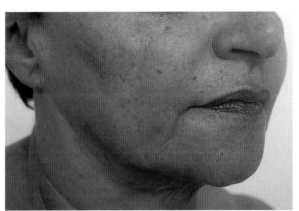

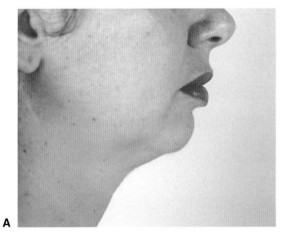
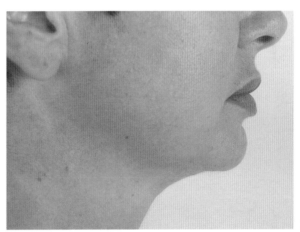

FIG. 23-1. *Continued.*

FIG. 23-2. **A:** This 39-year-old patient wanted fat suction of her neck. She was advised that the result would be further enhanced by chin augmentation. If I feel that facial harmony will be achieved by a chin prosthesis, I will suggest the procedure. **B:** Six years postoperatively, after syringe aspiration of the submental area and a chin implant.

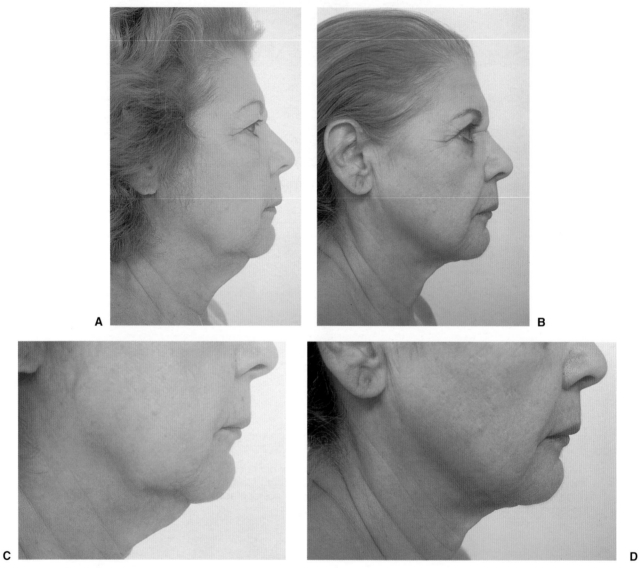

FIG. 23-3. A, C: A 73-year-old patient who wanted rejuvenation without a face-lift. Older patients who do not want rhytidoplasty will still have excess skin after the operation. **B, D:** A six-month postoperative result with a good definition of the jawline and neck. There is excess skin, which can be removed or not, depending on the patient's wishes.

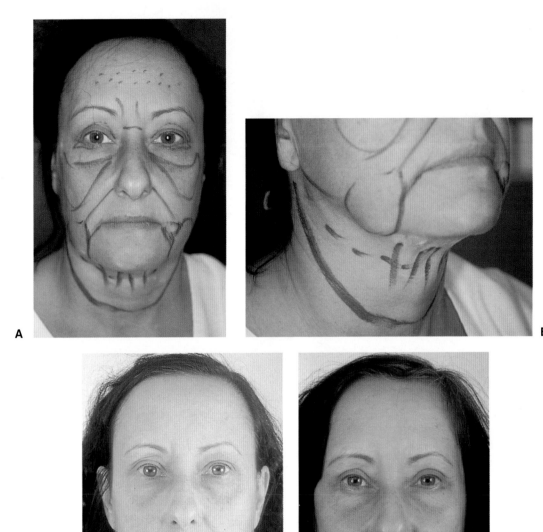

FIG. 23-4. A, B, C, E, G: Preoperative photos of a 54-year-old patient with excess fat on the neck and jowls. *Blue* marks the areas of fat suction, and *red,* fat injection. The jowls are one of the areas where I perform suction on the face. The patient's major complaint was the strong marionette lines running down from the corners of the mouth. **D F, H:** Six months postoperatively, with good retraction of the neck and jowl and improvement of the marionette lines without stretching the skin. The patient also had a blepharoplasty. *Figure continues on next page.*

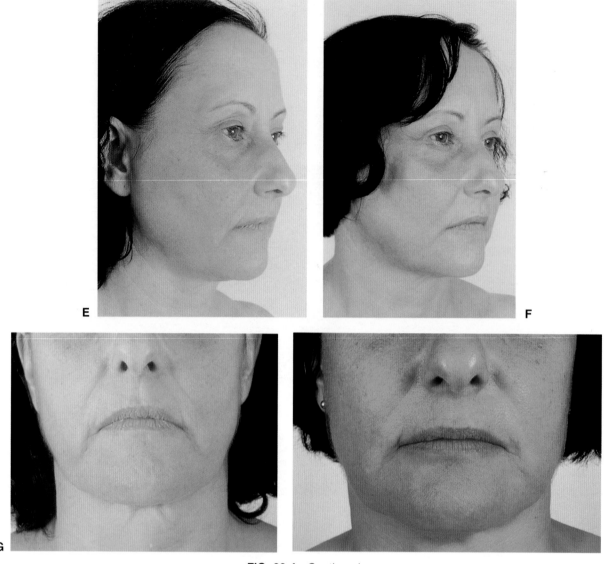

E   F

G   H

FIG. 23-4. *Continued.*

FIG. 23-5. **A, C, E:** A 62-year-old patient needed definition between her face and neck. **B, D, F:** One-month postoperative photos show there was a clear definition in her facial features. 60 cc of fat was removed from the neck, jowls, nasolabial, and preauricular area. Although her weight did not change, she looked as though she had lost weight.

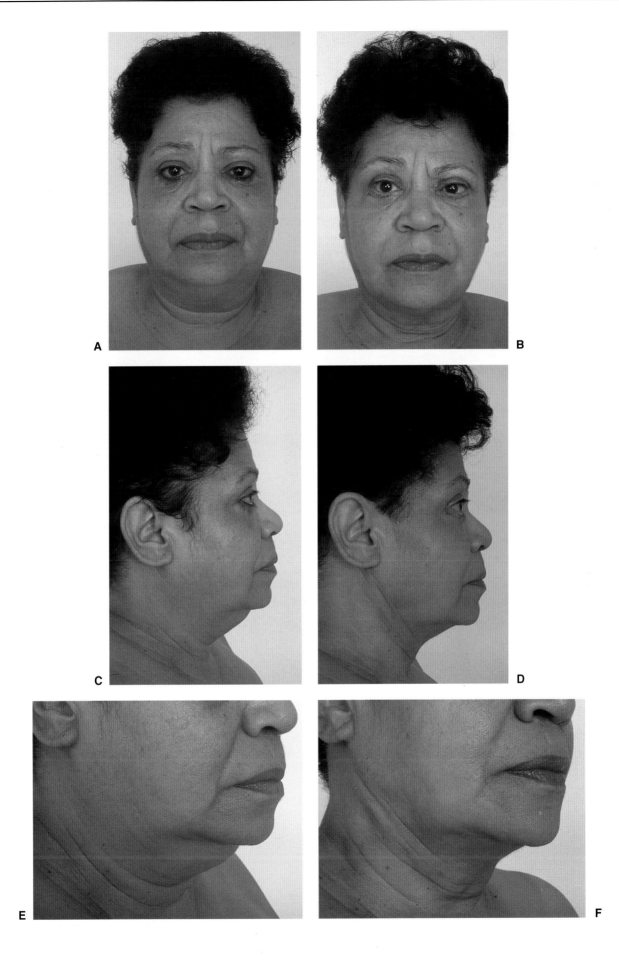

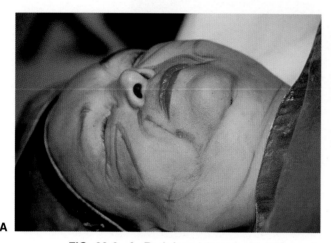
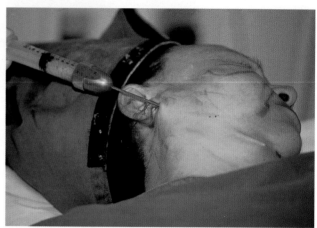

A

B

FIG. 23-6. A, B: A face injected with 150 cc of my local anesthesia formula. The technique creates an essentially bloodless field and decreased surgical morbidity. Aspirated fat is usually yellow and bloodless.

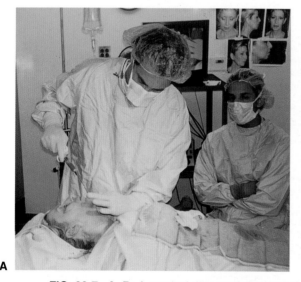
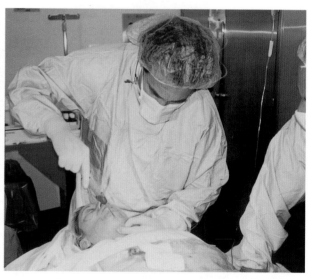

A

B

FIG. 23-7. A, B: A surgical demonstration at Johns Hopkins University with Dr. Oscar Ramirez, showing facial liposculpture of the neck. I insert a 3-mm-gauge Pyramid-tip 15-cm-long cannula connected to a 10-cc syringe into the submental incision for aspiration of the neck in the submental area.

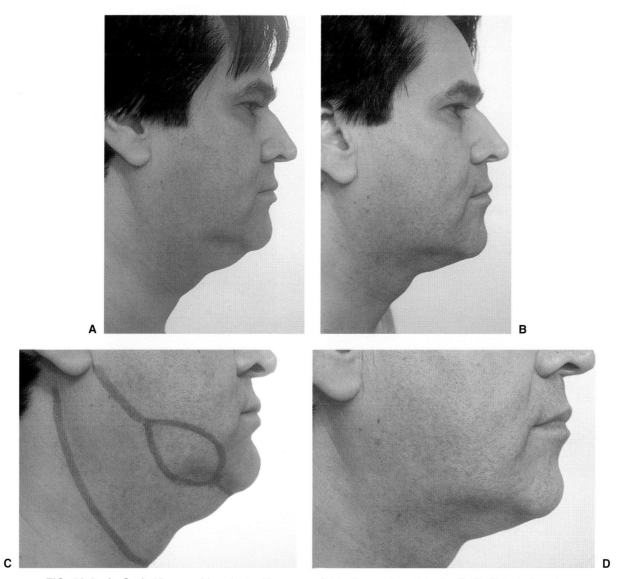

FIG. 23-8. A, C: A 42-year-old patient with excess fat in the neck and jowls. **B, D:** This is the six-month result after deep liposculpture of the neck and jowl. The patient had a good skin tone and did not need superficial suction. There was retraction and a rejuvenating effect.

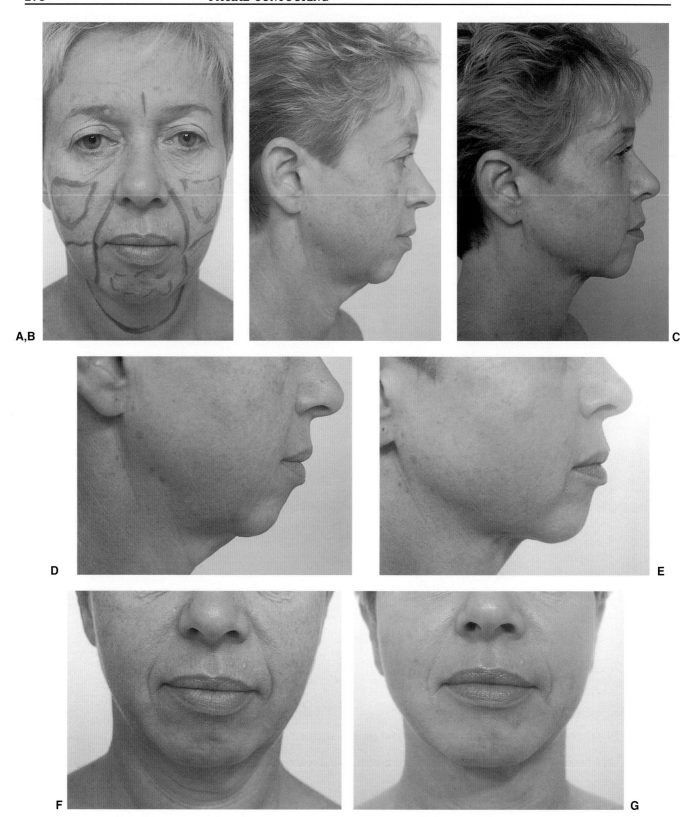

FIG. 23-9. A, B, D, F: Preoperative photos of a 60-year-old patient about to undergo facial liposculpture with superficial suction of the neck and jowls. **C, E, G:** Six months postoperatively. I injected 6 cc of fat into the chin and, after the initial absorption, it is still showing some projection. Fat was also injected into the malar and nasolabial area.

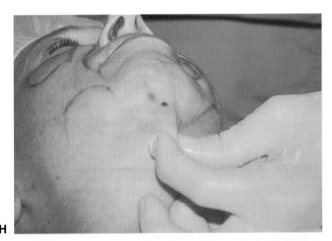

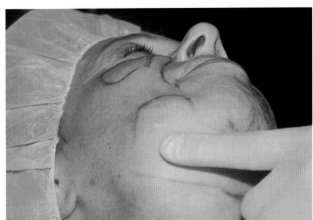

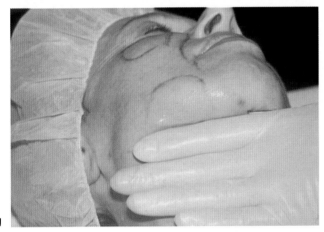

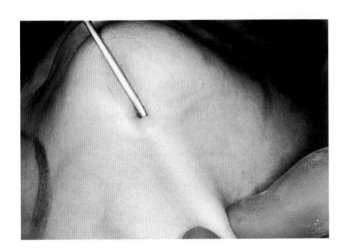

FIG. 23-9. *Continued.* **H, I:** After removing the neck adiposity, thinning the cervical flap allows for its retraction and adaptation to the new neck angle. Finally, the jowl deformities are treated with a 1.5-mm two-holed flat-tipped 15-cm-long cannula, adapted to a 10-cc syringe. **J:** Treating the jowls and the submental area. The left hand is imitating the effect of gravity in the standing position. By pulling the skin down the neck, it is possible to see any irregularities.

FIG. 23-10. Aspiration of fat close to the platysma muscle. A pinch test with the other hand helps to regulate the depth of the tunnels and reveals any irregularities that need treatment. After fat suction, the cannula is turned with the holes facing the dermis to scrape the skin gently, provoking an even, controlled retraction of the area.

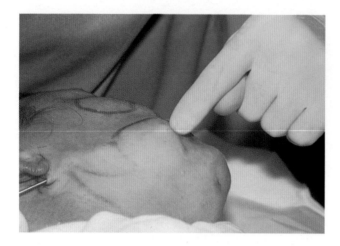

FIG. 23-11. By wetting the skin and constantly testing the cannula depth, it is possible to avoid sequelae of superficial suction of the face and neck.

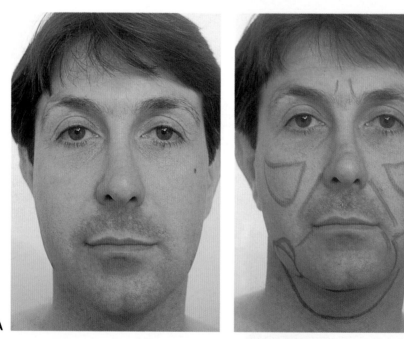

A   B

FIG. 23-12. A, B: Preoperative photos, with and without markings, of a 42-year-old patient who wants to look good for his age. Areas in *blue* are for suction and *red* for injection of fat. **C, D:** Pre- and one-year postoperative photos. The patient wanted more retraction of the skin, so I performed a second suction and the third fat injection at this stage. **E, G:** Preoperative pictures. **F, H:** Three years post-operatively, two years after the last procedure. There was a lasting result with a uniform retraction of the skin. This fulfilled the patient's wishes—a maintenance as well as a rejuvenation procedure.

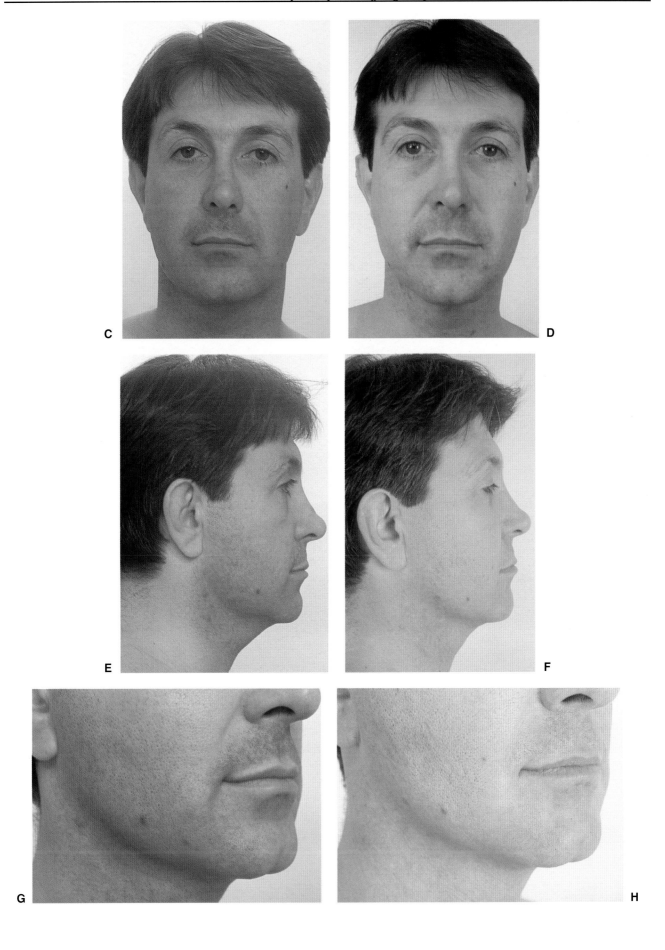

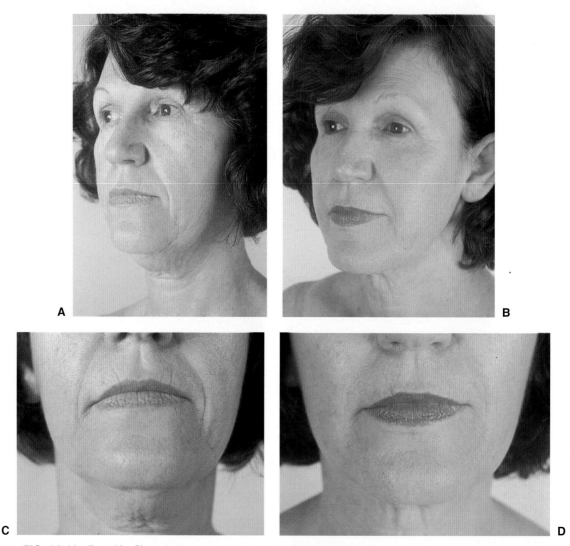

FIG. 23-13. Pre- (**A, C**) and six-year postoperative (**B, D**) photos. The patient is shown at 52 and 58 years old. I performed two aspirations of fat from her neck and jowls at a six-month interval. The result is 5½ years after the last procedure. The patient was also put on a skin care program.

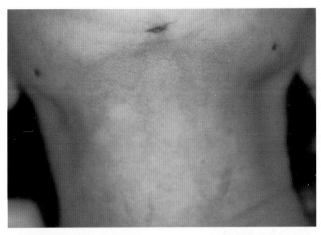

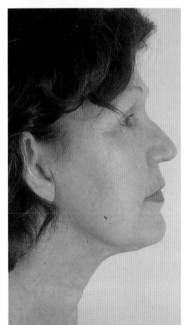

FIG. 23-13. *Continued.* **E:** The skin of the neck immediately after the second fat aspiration. If we leave a regular flap, we will have an even retraction. **F, G:** The patient six years postoperatively. Since skin was not removed, the neck area looks good when the face is at right angles or looking upwards.

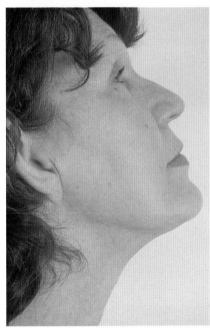

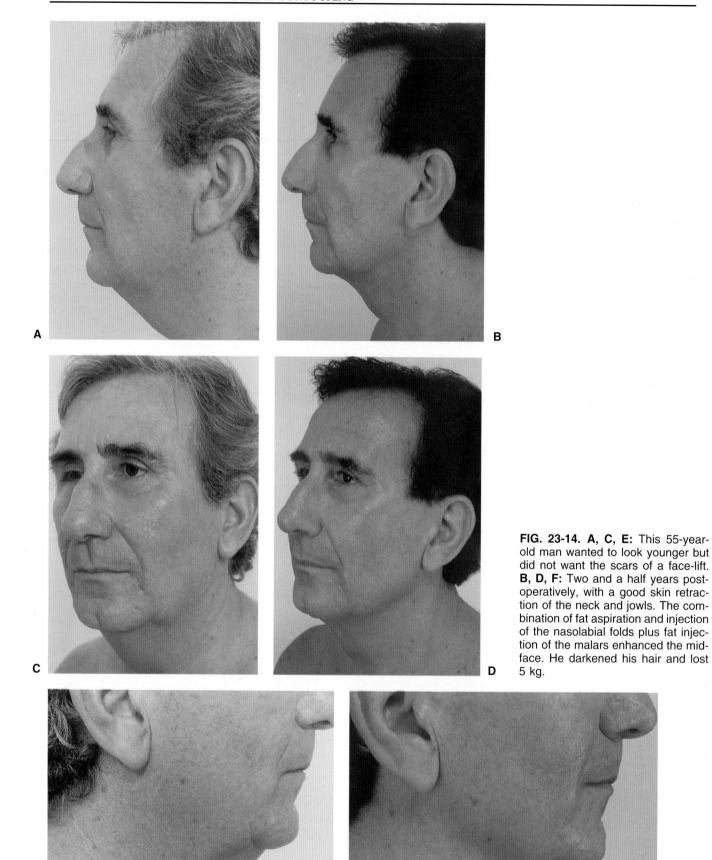

FIG. 23-14. A, C, E: This 55-year-old man wanted to look younger but did not want the scars of a face-lift. **B, D, F:** Two and a half years postoperatively, with a good skin retraction of the neck and jowls. The combination of fat aspiration and injection of the nasolabial folds plus fat injection of the malars enhanced the midface. He darkened his hair and lost 5 kg.

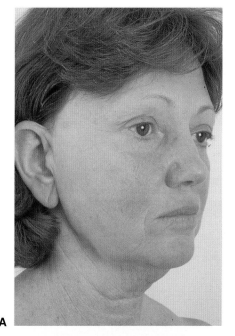

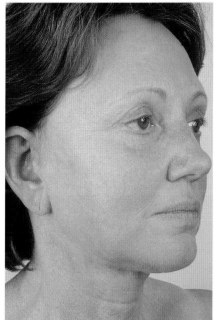

A

B

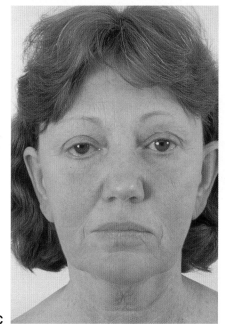

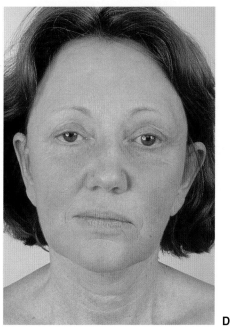

C

D

FIG. 23-15. A, C, E: Preoperative photos of a 60-year-old patient with flaccid wrinkled skin and fat deposits in the neck and jowls. **B, D, F:** Six months postoperatively, after a cervical rhytidoplasty plus liposculpture of the face. First the excess fat is aspirated (the syringe looses pressure once an incision is made in the area), then the excess skin is removed. Skin resection was necessary to obtain a good contour and eliminate flaccidity, wrinkles, and folds.

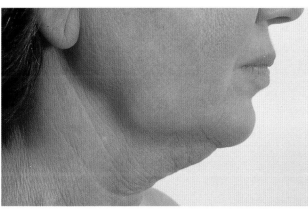

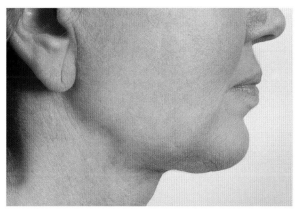

E

F

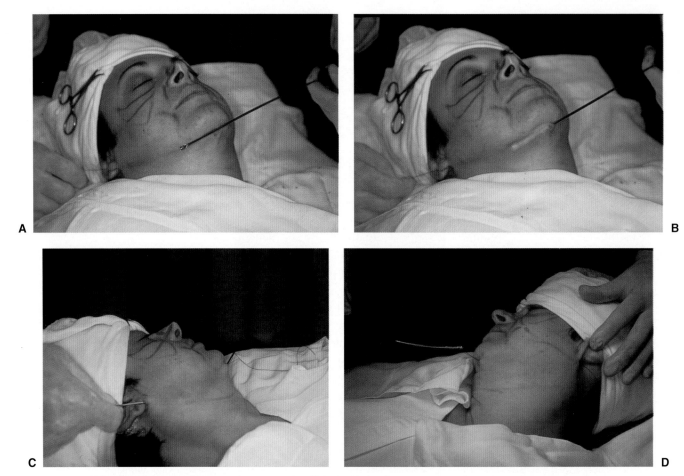

FIG. 23-16. A, B: After suction I use the Toledo V-tip dissector cannula to free the subcutaneous tissue and create a passage for the thread. **C, D:** The Gore-Tex thread is attached to the periosteum of the mastoid, and with the help of a thread passer, I pass this thread from one mastoid to the other. An endoscope helps with the dissection of the skin and in locating any bleeding vessels that need to be cauterized. This suture enhances the neck angle and helps to highlight the mandibular border.

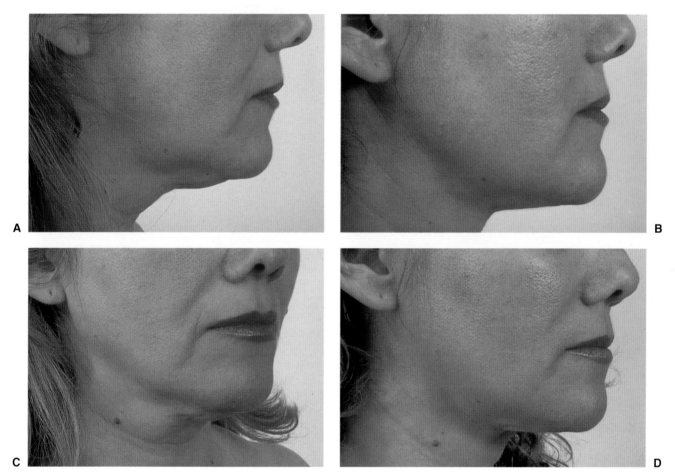

FIG. 23-17. A, C: Preoperative photos of a 41-year-old patient. **B, D:** Six months postoperatively, after an endoscopically assisted face-lift combined with facial liposculpture with no skin resection. There is a good repositioning of the midface and neck.

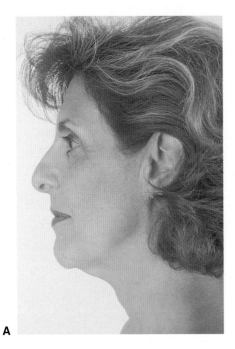

A

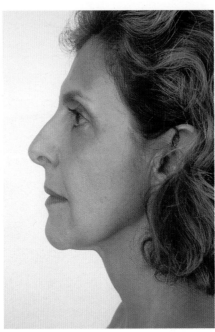

B

FIG. 23-18. A: Preoperative photo of a 52-year-old patient. **B:** One year postoperatively, after endoscopic elevation of the malars and cervical mental angle. Aspiration of fat from the neck and jowls completed the effect.

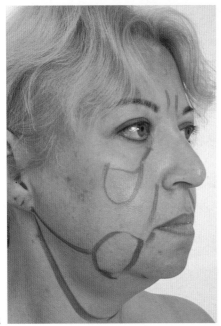

A

FIG. 23-19. A, B, D, F: Preoperative photos of a 48-year-old patient with ptosis of the malar and cervical areas. **C, E, G:** One year postoperatively, after facial liposculpture combined with endoscopic cervical and malar elevation. The patient began a skin care program that included 70% glycolic acid peels in the clinic plus a range of home products. She changed her hairstyle and starting using makeup.

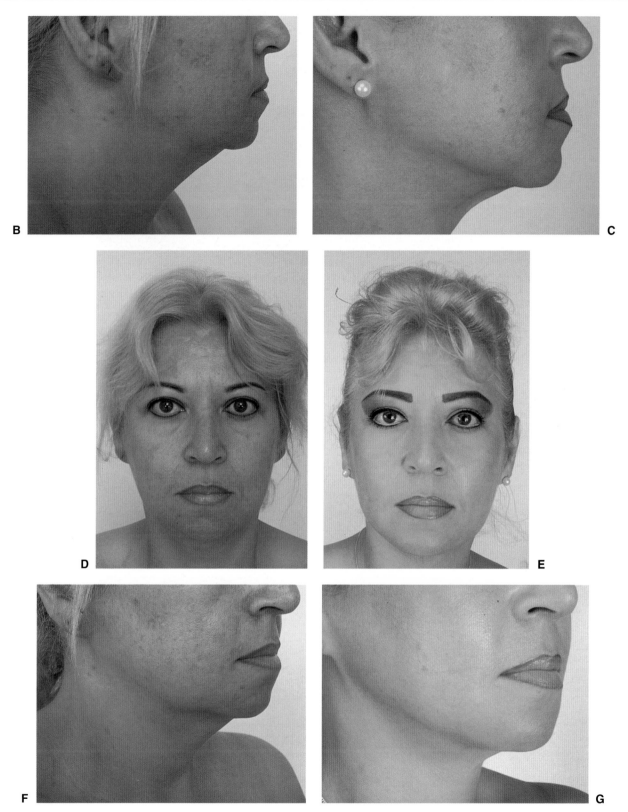

FIG. 23-19. *Continued.*

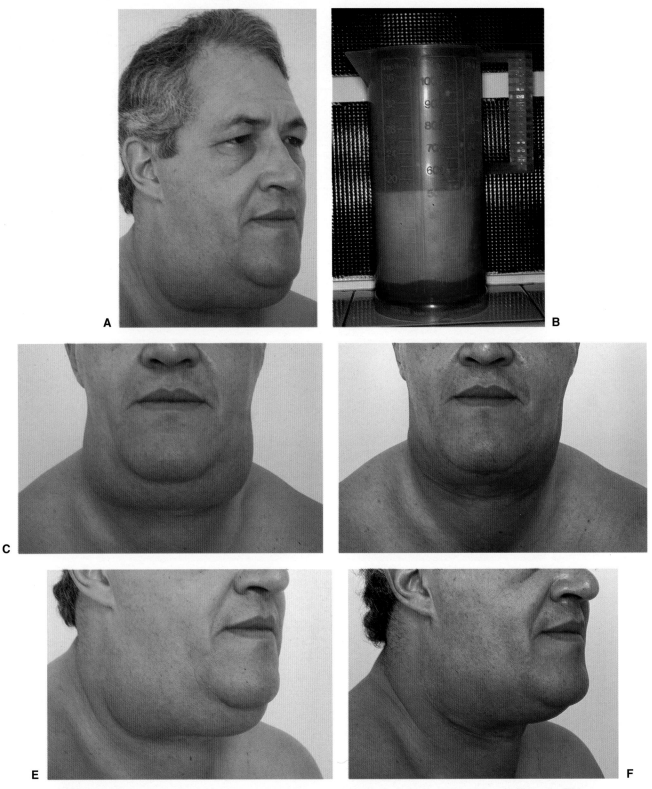

FIG. 23-20. A: Preoperative photo of a patient with Launois-Bensaude, or Madelung's disease. This patient had already had open resection for this disease two years before. **B:** We aspirated a total of 600 cc of fat from the face and cervical region. **C, E, G:** Preoperative condition. **D, F, H:** Six months postoperatively, after syringe aspiration with a good skin retraction.

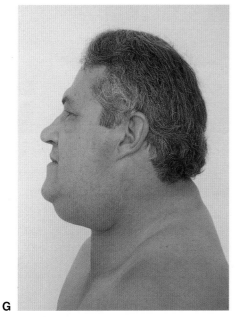

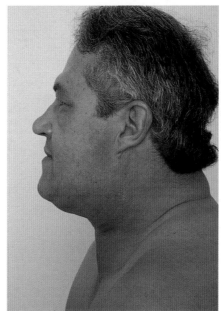

G · H · **FIG. 23-20.** *Continued.*

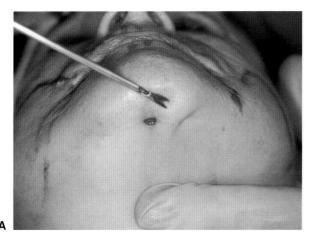

A · B

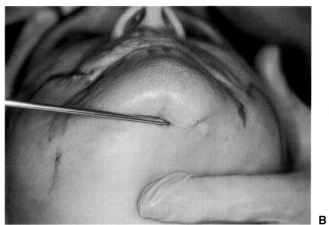

C

FIG. 23-21. A: The Toledo V-tip dissector cannula being used to free a submental retracted scar. **B:** With in-and-out movements, I cut the adhesions that retract the scar. **C:** After the scar is free, I inject 1 or 2 cc of fat to avoid its reattachment to the same position.

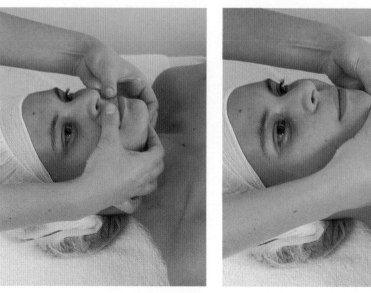

FIG. 23-22. A, B: Facial manual lymphatic drainage can be prescribed from the first postoperative day to reduce edema and increase comfort.

24

Facial Liposculpture

Fat Injection

For young patients in their twenties and early thirties, we generally inject fat only in the nasolabial folds. The next step will include a second site: fat injection of the malar region. Toward the mid-thirties, the original malar fat pad has already started to be reabsorbed or displaced by gravity. This injection will also enhance the nasolabial area, restoring the continent support the skin has lost. The glabellar region is next, with a frown or two forming between the eyebrows. By the late thirties, suction of the jowls and submandibular area, can be performed redefining the ''lost'' jawline. Suction is usually performed once and fat injection three times, following the Fournier principle: ''Overinject in time, not in space.'' Injection is repeated after 35 days. This means that facial liposculpture patients may return to normal activities the following day, if they had only fat injection, and in two to three days if they had suction, depending on the amount of fat removed and on the patients' predispositions to bruising. Corrective makeup is useful when clients wish to maintain a busy schedule.

INSTRUMENTS

I use 10-cc luer-lock syringes, cannulas, needles in varying gauges, transfers, and a fat injection precision pistol.

SEDATION

The objective of this technique is not to frighten the patient by provoking unnecessary pain, swelling, or bruising. The process is designed to avoid stress and discomfort. If patients are uncomfortable in a dentist's chair, this indicates that they will prefer and probably need sedation. I reserve local anesthesia without sedation for the brave, or for a patient already accustomed to the surgical environment. Patients who ''don't want to know'' are treated with intravenous (IV) sedation; there is also the option of a lighter oral sedation. The patients are asked their preference. For fat injection of the face, most patients will prefer only local anesthesia without sedation, and because it is a fast procedure of 20 minutes, they can drive themselves home after the operation. Others prefer oral sedation, and we use 15 mg midazolam taken 20 minutes prior to the surgery. These patients stay in the clinic for at least one hour after the procedure. IV sedation can also be used, and it is administered by the anesthesiologist. The stay in the recovery room will be a few hours after the 20-minute procedure, and the patient will have to be driven home. There is a late sedative effect that can vary between one and three days. Patients who do not want sedation are asked to apply lidocaine 2.5% and prilocaine 2.5%, anesthetic cream (EMLA cream, Astra USA, Westboro, MA), covered with Micropore tape, to the donor and recipient areas one hour prior to the procedure, so that they will not feel the first injection. Topical EMLA cream is a transdermal anesthetic that penetrates intact skin (1).

ANESTHESIA AND FAT ASPIRATION OF THE DONOR AREA

I use a 27×40 fine needle connected to a carpule with lidocaine 2%, 1:100.000 adrenaline to inject the dermal buttons where I am going to introduce the thicker needles. I puncture the skin with a 16-gauge needle, or a no. 11 blade. I use the 2-mm-gauge 15-cm-long multiholed blunt needle connected to a 10-cc luer-lock syringe to inject our tumescent formula. The formula is the same as the one we use for facial and body anesthesia. In the donor area for fat grafting of the face I slowly inject 100 ml of the tumescent formula at body temperature and wait 15 minutes before suctioning. I use a 10-cc luer-lock syringe connected to a 2- or 3-mm-gauge Pyramid-tip cannula to aspirate between 20 and 30 ml of pure fat for reinjection. The plunger of the syringe must be pulled manually (instead of using a lock) to regulate the negative pressure at the minimum necessary to produce the aspirate. One of the keys to a successful fat injection is delicate tissue handling and careful distribution into the recipient tissues. Aspiration under maximum negative pressure can cause partial breakage and vaporization of the fatty tissue (2).

CENTRIFUGING

The syringes with fat are centrifuged at 1,500 r/min for one minute. The anesthetic fluid is separated from the fat cells, and the pure fat is gently transferred to a syringe attached to the pistol for injection.

ANESTHESIA OF THE RECIPIENT AREA

Anesthesia of the area to receive the fat graft is important to eliminate pain and to measure the amount of fat that will be required to fill the depression adequately. The areas are marked with the patient in the standing position. A dermal button is injected with the carpule (Fig. 24-1). The skin is then perforated with a 16-gauge needle (Fig. 24-2). A blunt, multiholed needle is used to inject the diluted tumescent formula (Fig. 24-3). By not using sharp instruments, I avoid ecchymosis. I inject an amount of anesthesia that is sufficient to correct the depression, and this will be the amount of fat to be injected. After 24 hours the anesthesia will be reabsorbed, and only the injected fat will stay, in the amount calculated to provide a natural result. Over the next 35 to 60 days, 50% to 60% of this graft will be reabsorbed. Subsequent procedures will follow the same format.

AREAS AND DEPTH OF INJECTION

Some studies show that fat grafts survive better if placed into the muscle. In the face, however, there is little opportunity for that technique. Although it does even better when placed intramuscularly (3), fat will grow on fat. The fat that remains after two years is viable and permanent. It is injected into the subcutaneous tissue of the face. A few areas of the face have muscle that can be injected, for example, around the mouth.

Malar

We start by injecting deep in the malar area, below the superficial musculoaponeurotic system (SMAS), piling up layers of fat graft threads (Fig. 24-4). These fat threads should be no thicker than 3 mm. I start close to the malar bone and finish close to the skin. From one incision point, I inject medially and laterally towards the zygoma. The same incision point can be used to inject the nasolabial fold perpendicularly. Sometimes another incision in the oral comissure is necessary to inject the fold and the lips.

Nasolabial

The nasolabial fold has hardly any muscle to inject into (Fig. 24-5). I do not inject above, or cephalic, to the fold; this would increase the weight of it. Sometimes it is necessary to aspirate fat from this region. Although fat suction is rarely performed above the mandible line, this is one exception, together with the jowls and the preauricular region. I inject parallel threads subcutaneously, perpendicular to the nasolabial fold, trying to smooth this line and also injecting some fat on the upper lip muscle, if it is too thin, to help support the area.

Glabella and Forehead

On the glabella I perform fat injection as in other parts of the body. In the frontal horizontal wrinkles, I inject parallel and perpendicular to the lines. Fat injection in the glabella and the periorbital area should be performed with great care, without the use of sharp instruments (Fig. 24-6). There have been cases of unilateral blindness (1) and one case of severe damage to the central nervous system reported after fat injection into the glabellar frown lines. The probable cause was fat embolism in the central retinal artery and in the cerebral arteries, respectively.

Orbital Area: Nasojugal Fold and Supraorbital Fold

In areas like the eyelids and nasojugal and supraorbital folds, injection under the orbicular muscle (Fig. 24-7) is mandatory, because the skin is so fine that any graft placed between the skin and the muscle will show by transparency and can probably form an unaesthetic lump that is very difficult to remove after it gets fibrotic (Fig. 24-8) (see Appendix 2, Example Case 1).

Lips and Perioral Area

After the injection of the anesthesia dermal button, I perforate the skin with a sharp no. 16 needle and insert the multiholed blunt-tip 1-mm-gauge needle with the tumescent anesthesia formula. As in the other areas of the face, I measure the amount of fat I will inject by the anesthesia. The blunt needle will avoid unnecessary ecchymosis. The lips are one of the more sensitive areas for injection and one of the areas of the face that get most swollen. I inject very slowly with the least possible trauma to the tissues. Then, with the blunt fat injection needle, I inject the fat into the muscle in parallel threads. I treat the upper and lower lips from the two incision points in the oral comissure. (Figs. 24-9–24-11).

Earlobes

Fat injection into the ear lobes is a very useful procedure, especially for patients whose fat is being absorbed. The weight of heavy earrings tears the earlobe. Fat injection into the area is a small detail that not only makes the ear look younger, but also makes wearing earrings more comfortable. The procedure can be combined with partial resection of the earlobe (Fig. 24-12).

Chin

Fat can be injected into the chin to solve soft tissue problems. It is better to insert a silicone prosthesis as a substitute for bone.

Nose

Fat can be injected into the nose to cover defects of previous rhinoplasty or to increase the skin thickness in cases where the nose is skeletonized. Fat injection into the nose is an easy, cheap option to solve small depressions, and should be used before attempting to redo a rhinoplasty, which may increase scarring and provoke retraction on the operated nose. It is also easier to convince the patient to undergo small sessions of fat grafting under local anesthesia (Figs. 24-13, 24-14).

Temporal Region

Some patients complain of what they call "runner's face." There is a loss of the subcutaneous fat of the face, and the patient must either stop running or have fat injected into the face to improve the contour. It is difficult to find fat for reinjection in runners. Sometimes we have to harvest from two or three different regions to find 20 or 30 cc. But the implant of fat into the face gives a good result, and it is not reabsorbed as much as the original fat, possibly because it has more fibrotic tissue with the fat. One of the areas that gets thin is the temporal area, and the lack of fat on the face can give the impression of illness (Fig. 24-15).

DISCUSSION

The fat graft's ability to obtain nutrition through plasmatic imbibition occurs approximately 1.5 mm from the vascularized edge. The percentage of graft viability depends on the thickness and the geometrical shape (cylindroid) and is inversely proportional to the graft diameter in grafts with a diameter greater than 3 mm. The alterations found in fat grafts demonstrate a Type I collagen capsule circumscribing the graft, besides several alterations in the synthesis, degradation, and remodeling of Type I and Type III collagen within the transplanted tissue. Bands are formed from the periphery to the central region of the graft. The completion of this process, from the collagen synthesis to its degradation, depends on the total volume injected at a single point and may take a few months to one year or more (4).

We use Ringer's lactate instead of saline in our tumescent anesthesia formula because fat is better preserved in Ringer's than in saline. Fat is centrifuged at 1,500 r/min for one minute to separate it from the anesthetic fluid, because the slow-rotation centrifuging for only one minute does not break the cells. If the speed is faster or the centrifuging time longer, fat cells will break and the oil will separate from the cell frame. This can be used as autocollagen for dermal injection, but it is a different technique from fat injection, when you want the fat cell to live and take as a graft. Fat is injected in 3-mm-thick threads with a blunt needle of the same gauge as the aspirating cannula to avoid cell destruction. Following this technique, up to 50% of the injected fat should take.

Follow-up of 10 patients showed a particularly high volume loss of 49% at three months after the procedure. Further follow-up at six months showed that average volume decline had risen to a total of 55%, whereas at nine months as well as 12 months, no further loss could be detected (5) (Figs. 24-16–24-20). Another study shows that the grafted tissue of all groups was surrounded by a collagen capsule. The viable tissue was observed in the peripheral zone approximately 1.5 ± 0.5 mm from the edge of the graft. A loss of approximately 60% of the grafted tissue was still observed in this viable zone (6).

Since we do not overinject fat into the face, patients can return to normal activities in a few days. Two months after the procedure, when reabsorption is completed, they are ready for the second procedure. After two more months, the third and last injection will complete the result. At that stage we tell our patients that they should keep their new looks for one to three years, depending on a series of factors—their age, type of skin, food habits, sun exposure, hormones, etc. This procedure can be repeated as needed, but patients should be informed that at the point when skin excess becomes apparent, skin removal through a rhytidoplasty will be necessary to maintain the younger look. But before that, we can indicate smaller procedures such as liposculpture, combining fat grafting with fat suction, blepharoplasty, laser skin resurfacing, and skin care (see Appendix 2, Example Case 3).

There is a great number of patients who want to have "something done" to improve their appearance but are afraid to be "cut." Our philosophy has allowed many patients to improve their features but postpone a rhytidoplasty until they feel they are ready for the procedure. By then, they may have lost any fear of surgery, there will be a better relationship between surgeon and patient, and the indication for a face-lift will be accepted.

REFERENCES

1. O'Connell JB. EMLA cream in dermabrasion [letter]. *Plast Reconstr Surg* 1994;93:1310.
2. Niechajev I, Sevcuk O. Long-term results of fat transplantation: clinical and histologic studies. *Plast Reconstr Surg* 1994;94:496–506.
3. Nguyen A, Pasyk KA, Bouvier TN, Hassett CA, Argenta LC. Comparative study of survival of autologous adipose tissue taken and transplanted by different techniques. *Plast Reconstr Surg* 1990;85:378–386.
4. Carpaneda CA. Collagen alterations in adipose autografts. *Aesthetic Plast Surg* 1994;18:11–15.
5. Horl HW, Feller AM, Biemer E. Technique for liposuction fat reimplantation and long-term volume evaluation by magnetic resonance imaging. *Ann Plast Surg* 1991;26:248–258.
6. Carpeneda CA, Ribeiro MT. Study of the histologic alterations and viability of the adipose graft in humans. *Anesth Plast Surg* 1993;17:43–47.

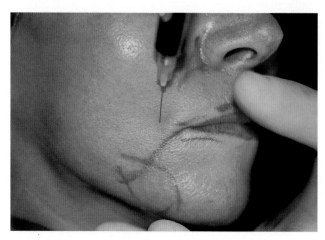

FIG. 24-1. Injecting a dermal button with the carpule.

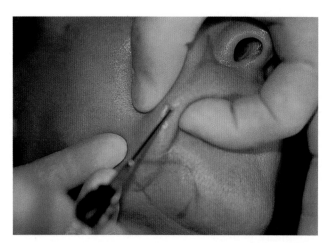

FIG. 24-2. Perforating the skin with a 16-gauge needle.

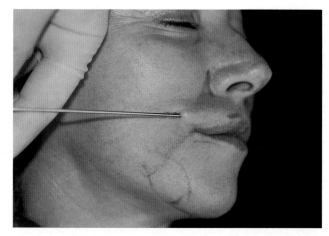

FIG. 24-3. Injecting the diluted tumescent formula with the blunt multiholed needle. I inject the amount of anesthesia that is sufficient to correct the depression. The same amount of fat will be injected.

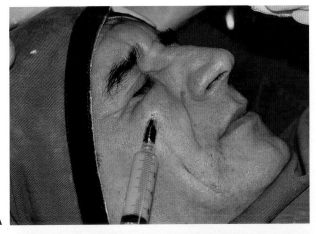

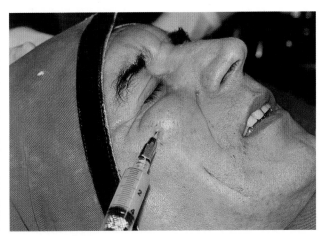

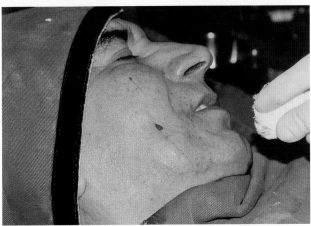

FIG. 24-4. A: I start injecting deep into the malar area, below the superficial musculoaponeurotic system, piling up layers of fat graft threads. I inject fat as I remove the needle. **B:** Fat threads should not be thicker than 3 mm. I start injection close to the malar bone and finish close to the skin. I inject medially and laterally from one incision point, towards the zygoma. **C:** The immediate aspect after fat injection. The anesthesia will be reabsorbed in the first 24 hours.

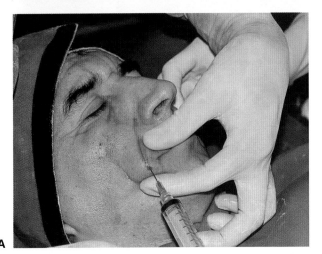

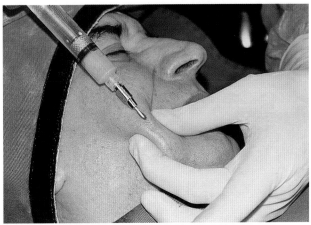

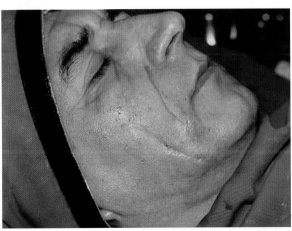

FIG. 24-5. A: Sometimes another incision in the oral commissure is necessary to inject the fold, or I can use the same incision point from the malar to inject the nasolabial fold perpendicularly. **B:** Sometimes the nasolabial fold reaches the mandibular border. **C:** Immediately postoperatively.

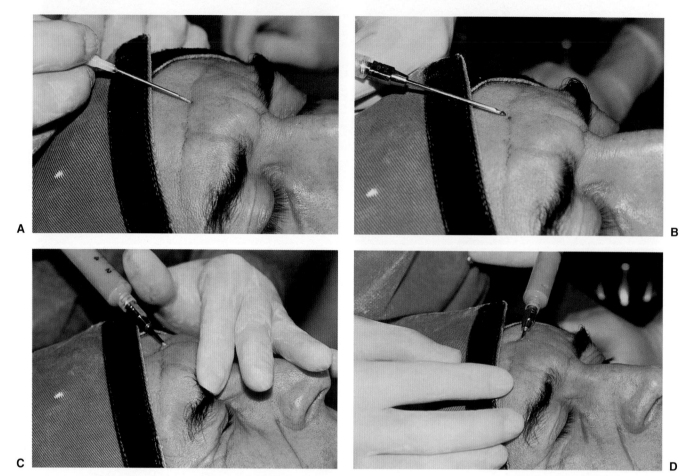

FIG. 24-6. A: I do not use sharp instruments on the forehead. I perforate the skin with a no. 16 needle. **B:** The blunt needle for injection is introduced. (Richter-Hodara). **C, D:** Fat is injected slowly, in threads. The needle will go parallel and perpendicular to the wrinkles.

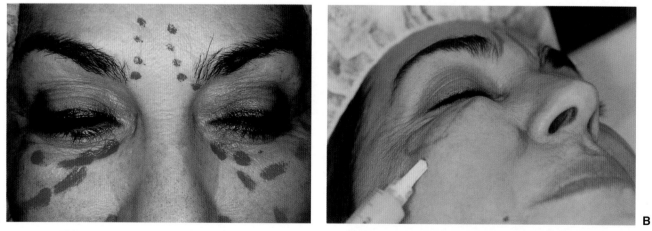

FIG. 24-7. A: The markings for fat injection in the eyelids, and nasojugal and supraorbital folds. **B:** The injection should be under the orbicular muscle.

FIG. 24-8. A–F: The sequence for fat injection in the eyelids, and nasojugal and supraorbital folds. Puncture the skin with a sharp needle, but inject the fat under the muscle with a blunt needle. Do not overinject.

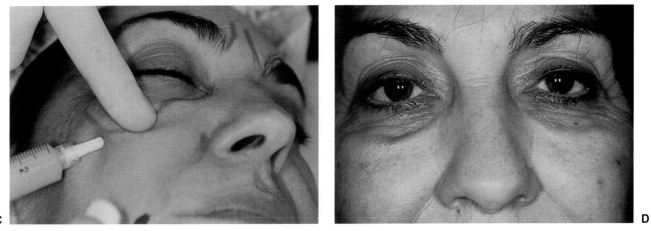

FIG. 24-7. *Continued.* **C:** I feel the depth of the needle with the fingertip. The skin is so fine and transparent that any graft placed between the skin and the muscle will show. **D:** Immediately postoperatively.

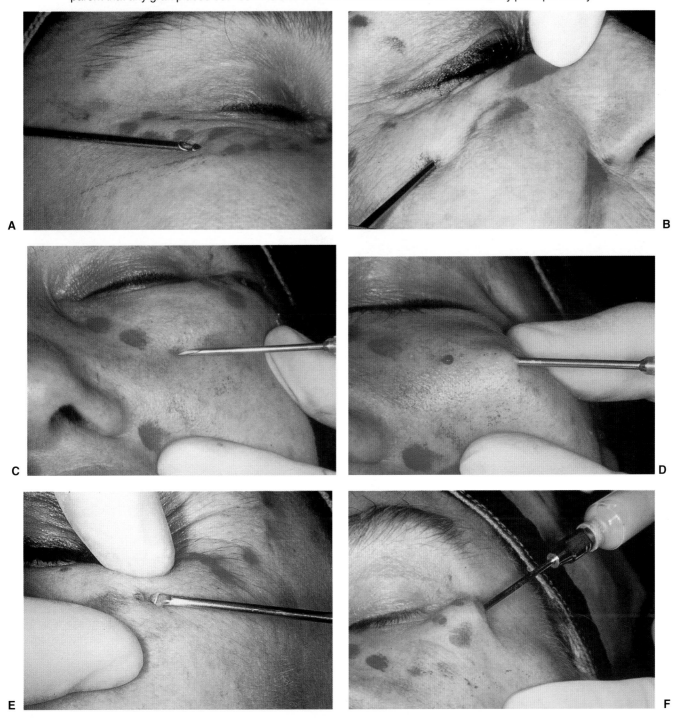

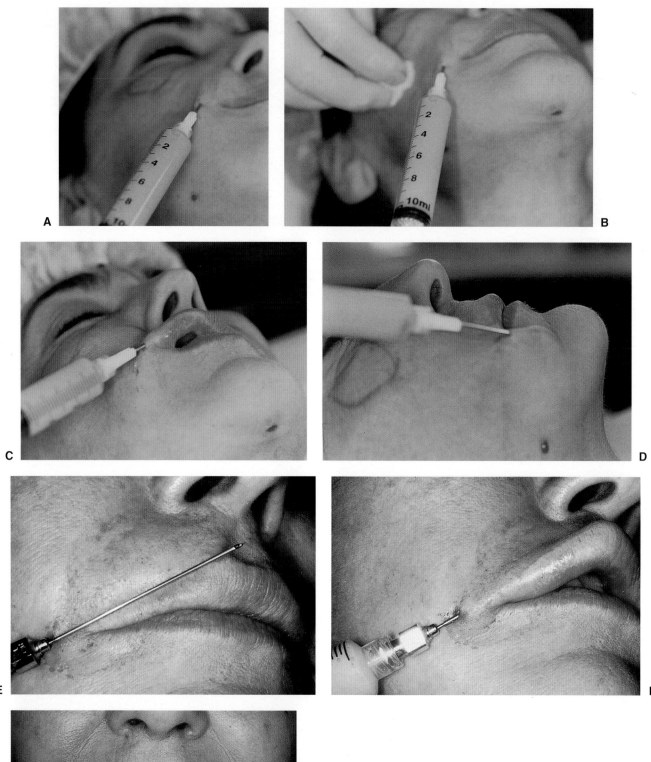

FIG. 24-9. A: Fat injection in the lips. The lips are one of the more sensitive areas for injection and one of the areas of the face that get most swollen. **B:** I inject very slowly with the least possible trauma to the tissues. I fill the upper lip from the oral commisure and also from the malar incision. **C:** With the blunt fat injection needle, I inject the fat into the muscle in parallel threads. **D:** From the two incision points in the oral comissure, I treat the upper and lower lips. **E, F:** I also use fat aspirated with 1-mm-gauge cannulas to inject finer threads subdermally, especially under the cupid's bow. **G:** Immediately postoperatively.

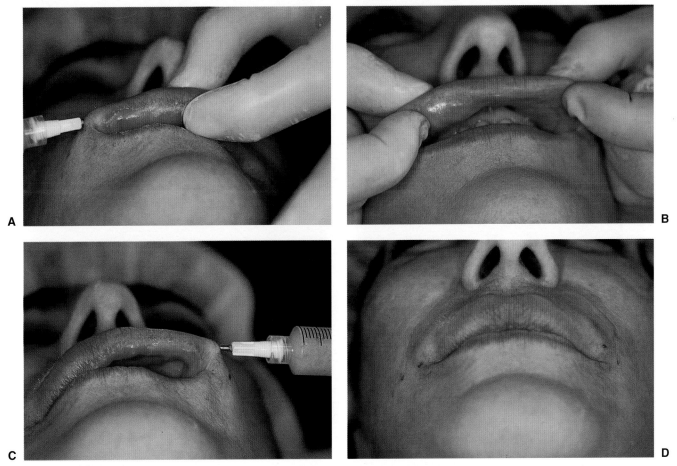

FIG. 24-10. A: Fat injection on the right side of the upper lip. **B:** Comparison of the thickness between the injected side and the left side. **C:** The left side is injected. **D:** Immediately postoperatively. The lips are fuller and projected.

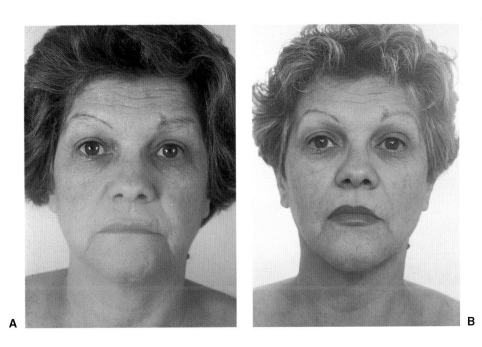

FIG. 24-11. A, B: Pre- and postoperative photos of fat injection.

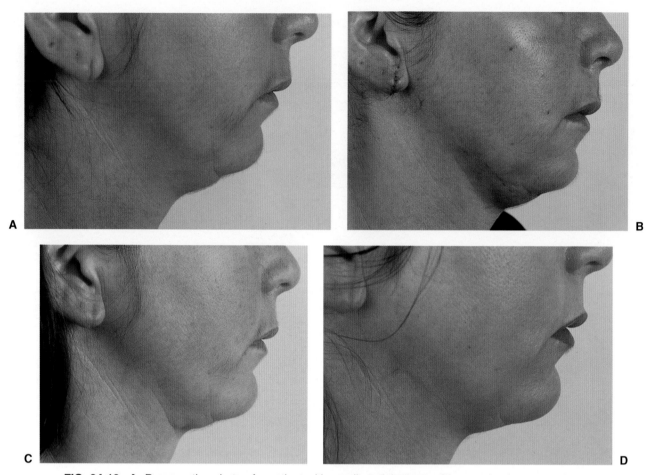

FIG. 24-12. A: Preoperative photo of a patient with a split earlobe caused by wearing heavy earrings. **B:** Three days postoperatively. I have sutured the lobe and injected fat to thicken it. **C:** Two months postoperatively. Fat injection into the area not only makes the ear look younger, but also makes wearing earrings more comfortable. **D:** Four months postoperatively.

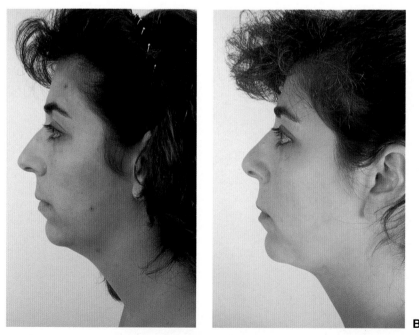

FIG. 24-13. A, C: Preoperative photos of rhinoplasty. **B, D:** Two-month postoperative photos of rhinoplasty. The patient complained of a small depression on the right side of her nose. **E:** I injected 3 cc of fat into the area under local anesthesia to cover the defect. **F, G:** Pre- and six-month postoperative photos, after fat injection in the right side of the nose.

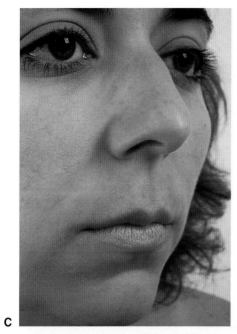

C

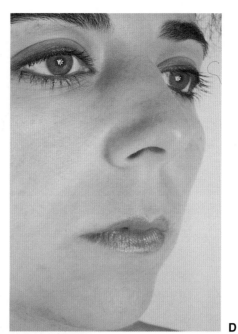

D

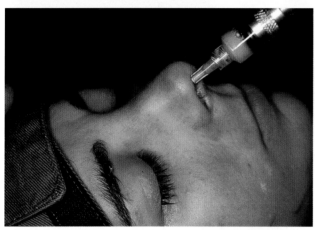

E

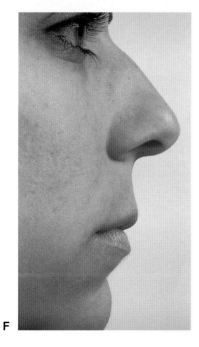

F

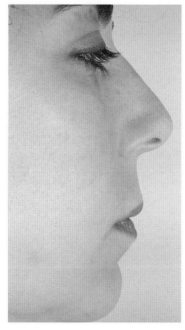

G **FIG. 24-13.** *Continued.*

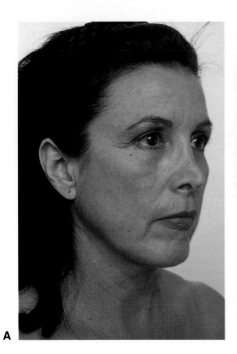

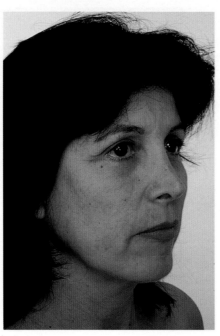

FIG. 24-14. A, B: Pre- and six-month postoperative photos of fat injection into the nose, after a previous rhinoplasty, to increase the skin thickness, because the nose had attained a skeletonized look.

A

B

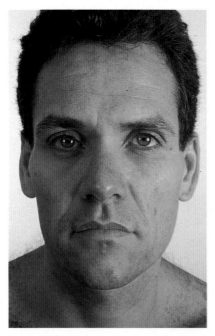

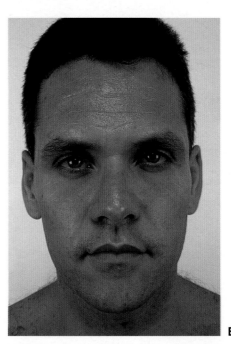

A

B

FIG. 24-15. A, C, E, G: This 34-year-old patient complained of having a "runner's face." There was a loss of subcutaneous fat from the face. This provoked frequent questions about his health. **B, D, F, H:** One year postoperatively after two sessions repeated after two and four months. The amounts were 3.5 cc on each malar, 2 cc on each nasolabial fold, and 1 cc on each cheek depression. On the second procedure I injected, apart from the above, 5 cc on each temporal area.

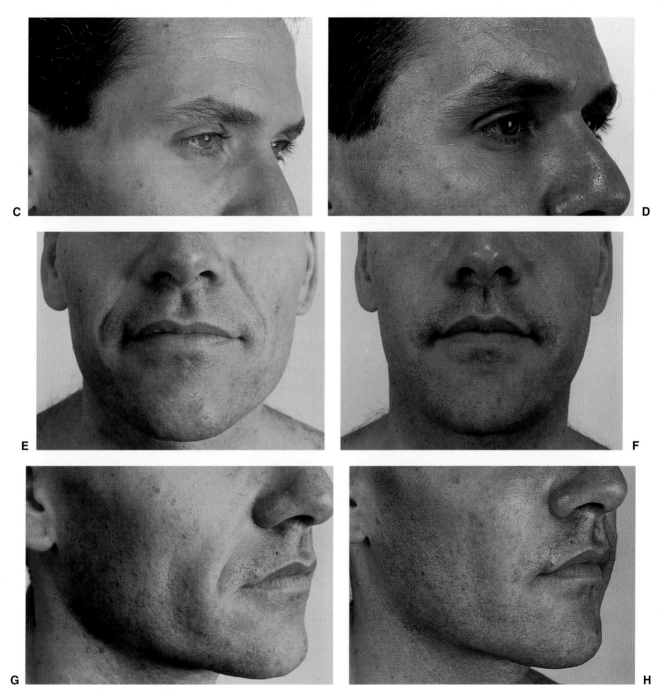

FIG. 24-15. *Continued.*

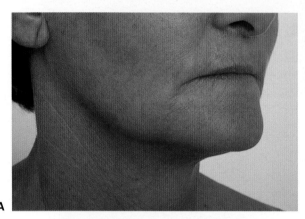
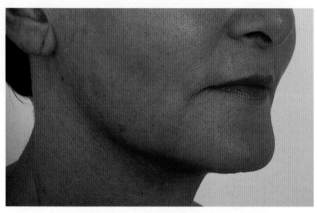

A   B

FIG. 24-16. A, B: Pre- and one-year postoperative photos of a 54-year-old patient who had an endoscopic neck rejuvenation and facial liposculpture. Fat was injected three times into the malars, nasolabial area, and lips. The last injection was eight months earlier. The lip wrinkles were smoothed, and they gained more projection and a more youthful look.

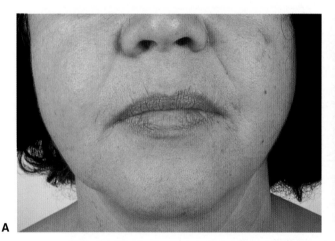
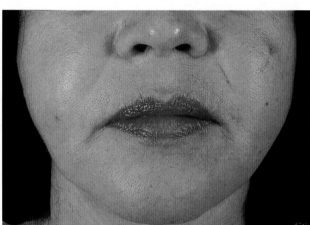

A   B

FIG. 24-17. A, B: Pre- and one-year postoperative photos of a 53-year-old patient who had facial liposculpture. Fat was injected three times into the malars, nasolabial fold, and lips. The last injection was six months earlier. The lip lines have been improved.

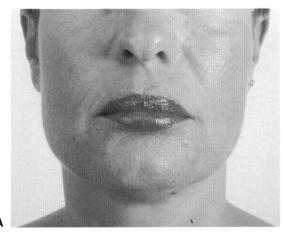
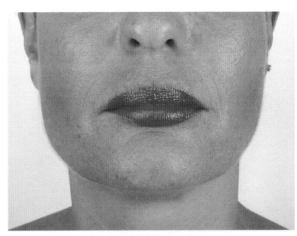

A   B

FIG. 24-18. A, B: Pre- and one-year postoperative photos of a 44-year-old patient who had facial liposculpture. Fat was injected three times into the malars, nasolabial fold, and lips. This patient wears lipstick constantly and complained about the lipstick running through the vertical lines. Her lips got fuller and the cupid's bow smoother.

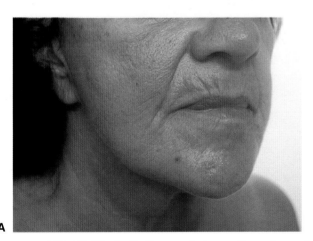
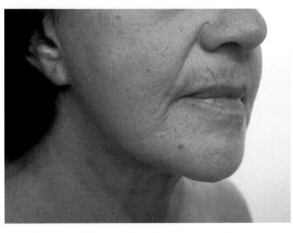

A   B

FIG. 24-19. A, B: Pre- and six-month postoperative photos of a 58-year-old patient who had facial liposculpture. Fat was injected twice into the lips. The last injection was four months earlier. This type of lips need more than fat injection, but this is all the patient wanted.

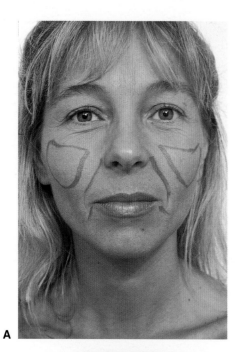

A

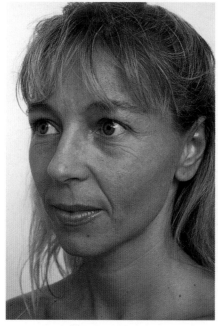

B

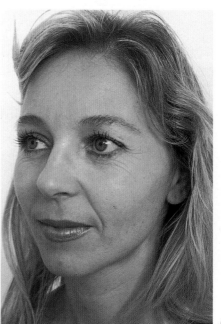

C

FIG. 24-20. A: Preoperative view with markings of a 42-year-old patient. Areas for fat injection are marked in red. Pre **(B)** and two-months postoperative **(C)** photos of fat injection of 5 cc into each malar and 2 cc into each nasolabial fold.

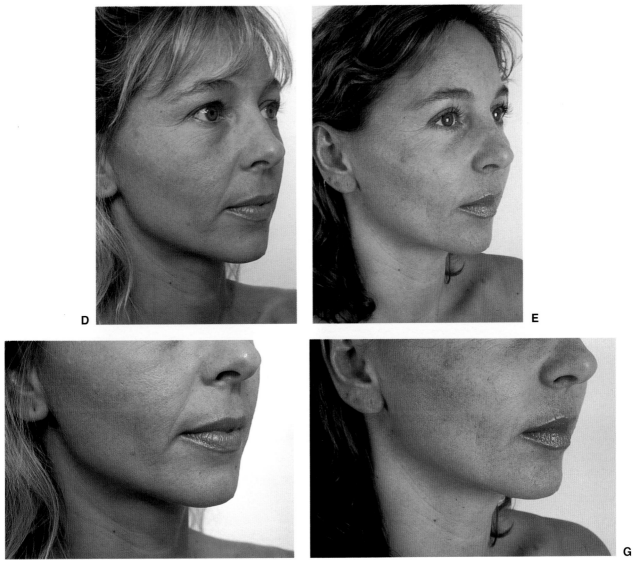

FIG. 24-20. *Continued.* **D, F:** Preoperative photos of fat injection into the malar and nasolabial fold areas. **E, G:** Three years postoperatively. The patient had three injections of the same amount of fat in the same areas, with an interval of two months between the procedures. The last procedure was 21/2 years earlier.

25

The Nasolabial Fold

CONSIDERATIONS IN CHOOSING THE APPROPRIATE TREATMENT

The deepening of the nasolabial fold with age is caused by changes in the cheek mass and its support (1). With aging there is anterior, lateral, and inferior displacement of the cheek mass and deepening of the nasolabial fold. Microscopic studies have shown the fold to be made of dense fibrous tissue, muscle fibers from the elevator muscles of the upper lip, and striated muscle bundles in the fold fascia (2). Other causes may be excessive exposure to the sun, disease, or a genetic disposition (3). There are three main variations in the nasolabial fold: convex, concave, and straight (4). The smiling muscles are considered to be responsible for the shape and depth of the fold. In facial palsy, the nasolabial fold disappears with the absence of muscle function. Cadaver and clinical studies confirm the consistent presence of a localized subcutaneous malar fat pad overlying the body of the zygoma and maxilla (5). The displacement of the infra-orbital skin and malar fat pad causes an increased prominence of the nasolabial fold.

Other factors that influence the nasolabial fold are thinning of the skin, ptosis or deposition of fat laterally, and presence of excess skin (6). Anatomic and histologic evaluation of the fold tissues show a fascial-fatty layer in the superficial subdermal space extending from the upper lip across the nasolabial fold to the cheek mass (7). The superficial musculoaponeurotic system (SMAS) is present in the upper lip as the superficial portion of the orbicularis oris muscle. Traction on the SMAS or periosteum lateral to the nasolabial fold can deepen the fold, while traction on the fascial-fatty layer lessens the fold.

Other cadaver studies have shown that the levator alae muscle is the primary facial muscle responsible for creating the medial nasolabial fold, and the levator labii superioris muscle was found to define the middle nasolabial fold (8). Together, these two muscles may be significant in the etiology of the prominent nasolabial fold that occurs with aging. Other factors are flaccidity and thinning of the skin and subcutaneous tissue, with consequent displacement of the area caused by gravity.

FORMS OF TREATMENT

The ideal procedure for treating this undesirable change caused by aging would be to eliminate the excess skin, add to the thickness of the skin under the crease, and shield the bands from adherence to the dermis, with or without repositioning or resection of fat laterally (6). The combination of removal of the maximum amount of skin, injection of fat immediately under the fold in the subcutaneous plane, and removal of the fat lateral to the fold is perhaps the ideal form of treatment (9). However, under certain conditions, the patient or physician may choose alternative techniques, according to the needs of the patient. These include injection of fat or fat graft, or direct excision. Patients with extremely thin skin are better candidates for direct excision, whereas those with thicker skin may benefit more from fat injection or fat graft.

Selective myotomy, myectomy, and neurotomy of the responsible mimetic muscles has also been advocated, exclusively or in combination with blepharoplasty, rhytidectomy, or other procedures (3). Resecting the levator labii superioris alaeque nasi muscle has been advocated as an ancillary procedure to improve nasal symmetry (10).

In rhytidectomy, the nasolabial fold can be enhanced by undermining the malar fat pad and advancing it laterally (5). Suturing the fat pad to the subcutaneous fascia at the lateral malar eminence eliminates the traction on the skin flap.

However, in composite rhytidectomy and other techniques that elevate a muscle-fat flap in the malar region, all of the deep aging anatomic components of the midface are elevated in the skin flap (11–13). The platysma muscle, cheek fat, and orbicularis oculi muscle are repositioned in this bipedicled musculocutaneous flap, which very effectively improves the nasolabial fold. It is believed that the key to nasolabial fold correction is the complete release of the anterior SMAS from the zygoma and zygomaticus major muscle (14). This would allow the mobilization of the nasolabial fold without tension, advancing the SMAS and reattaching it to the zygomatic periosteum with permanent sutures to correct the nasolabial region, including the jowl.

FACIAL LIPOSCULPTURE

When patients do not want or are not ready for a face-lift but wish to improve these folds, we propose three sessions of fat injection, one every 50 or 60 days (15,16). Sometimes liposuction of the malar area, cephalic to the fold, is also necessary to flatten the area even more.

It has been proposed that, to improve the results of fat injection in the nasolabial folds, the adjacent tissues should be radically undermined before using fat grafts or injections to place the fat in the proper locations (17). Every time I tried this undermining of the fold with sharp instruments, it resulted in a hematoma or long-lasting edema, which is contrary to the main indication for this procedure when it is performed alone: the fast recovery. This technique did not improve my facial liposculpture results. However, when used in conjunction with other procedures that involve skin resection and a longer recovery time, such as a rhytidoplasty, this dissection may provide easier and more direct access to the dermal attachments. It is safer than extending the rhytidoplasty skin dissection to the nasolabial fold and reducing the fat of this fold by excision (18). The removal of the superficial fat by curettes has also been proposed (19), but complications include small hematomas and visible depressions in the sculpted areas.

If patients are from out of town or if they do not want to undergo repeated procedures, the inclusion of a permanent prosthesis, such as Gore-Tex [expanded polytetrafluoroethylene (EPTFE)], has been suggested. I have used no. 0 threads instead of the 2-mm strips because they are easier to place and, if necessary, to remove (20,21).

I do not recommend inclusion of fat and aponeurotic galea strips, fat-dermal and dermal autologous grafts by intraoral access (22). I find inclusion of dermis very unpredictable. I have seen many complications related to misplacement and irregularities that are difficult to treat. There is another option before excess skin is stretched and removed. It is possible to elevate the malar area through an endoscopic midface lift, plicating the SMAS and premalar fat pads to the temporal fascia to treat the nasolabial fold and the jowl (23), but when laxity reaches a certain point, it is necessary to remove skin.

RHYTIDOPLASTY

During a rhytidoplasty, a combination of repositioning fat by suction and by injection can be used. The SMAS/platysma can be repositioned, and excess skin can be resected. In comparisons of patients who had rhytidectomy alone and those who underwent rhytidectomy with liposuction of the nasolabial folds, the latter group had better results (24). This is due to the reduction not only in the length but also in the depth of the fold, suggesting that fat aspiration consistently improves the results of rhytidectomy in the region of the nasolabial fold.

It must be remembered that in select patients, direct excisions of nasolabial folds and secondary malar festoons may be appropriate (25).

REFERENCES

1. Yousif NJ, Gosain A, Sanger JR, Larson DL, Matloub HS. The nasolabial fold: a photogrammetric analysis. *Plast Reconstr Surg* 1994;93:70–77.
2. Rubin LR, Mishriki Y, Lee G. Anatomy of the nasolabial fold: the keystone of the smiling mechanism. *Plast Reconstr Surg* 1989;83:1–10.
3. Muhlbauer W, Fairley J, van Wingerden J. Mimetic modulation for problem creases of the face. *Aesthetic Plast Surg* 1995;19:183–191.
4. Zufferey J. Anatomic variations of the nasolabial fold. *Plast Reconstr Surg* 1992;89:225–231.
5. Owsley JQ. Lifting the malar fat pad for correction of prominent nasolabial folds. *Plast Reconstr Surg* 1993;91:463–474; discussion 475–476.
6. Guyuron B. The armamentarium to battle the recalcitrant nasolabial fold. *Clin Plast Surg* 1995;22:253–264.
7. Yousif NJ, Gosain A, Matloub HS, Sanger JR, Madiedo G, Larson DL. The nasolabial fold: an anatomic and histologic reappraisal. *Plast Reconstr Surg* 1994;93:60–69.
8. Pessa JE, Brown F. Independent effect of various facial mimetic muscles on the nasolabial fold. *Aesthetic Plast Surg* 1992;16:167–171.
9. Guyuron B, Michelow B. The nasolabial fold: a challenge, a solution. *Plast Reconstr Surg* 1994;93:522–529; discussion 530–532.
10. Pessa JE, Crimmins CA. The role of facial muscle resection in reconstruction of the paralyzed face. *Ann Plast Surg* 1993;30:537–540.
11. Hamra ST. Composite rhytidectomy and the nasolabial fold. *Clin Plast Surg* 1995;22:313–324.
12. Le Louarn C. The malar musculo-fatty flap. *Ann Chir Plast Esthet* 1989;34:510–525.
13. Le Louarn C, Cornette de Saint-Cyr B. Cutaneous incision in facelift. Oblique cervicomalar SMAS flap and malar facelift. *Ann Chir Plast Esthet* 1994;39:756–764.
14. Mendelson BC. Correction of the nasolabial fold: extended SMAS dissection with periosteal fixation. *Plast Reconstr Surg* 1992;89:822–833.
15. Matsudo PK, Toledo LS. Experience of injected fat grafting. *Aesthetic Plast Surg* 1988;12:35–38.
16. Toledo LS. Syringe liposculpture. A two year experience. *Aesthetic Plast Surg* 1991;15:321–326.

17. Loeb R. Nasolabial fold undermining and fat grafting based on histological study. *Aesthetic Plast Surg* 1991;15:61–66.

18. Millard DR Jr, Yuan RT, Devine JW Jr. A challenge to the undefeated nasolabial folds. *Plast Reconstr Surg* 1987;80:37–46.

19. Ellenbogen R, Wethe J, Jankauskas S, Collini F. Curette fat sculpture in rhytidectomy: improving the nasolabial and labiomandibular folds. *Plast Reconstr Surg* 1991;88:433–442.

20. Mole B. The naso-labial fold: analysis and proposed techniques for correction. *Ann Chir Plast Esthet* 1990;35:191–200.

21. Lassus C. Expanded PTFE in the treatment of facial wrinkles. *Aesthetic Plast Surg* 1991;15:167–174.

22. Horibe EK, Horibe K, Yamaguchi CT. Pronounced nasolabial fold: a surgical correction. *Aesthetic Plast Surg* 1989;13:99–103.

23. Toledo LS. Video-endoscopic facelift. *Aesthetic Plast Surg* 1994;18:149–152.

24. McKinney P, Cook JQ. Liposuction and the treatment of nasolabial folds. *Aesthetic Plast Surg* 1989;13:167–171.

25. Netscher DT, Peltier M. Ancillary direct excisions in the periorbital and nasolabial regions for facial rejuvenation revisited. *Aesthetic Plast Surg* 1995;19:193–196.

26

CO$_2$ Laser Blepharoplasty

Accurate patient evaluation, correct preoperative diagnosis, knowledge of the anatomy of the eyelid, plus a meticulous surgical technique are all fundamental in performing a successful blepharoplasty (1–6).

The CO$_2$ laser has frequently been employed for medical surgical resections and more recently been used in the field of plastic surgery. In blepharoplasties, the main advantages of using the laser are the possibility of resecting skin, fat, and muscle with no bleeding, and cauterizing the blood and lymphatic vessels without damaging the surrounding tissue. Comparison studies using the CO$_2$ laser on one side and standard cold-steel surgery and electrocautery on the contralateral side, performed by surgeons who advocate the laser procedure, have shown reduced intraoperative time and bleeding, and less postoperative ecchymosis and edema on the laser-treated side (7), superior intraoperative visibility, less bruising and swelling, no pain or discomfort, and a shorter recuperation period (8).

I have observed that, once initial difficulties with a new instrument have been mastered, the CO$_2$ laser procedure shows reduced intraoperative time largely because the lack of bleeding allows for a far superior intraoperative visibility. It is faster and safer, with much less postoperative edema and ecchymosis, and no pain or discomfort, leading to a faster recovery time. Long-term follow-up showed no cosmetic difference when comparing results and scarring (7).

Preoperative tests include complete blood count (CBC), coagulation, blood sugar, human immunodeficiency virus (HIV), electrocardiogram (EKG) for patients over 45 years of age, a screening for hypertensive patients, plus a complete ophthalmologic exam to confirm any preoperative visual impairment. Preoperative photographs are displayed in the operating room for evaluation during the procedure.

MARKINGS

Lower Eyelid

I mark the fat pockets on the skin of the lower eyelids with the patient in the standing position (Fig. 26-1). The excess skin is measured using forceps (Fig. 26-2). If skin elasticity is present, I use the transconjunctival approach and do not remove any skin. If the pinch test shows that the skin has lost its retraction capability and does not return quickly to its original position, I will combine skin removal with the transconjunctival procedure.

Upper Eyelid

Excess skin on the upper eyelid is marked with the patient in the standing position. The length of the caudal incision varies according to the fold, never exceeding its length (Fig. 26-3). The incision line is marked parallel to the sulcus, approximately 8 mm from the ciliary margin in the medial portion of the eyelid (Fig. 26-4).

The excess skin is measured with forceps, and the cephalic incision is marked conservatively (Fig. 26-5). I prefer to remove a little more skin, if necessary, in a second procedure rather than remove too much skin initially. I do believe that the eyelid should be slightly open at the end of the surgery, but I prefer that the eye close naturally when the excess skin is pinched preoperatively and after suture. To locate the fat pads, we lightly press the globe of the eye and mark their position on the skin surface. The number of fat pads in the upper eyelid varies; in 56% of the cases there are two fat pads, and in 44%, there are three. The third fat pad is anatomically and histologically an accessory medial extension of the lateral fat pad (9).

ANESTHESIA

The preanesthetic sedation is 15 mg oral or IV midazolam. After one drop of tetracaine hydrochloride ophthalmic solution (Pontocaine, Sanofi Winthrop, New York, NY) 0.5% in each eye, I infiltrate locally with 2% lidocaine and adrenaline 1:100.000.

Lower Eyelid

Cases of ecchymosis are usually formed during the injection (10), and so the technique of injecting the anesthesia is crucial for a good postoperative result. I cover the eye globe up to the fornix with a Jaeger plate (Fig. 26-6) and pull down the lower lid with a modified Desmarres retractor (Fig. 26-7). I have modified this retractor because its original curve hid the ideal incision line. With our modification, the exact amount of conjunctiva is exposed and the fat compartments are now visible. Light pressure on the plate exposes the lower fat pockets. I feel for the orbital rim and inject 1 to 2 cc of anesthetic through a 0.3 x 21 mm needle, pulling the tip of the needle back 1 to 2 mm from the rim, and inject 1 cc subconjunctival.

Upper Eyelid

On the upper eyelid, taking care to avoid damaging the capillaries, I use a blunt needle (Fig. 26-8) with a lateral hole to distribute 2 to 3 cc of anesthetic under the marking lines (Fig. 26-9). We avoid any other punctures.

TECHNIQUE

Lower Eyelid

I use a 20 watt Luxar LX-20 CO_2 laser (Luxar Corp., Bothel, WA). The Luxar is a small laser with more than enough power to perform this procedure; it is also cost-effective for the solo practitioner. It can be moved easily from room to room or from one hospital to another. I incise the conjunctiva with a 10-mm-tip, 0.4-mm spot tip, at superpulse mode, regulated to 20 W (Fig. 26-10). For the removal of the lower eyelid fat pads, I perform the transconjunctival incision 5 mm from the tarsal border and of variable length, according to the fat compartments. The eyelid is exposed by the assistant with the Jaeger plate and the modified Desmarres retractor. After the conjunctival incision, I change to a 10-mm ceramic tip, 0.8-mm spot and the laser beam is regulated to 10 W (Fig. 26-11), continuous mode, to dissect and cut the fat pockets. With delicate one-tooth forceps, the excess fat is pulled out and placed against a wet cotton tip held by the assistant. The fat is cut by the laser beam and is easily removed. The resection is repeated in the three fat pads. The lateral fat pad may present some difficulty in its removal. Using the cotton tip, I pull through the skin, showing the excess fat through the incision (Fig. 26-12). This facilitates its identification and removal. I do not suture. If we have to remove skin (in 10% of cases), we do it through a separate incision without any damage to the septum orbitalis. We prescribe antibiotics and cold compresses for 72 hours. Analgesics are rarely needed. Figures 26-13–26-15 show pre- and postoperative images of patients who have undergone this procedure.

Upper Eyelid

A protective sheath is placed beneath the eyelid (Fig. 26-16), covering the eye globe and exposing the incision markings. I prefer the sheath because it does not have to be held and allows me to operate with only one assistant. The skin incision is made using the 10-mm, 0.4-mm spot tip at superpulse mode, regulated to 20 W (Fig. 26-17).

The laser tip is changed to a 10-mm ceramic tip, 0.8-mm spot tip and changed to continuous mode with power at 10 W to dissect the incised skin (Fig. 26-18) and continue with the procedure. We elevate the lateral angle of the incision, and the flap is dissected against a wet cotton tip held by the assistant. Wet gauze is placed over the patient's nose as protection against the laser beam (Fig. 26-19). The temperature of the upper eyelid conjunctiva has been monitored and recorded during laser surgery. A minimal increase in temperature has been noted, confirming the absence of thermal injury at a distal site from the laser application and the safety of the laser procedure (11). Hemostasis is checked (Fig. 26-20). If cauterization of blood vessels is necessary, we use the out-of-focus laser beam. Usually, hemostasis is performed throughout the surgery with one or two cotton tips. The orbicular muscle is incised and, by gently pressing the eye globe with the protector, the fat compartments are exposed (Figs. 26-21, 26-22). Bleeding is practically nonexistent, because the laser beam cuts and cauterizes simultaneously. With the help of delicate forceps, the assistant holds a wet cotton tip for protection, and we excise the excess fat with the laser beam. Skin and fat are then placed on a Sheen grid for comparison with the opposite side (Fig. 26-23). We use a running 5–0 mononylon suture, bearing in mind that every suture placed and every maneuver performed, can increase the possibility of edema or ecchymosis (Fig. 26-24). No dressings are required. If there is a lack of fat in the nasojugal fold, I inject fat (Fig. 26-25). If there are crow's-feet, I resurface the area (Fig. 26-26). Figures 26-27–26-32 show pre- and postoperative images of patients who have undergone this procedure.

DISCUSSION

Besides the "marketing factor," the advantages of the CO_2 laser are the precision of resection and cauterizing, a fast procedure with almost no bruising or edema postoperatively, since the CO_2 laser seals the capillary and lymphatic vessels as they are cut, with little need for additional hemostasis (12). It is known that bleeding, with ecchymosis and hematoma, are among the serious blepharoplasty complications. A complete patient evaluation before a blepharoplasty confirms the diagnosis and indication for surgery and identifies any potentially complicating factors. Accurate examination, proper diagnosis, and meticulous surgical technique should prevent complications (4).

Cutting the septum almost always provokes a certain degree of scleral show, at least for one or two months. Preoperative analysis of the periorbital anatomy and a good medical history can identify patients predisposed to postoperative eyelid malposition (13), which is the most common complication associated with transcutaneous blepharoplasty (14). Transconjunctival blepharoplasty reports have found no cases of lid retraction, ectropion, entropion, inferior oblique palsy, or overexcision of fat. The main advantage of this technique is that it avoids the most common complications of transcutaneous lower eyelid blepharoplasty, lower eyelid retraction (15), ectropion, and scleral show (16). The transconjunctival approach offers many advantages for lower blepharoplasty. It addresses bulging fat directly, minimizes late lid retraction problems, permits skin resection if indicated, and retains a natural appearance (17). The technique is straightforward, and is easily mastered once the anatomy is understood. Exposure of the central and medial fat compartments is excellent. The lateral fat pad area is not as easy to visualize, and care must be taken to assure that adequate fat removal is achieved (18). As a rule, we do not remove skin from the lower eyelids; the skin will generally retract sufficiently within two months following the surgery. Although skin excision may be required during the initial procedure or at a later stage, patients with apparent skin excess need not be excluded from consideration for transconjunctival lower lid blepharoplasty (18). When there is obvious skin excess, I can perform skin resection immediately. When skin and fat are removed from the lower eyelid during the same procedure, I first remove the excess fat through the transconjunctival incision and then remove skin with a simple skin-pinch technique, very conservatively, without incising the septum orbitalis. Secondary skin removal, if necessary, is a straightforward procedure that can be done under local anesthesia at a later date (19)—a simple excision of a skin wrinkle, avoiding incision of the septum orbitalis. Another option for lower lid blepharoplasty has been described to correct the problems of fine wrinkling, fat herniation, and mild skin excess. Fat is removed through a transconjunctival approach, and the lower lid is peeled using full-strength Baker's phenol solution (20). Chemical peeling promotes formation of new epidermis and new dermal collagen, resulting in skin shrinkage, reduction of wrinkling and "crepe paper" skin, softening of crow's-feet, and, when desired, lightened eyelid color (21). I prefer repeated 70% glycolic acid peels, which are not as strong and dramatic as the Baker's formula, but safer. The disadvantages of using the laser compared with the steel scalpel include the cost of purchasing and maintaining the laser equipment and the need for additional training for surgeons and assistants. Long-term follow-up (8) shows no difference between the two sides when the cosmetic result and scars are compared. Surgeons opposed to this procedure found that the possibility of adverse safety factors or accidents increased with use of the laser. They have found no significant difference in immediate and late postoperative pain, swelling, ecchymosis, and scarring on the two sides. They claim, however, that a positive marketing factor could be demonstrated with use of the carbon dioxide laser for blepharoplasty (12). However, practice enhancement or the surgeon's personal economic gain should not be considered reasons to use a technique; only the benefit of patients is a valid concern (22). I personally have found CO_2 laser blepharoplasty to be a major contribution to my patients' safety and it has also improved economic gain, because I started performing better procedures and producing better results—at the end of the day, this is the goal of our profession.

LEARNING

Surgeons can practice using the CO_2 laser on chicken legs, cutting and removing skin, learning to use the instrument with precision, and finding the ideal distance for cutting and cauterizing. Additional precautions should be taken while using the CO_2 laser, such as the use of protective glasses, and the regions around the surgical field must be protected with wet gauze, particularly the nose, which can be burned during the dissection of the upper eyelid. Adequate protection of the patients' eyes avoids risks to the eyeballs and eyesight. The only disadvantage is the price of the machine; however, the instrument has other uses besides blepharoplasty, which helps to make it more cost-effective.

When we started performing this procedure, we used to inject the anesthetic solution in a ''bubble.'' Using the fingertips, this ''bubble'' is pushed under the markings of the skin to be resected. Our complications to date are minor, and occurred during the first procedures performed, while we were adapting to the machine. It takes 40 minutes to perform a four-eyelid blepharoplasty. It is important to inject the anesthetic solution where there are no apparent blood vessels and with as little movement of the needle as possible. One of the cases requiring a second injection in the upper eyelid showed, at the dissection time, an ecchymosis that took three weeks to disappear. Two patients had superficial burns (2 mm width) in the lateral region of the nose due to inadequate skin protection. Two patients had prolonged edema (one week) of the lower eyelids due to excessive manipulation and incorrect presentation. We used a Desmarres retractor that hid the ideal incision line, making it difficult to remove fat and increasing unnecessary manipulation. I consequently designed a retractor for a similar purpose with a smaller curve at the tip, which makes the presentation easier.

Patients' return to normal activity is rapid because of decreased bruising and swelling. The laser procedure is well-suited to the office-based practice but requires a high degree of skill in CO_2 laser excisional surgery. In the hands of the inexperienced surgeon, new and serious complications may occur (23).

COMPLICATIONS

To avoid complications of blepharoplasties, the surgeon must first communicate with the patient. Once a rapport is established, the expectations of the patient can be determined and the realistic results that can be achieved from surgery can be explained (24). Proper surgical technique is essential for good postoperative results. If complications do occur, correct diagnosis of the etiology of the problem usually leads to a satisfactory resolution.

Inadequate fat removal is reported to be the most common complication when the transconjunctival method is used (14). It can be avoided by the careful, graded, and thorough removal of herniated lower lid fat. One study showed the main complication was underexcision of fat (7.4%), and moderate postoperative wound hemorrhage without hematoma formation occurred in one patient (0.8%) (14).

Edema is usually due to unnecessary trauma, the excessive use of cautery for hemostasis, or is a reaction to a foreign body such as a suture. The use of traditional instruments and techniques may increase the possibility of trauma and bleeding and extend the postoperative recovery period. The use of electrocautery provokes burns and additional trauma to the surgical field and to the surrounding delicate tissues. The possibility of blindness after eyelid surgery is 0.04% (25). The 68 registered cases of blindness postblepharoplasty are all related to bleeding (26). Bleeding after blepharoplasty is usually due to three anatomic components: the individual tissue vascularity, the major arterial trunks in the region, and the connective tissue support of the arteries (27).

CONCLUSION

CO_2 laser blepharoplasty has the advantage of being a simple procedure for the patient, with less postoperative pain, edema, or ecchymosis and a return to normal activities within three to five days. For surgeons, once they have adapted to the new instrument, the technique is fast and dry, with good visualization of all structures.

REFERENCES

1. Dailey RA, Wobig JL. Eyelid anatomy. *J Dermatol Surg Oncol* 1992;18:1023–1027.
2. Siegel RJ. Essential anatomy for contemporary upper lid blepharoplasty. *Clin Plast Surg* 1993;20:209–212.
3. de Castillo HT, Andrews J de M, Zani R. Eyelid pouches: anatomical study of the orbital fat applied to surgery. *Rev Paul Med* [Brazil], 1991;109:217–220.
4. Holt JE, Holt GR. Blepharoplasty. Indications and preoperative assessment. *Arch Otolaryngol* 1985;111:394–397.
5. Meyer DR, Linberg JV, Wobig JL, McCormick SA. Anatomy of the orbital septum and associated eyelid connective tissues. Implications for ptosis surgery [see comments]. *Ophthal Plast Reconstr Surg* 1991;7:104–113. Comments in: *Ophthal Plast Reconstr Surg* 1993;9:150–151.
6. Siegel R. Surgical anatomy of the upper eyelid fascia. *Ann Plast Surg* 1984;13:263–273.
7. David LM, Sanders G. CO_2 laser blepharoplasty: a comparison to cold steel and electrocautery. *J Dermatol Surg Oncol* 1987;13:110–114.
8. Morrow DM. Re: Carbon dioxide laser blepharoplasty—advantages and disadvantages [Letter] *Ann Plast Surg* 1992;28:397–399. Comment in: *Ann Plast Surg* 1990;24:1–6.
9. Niechajev IA, Ljungqvist A. Central (third) fat pad of the upper eyelid. *Aesthetic Plast Surg* 1991;15:223–228.
10. David LM, Abergel RP. CO_2 laser blepharoplasty—advantages and disadvantages. *Ann Plast Surg* 1990;24:1.
11. David LM, Abergel RP. Carbon dioxide laser blepharoplasty: conjunctival temperature during surgery. *J Dermatol Surg Oncol* 1989;15:421–423.
12. Mittelman H, Apfelberg DB. Carbon dioxide laser blepharoplasty—advantages and disadvantages. *Ann Plast Surg* 1990;24:1–6. Comments in: *Ann Plast Surg* 1990;25:159; *Ann Plast Surg* 1991;27:180n181; *Ann Plast Surg* 1992;28:397–399.
13. Dubayle P, Zenatti C, Benelli L. [Transconjunctival approach in lower blepharoplasties]. *Bull Soc Ophtalmol Fr* [French] 1986;86:67–69.
14. Palmer FR III, Rice DH, Churukian MM. Transconjunctival blepharoplasty. Complications and their avoidance: a retrospective analysis and review of the literature. *Arch Otolaryngol Head Neck Surg* 1993;119:993–999.

15. Baylis HI, Long JA, Groth MJ. Transconjunctival lower eyelid blepharoplasty. Technique and complications. *Ophthalmology* 1989;96:1027–1032.

16. Mahe E, Harfaoui-Chanaoui T, Banal A, Chappey C, Tran quoc chi. Different technical approaches for blepharoplasty in eyelid rejuvenation surgery. *Arch Otorhinolaryngol* 1989;246: 353–356.

17. Zarem HA, Resnick JI. Minimizing deformity in lower blepharoplasty. The transconjunctival approach. *Clin Plast Surg* 1993;20:317–321.

18. Zarem HA, Resnick JI. Expanded applications for transconjunctival lower lid blepharoplasty *Plast Reconstr Surg* 1991;88:215–220;discussion, 221. Comments in: *Plast Reconstr Surg* 1992;89:764, 765; *Plast Reconstr Surg* 1992;89:1176; *Plast Reconstr Surg* 1992;90:731–732.

19. Zarem HA, Resnick JI. Operative technique for transconjunctival lower blepharoplasty. *Clin Plast Surg* 1992;19:351–356.

20. McKinney P, Zukowski ML, Mossie R. The fourth option: a novel approach to lower-lid blepharoplasty. *Aesthetic Plast Surg* 1991;15:293–296.

21. Morrow DM. Chemical peeling of eyelids and periorbital area. *J Dermatol Surg Oncol* 1992;18:102–110.

22. Fredricks S. Carbon dioxide laser blepharoplasty [Letter]. *Ann Plast Surg* 1990;25:159. Comment in: *Ann Plast Surg* 1990;24:1–6.

23. David LM. The laser approach to blepharoplasty. *J Dermatol Surg Oncol* 1988;14:741–746.

24. Wilkins RB, Byrd WA. Complications of blepharoplasty. *Ophthal Plast Reconstr Surg* 1985;1: 195–198.

25. DeMere M, Wood T, Austin W. Eye complications with blepharoplasty or other eyelid surgery. *Plast Reconstr Surg* 1974;53:634–636.

26. Callahan M. Prevention of blindness after blepharoplasty. *Ophthalmology* 1983;90:1047–1051.

27. Gurdin MM. Caution advised regarding transconjunctival lower lid blepharoplasty [Letter]. *Plast Reconstr Surg* 1992;90:731–732. Comment in: *Plast Reconstr Surg* 1991;88:215–220; discussion, 221.

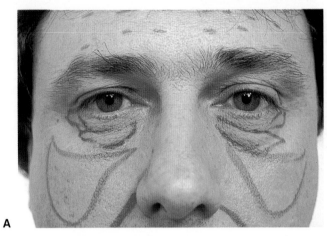

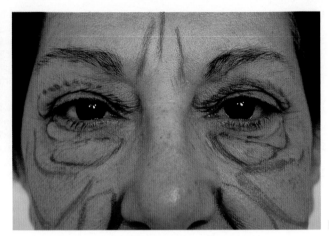

A

B

FIG. 26-1. A, B: With the patient in the standing position, I mark the fat pockets on the skin in the lower eyelids.

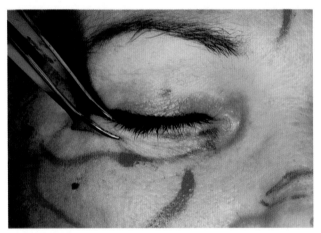

FIG. 26-2. Lower eyelid: The excess skin is measured using forceps.

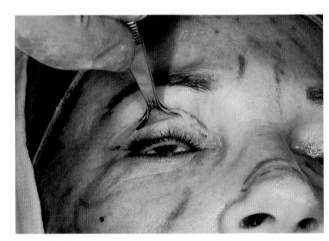

FIG. 26-4. Upper eyelid: The incision line is marked parallel to the sulcus, approximately 8 mm from the ciliary margin in the medial portion of the eyelid.

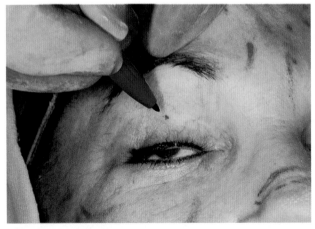

FIG. 26-3. Upper eyelid: The length of the caudal incision varies according to the fold, never exceeding its length.

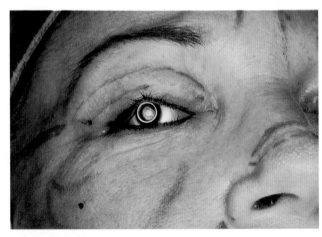

FIG. 26-5. Upper eyelid: The excess skin is measured with a forceps and the cephalic incision is marked conservatively.

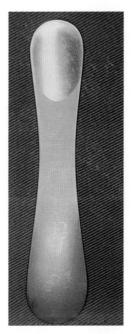

FIG. 26-6. A Jaeger plate.

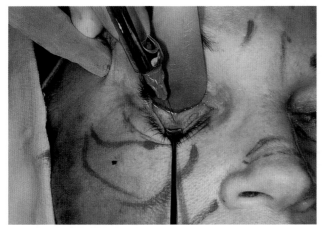

FIG. 26-7. A modified Desmarres retractor pulls down the lower lid.

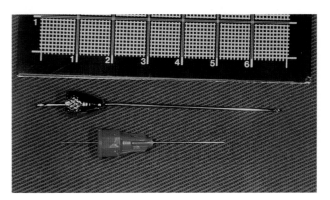

FIG. 26-8. For the upper eyelid, I use a blunt needle for anesthesia injection, taking care to avoid damaging the capillaries.

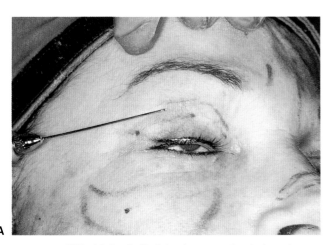

A

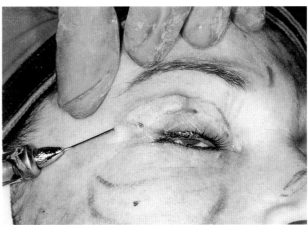

B

FIG. 26-9. A, B: Injecting anesthesia into the upper eyelid with a blunt needle with a lateral hole.

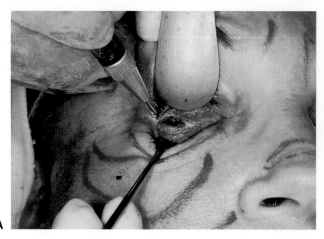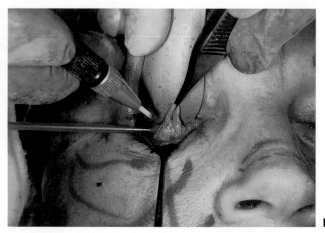

FIG. 26-10. A, B: For the removal of the lower eyelid fat pads, I perform the transconjunctival incision 5 mm from the tarsal border. I incise the conjunctiva with a 10-mm tip, 0.4-mm spot tip.

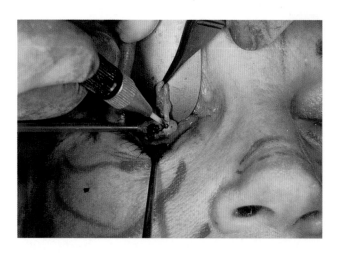

FIG. 26-11. I change to a 10-mm ceramic tip, 0.8-mm spot tip; the laser beam is regulated to 10 W, continuous mode, to dissect and cut the fat pockets.

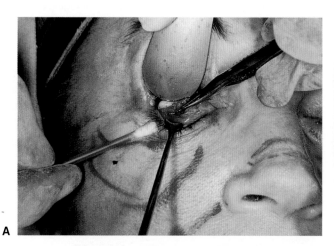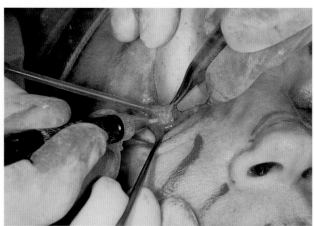

FIG. 26-12. A, B: Lateral pockets: With the cotton tip, I pull through the skin, showing the excess fat through the incision. I do not suture.

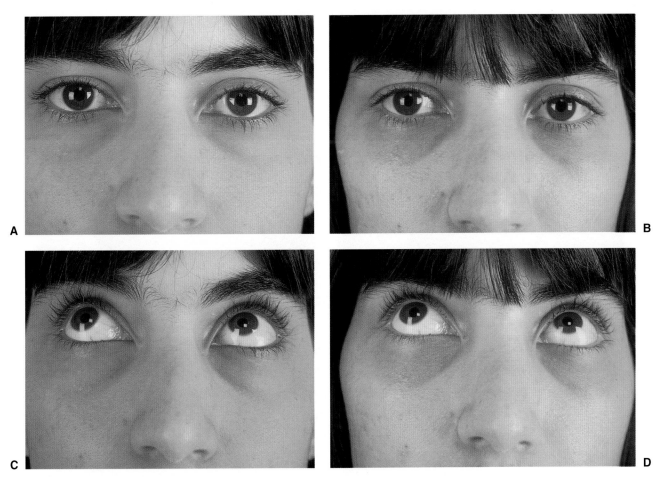

FIG. 26-13. Pre- **(A, C)** and 24-hour postoperative **(B, D)** photos of transconjunctival lower blepharoplasty of a 23-year-old patient.

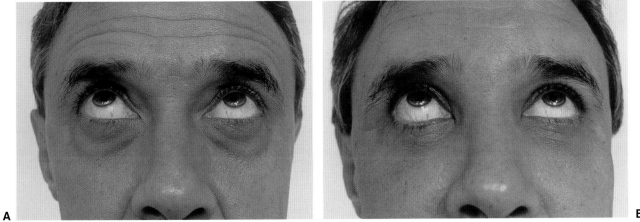

FIG. 26-14. Pre- **(A)** and one-year postoperative **(B)** photos of transconjunctival lower blepharoplasty of a 54-year-old patient.

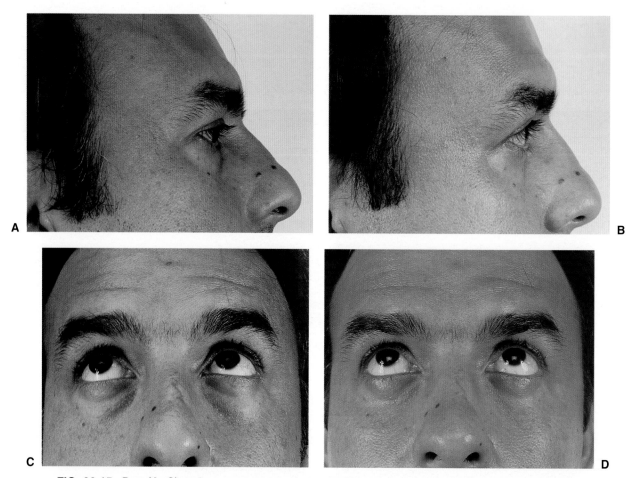

FIG. 26-15. Pre- **(A, C)** and one-year postoperative **(B, D)** photos of transconjunctival lower blepharoplasty of a 46-year-old patient.

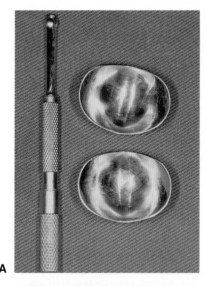

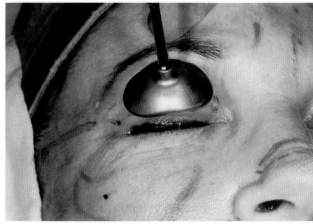

FIG. 26-16. A, B, C: Upper eyelids: A protective sheath is placed beneath the eyelid, covering the eye globe and exposing the incision markings.

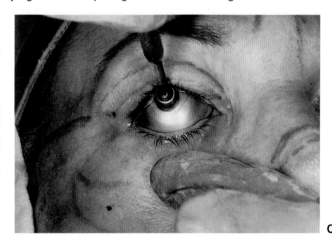

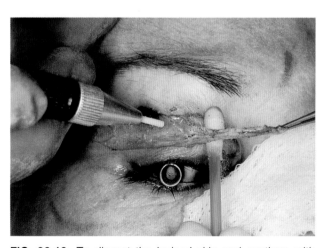

FIG. 26-17. Upper eyelids: The skin incision is made using the 10-mm, 0.4-mm spot tip at superpulse mode, regulated to 20 W.

FIG. 26-18. To dissect the incised skin and continue with the procedure, we change the laser tip to a 10-mm ceramic tip, 0.8-mm spot tip and change to continuous mode with power at 10 W.

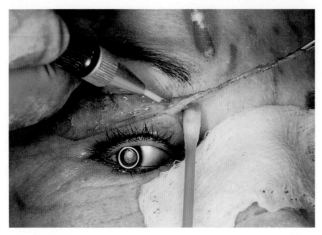

FIG. 26-19. Wet gauze is placed over the patient's nose as protection against the laser beam.

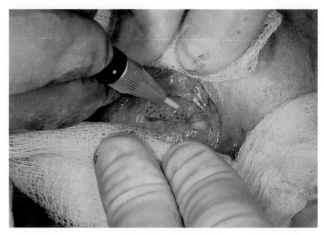

FIG. 26-22. By gently pressing the eye globe with the protector, the fat compartments are exposed.

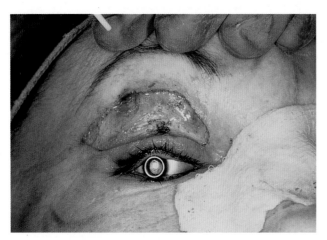

FIG. 26-20. Hemostasis is checked.

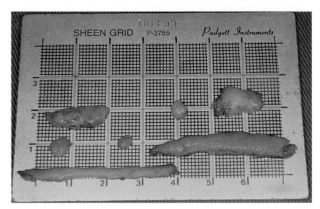

FIG. 26-23. Skin and fat are placed on a Sheen grid for comparison.

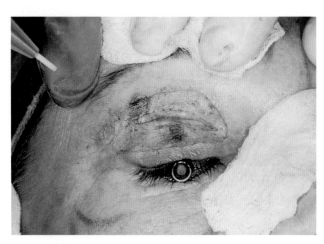

FIG. 26-21. The orbicular muscle is incised.

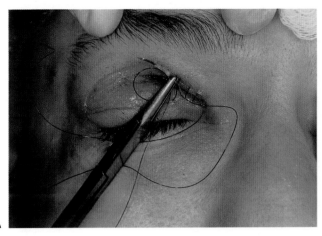
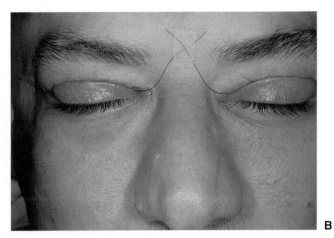

FIG. 26-24. A, B: A running 5–0 mononylon suture.

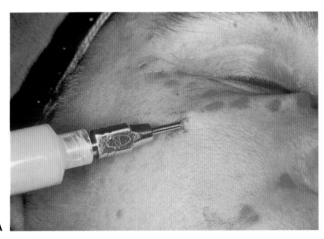
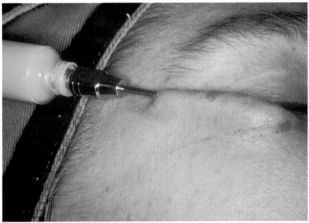

FIG. 26-25. A, B: If there is a lack of fat in the nasojugal fold, I inject fat.

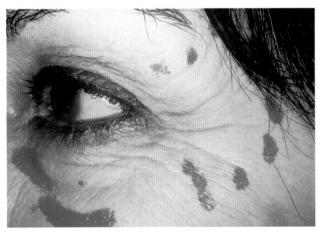
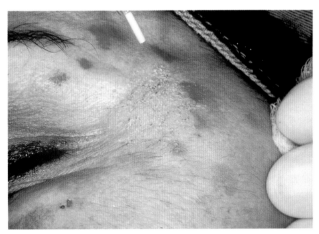

FIG. 26-26. A, B: If there are crow's-feet, I resurface the area.

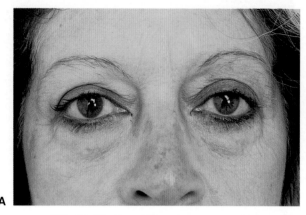
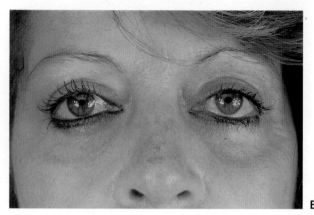

A   B

FIG. 26-27. Pre- **(A)** and one-year postoperative **(B)** photos of a 52-year-old patient who had upper blepharoplasty with skin, muscle, and fat removal and only transconjunctival lower blepharoplasty.

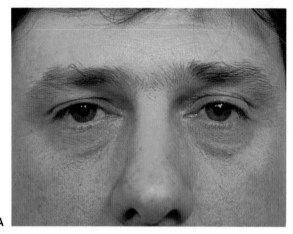
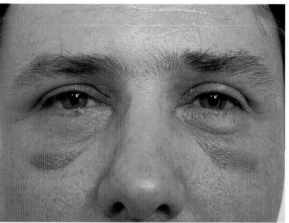

A   B

FIG. 26-28. Pre- **(A)** and five-day postoperative **(B)** photos of a 44-year-old patient who had upper blepharoplasty with skin, muscle, and fat removal and only transconjunctival lower blepharoplasty.

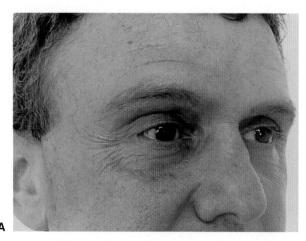
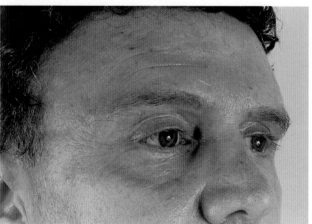

A   B

FIG. 26-29. Pre- **(A)** and one-year postoperative **(B)** photos of a 54-year-old patient who had upper blepharoplasty with skin, muscle, and fat removal and only transconjunctival lower blepharoplasty, plus glycolic acid peels and home treatment with 8% glycolic acid.

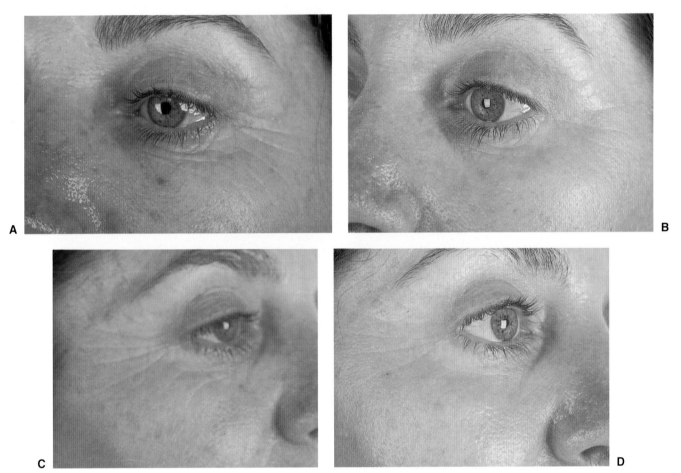

FIG. 26-30. Pre- **(A, C)** and two-month postoperative **(B, D)** photos of a superficial laser resurfacing of the lower eyelid.

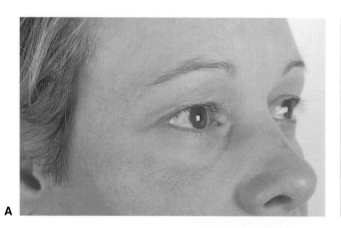

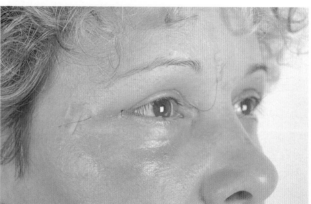

A

B

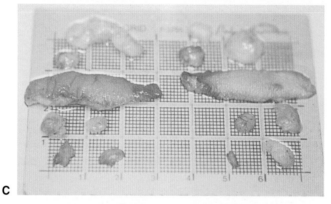

C

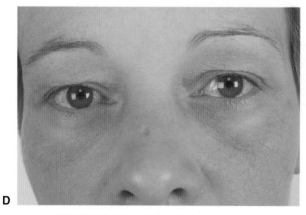

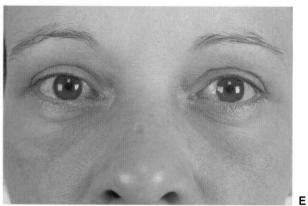

D

E

FIG. 26-31. Pre- **(A)** and two-week postoperative **(B)** photos of a 42-year-old patient who had upper blepharoplasty with skin, muscle, and fat removal and only transconjunctival lower blepharoplasty, plus laser resurfacing. **C:** The tissue is removed. **D, E:** Pre- and four-month postoperative photos.

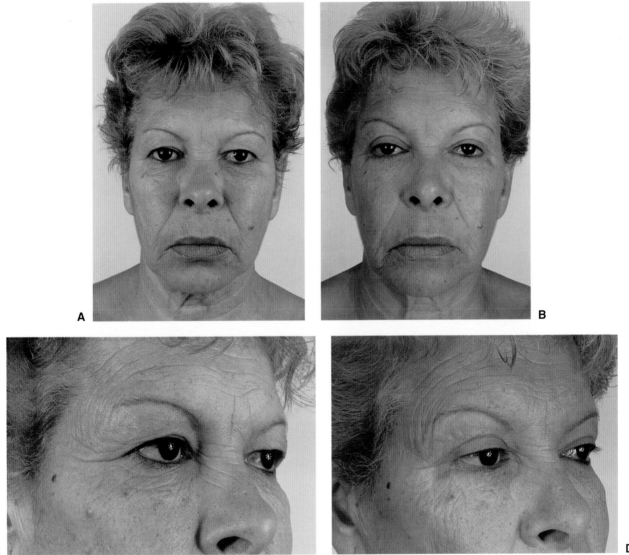

FIG. 26-32. Pre- **(A, C)** and five-month postoperative **(B, D)** photos of a 65-year-old patient who had upper blepharoplasty with skin, muscle, and fat removal, transconjunctival lower blepharoplasty, plus skin removal. No laser resurfacing was done.

APPENDIX 2

Combined Facial Liposculpture Procedures

EXAMPLE CASE 1

A 47-year-old patient (Fig. A2-1A) did not present much excess fat in the neck, but needed retraction in the area of the so-called platysmal bands and jowls (Fig. A2-1B). She needed fat injection in the malar, nasolabial and periorbital areas, and lips. She also wanted a light peel of her vertical lip wrinkles. Under local anesthesia, I performed superficial suction with a 1.5-mm-gauge cannula (Fig. A2-1C), with the holes first pointed towards the platysma and then pointed towards the dermis (Fig. A2-1D–F). I utilized three incisions (Fig. A2-1G, H): one submental and two submandibular, below the jawline. Total aspirated fat was only 17 ml, but we accomplished a good retraction of the skin (Fig. A2-1 I). The rejuvenation effect was completed with fat injection (Fig. A2-1J–N) of the malar region, nasolabial and nasojugal folds, upper eyelids, and earlobes plus a combination of fat injection on the lips and CO_2 laser peel of the vertical lines of the upper lip (Fig. A2-1O–Q). Preoperative photos and five-year postoperative photos (Fig. A2-1R–W) show this 52-year-old patient, still without a face-lift.

EXAMPLE CASE 2

A 39-year-old patient felt she was starting to look older, and decided to begin a facial rejuvenation program. We prescribed a chin prosthesis, aspiration of fat from the neck, and fat injection in the periorbital, malar and nasolabial areas, and lips (Fig. A2-2).

EXAMPLE CASE 3

A 33-year-old, prematurely aged patient wanted to rejuvenate without undergoing a rhytidoplasty (Fig. A2-3). I indicated several small procedures to be performed under local anesthesia with sedation, to provide a subtle change of her facial features with a fast recovery time. The diagnosis was aged and sun-damaged skin, submental and jowl fat deposits, receding chin, nasojugal folds, nasolabial folds, marionette lines, nasal dorsum hump, upper eyelid skin and fat excess, lower eyelid fat excess, and fine wrinkles.

Surgical Plan

First Procedure

My approach to these problems was to first prescribe a preoperative skin care program to eliminate the fine wrinkles as much as possible and to unify the color and texture of the skin. The first surgical session was planned accordingly. Using the syringe liposculpture technique, I would remove fat from the neck and jowls, obtaining a regular skin retraction of the area. Fat would be harvested from the flank area and injected into the nasojugal, nasolabial and marionette folds, the first of three injections over a four-month period. The chin would be augmented with an inclusion of Bioplastique. CO_2 laser upper and lower blepharoplasty would be performed. The nasal dorsum hump would be rasped.

Second Procedure

Two months after the first procedure we planned CO_2 laser resurfacing of the lower eyelids and crow's feet, and a second fat injection of the facial folds.

Third Procedure

Two months after the second procedure we planned a third fat injection of the facial folds.

First Procedure

Fat Suction

The first procedure was performed under IV sedation by the anesthesiologist and local anesthesia. For sedation, midazolam and fentanyl were used. The first areas to be treated were the neck and jowls. After skin prepping, I injected a dermal button of lidocaine 2% with adrenaline 1:100,000 behind the earlobes and in the submental crease. In these three points, I made small incisions with a no. 11 blade. I inserted the blunt multiholed needle through these incisions and injected 200 cc of the diluted anesthesia formula. After 10 minutes I began suctioning, referring to photos of the patient (Fig A2-4) and working within the premarked areas (Fig. A2-5).

Suction was initially performed with a 3-mm-gauge 15-cm-long Pyramid-tip cannula connected to a 10-cc luer-lock syringe. With this cannula I suctioned the deeper layer of fat, close to the platysma muscle. The suction with the thicker cannula improved the contour of the neck and the cervical-mental angle (Fig. A2-6). Then I changed to a 1.5-mm-gauge 15-cm-long two-holed flat-tip cannula with the same syringe (Fig. A2-7). This cannula induces skin retraction and can be used closer to the skin in the subdermal area. The holes can be turned towards the dermis when more retraction is necessary. The jowls are suctioned only with this fine cannula, and the area can be crisscrossed from the chin and earlobe incisions. If necessary, additional incisions can be placed in the oral comissures and submandibular area for better access.

I suctioned a total aspirate of 50 cc, of which 27 cc was pure fat. The incision was not sutured, just taped with Micropore. The neck was taped with Microfoam for 24 hours. After that, the patient began sessions of manual lymphatic drainage by the esthetician. There are usually five sessions, held every other day. The patient should wear an elastic bandage to sleep for seven nights.

Fat Injection

The second part of the same procedure was fat injection of the facial folds. I harvested fat from the flank area and centrifuged it for one minute at 1,500 r/min. This fat was anaerobically transferred to a syringe connected to a pistol (Fig. A2-8). The areas to be injected had been marked in red with the patient standing (see Fig. A2-5). When a patient does not wish to be sedated, I prepare the skin with lidocaine 2.5%, prilocaine 2.5% topical anesthetic cream (EMLA cream, Astra USA, Westboro, MA) for one hour before the procedure. As in the neck area, I injected intradermal anesthesia buttons in the places where the thicker needles were going to be introduced. Then I perforated the skin with a 40 x 16 sharp needle and inserted the blunt multiholed 1-mm-gauge needle to inject the diluted local anesthesia formula. This formula plays an important role, not only in anesthetizing the area, but also in measuring the amount of fat injection that will produce a natural result. Injection of the anesthesia and fat with a blunt needle prevents unnecessary ecchymosis and edema provoked during injection (Fig. A2-9). After measuring the amount of anesthesia injected, I injected the same amount of fat in each area.

I inject only the amount of fat necessary to recontour the face. After 24 hours the local anesthesia has usually been reabsorbed, and the face will look normal. I do not overinject fat on the face. I prefer to reinject again after two and four months. By repeating the injections in three phases, I avoid a longer postoperative recovery period. In this case, I injected 5 cc into each malar area, 4 cc into each nasolabial area, and 1 cc into each side of the marionette lines (Fig. A2-10). The fat graft can be molded immediately after injection (Fig. A2-11).

Chin Augmentation with Bioplastique

To augment the chin I injected 0.8 cc of Bioplastique into the chin area, also under local anesthesia (Fig. A2-12). I prefer this to the traditional solid silicone chin prosthesis for augmenting the chin by only a small amount. The procedure is simpler and the recovery time faster.

Upper and Lower Eyelid CO_2 Laser Blepharoplasty

The anesthesiologist controled sedation with midazolam and fentanyl. After 1 drop of 0.5% tetracaine hydrochloride opthalmic solution in each eye, I did a local infiltration with 2% lidocaine with adrenaline 1:100,000 (Fig. A2-13).

The technique for anesthesia injection is crucial to good postoperative results, because most ecchymosis is formed during anesthesia injection. I pulled the lower eyelid with a modified Desmarres retractor and the assistant covered the eyeball with a Jaeger plate. Light pressure on the plate exposed the fat pads. The 0.3 × 21 mm needle was introduced into the conjunctiva and stopped at the orbital rim, and I pulled it back by 2 mm and injected 1 or 2 cc of anesthetic solution. I pulled the needle back and injected 1 cc subconjunctivally (see Fig. A2-13).

I injected a dermal button of anesthetic into the lateral area of the upper eyelid, perforated the skin with a sharp needle, inserted a blunt 1-mm-gauge needle, and injected 2 or 3 cc of anesthesia. This bubble of anesthetic can be pushed with the fingertips under the markings of the skin to be resected from the upper eyelid, avoiding other punctures.

Lower Eyelids

I used the transconjunctival incision. The assistant with a Jaeger plate and the modified Desmarres retractor exposed the eyelid (Fig. A2-14). The curve angle of this retractor was modified, because the original curve hid the ideal incision line, 5 mm parallel to the tarsal border. With this modification, the instrument exposes the exact amount of conjunctiva and the fat compartments are visible under the conjunctiva. The incision should be 5 mm parallel to the tarsal border, and can be of variable length, according to the fat compartments. I always keep the electrocautery ready in case a thicker blood vessel is cut and cannot be cauterized by the laser. With delicate, one-toothed forceps, I pulled out the excess fat and placed it against a wet cotton tip. Fat is easily cut by the laser beam and placed on a Sheen grid for comparison with the opposite side (Fig. A2-15). I did not suture the conjunctiva. If it is necessary to remove skin, as it is in 10% of cases, I will do it through a separate incision, without any damage to the septum orbitalis.

Upper Eyelids

A stainless steel eye protector was placed on the eyeball beneath the upper eyelid (Fig. A2-16). Skin incision was performed with the laser in pulse mode (Fig. A2-17). After the skin was incised in the marked areas, the laser settings were changed to continuous mode. The forceps lifted the lateral angle of the incision, and I dissected the muscle cutaneous flap against the wet cotton tip held by the assistant. The nose was protected with wet gauze (Fig. A2-18). The septum was incised and the fat pockets exposed by gently pressing the eyeball (Fig. A2-19).

As with the lower eyelid, the fat pocket was exposed and cut with the laser beam against a wet cotton tip. Hemostasis was checked (Fig. A2-20). It is common that one or two cotton tips are used through an entire surgery to check hemostasis. If it is necessary to cauterize a blood vessel, I use the out-of-focus laser beam as electrocautery. For blood vessels thicker than 1 mm, I use electrocautery. Skin was sutured subcuticularly with a 5–0 mononylon, bearing in mind that every maneuver performed can provoke edema or ecchymosis. No dressings are required, but I prescribe wet compresses for the first 24 hours and oral antibiotics for 72 hours. Analgesics are rarely needed.

Rhinoplasty

With local anesthesia, I performed an intracartilaginous incision in the left nostril, dissected the dorsum periosteum, and rasped 2 mm of the dorsal hump (Fig. A2-21). No suture was needed. A tampon was left for 24 hours and a Micropore dressing was worn for five days (Fig. A2-22).

Postoperative Care

On the first postoperative day the patient returned to the office to remove the submental dressing and undergo the first session of manual lymphatic drainage

(Fig. A2-23). This French massage method helps to remove the edema by draining it to the pre- and retroauricular lymph nodes. There are usually five sessions of massage, applied every other day.

Second and Third Procedures

Two months after the first procedure, I performed CO_2 laser resurfacing of the lower eyelids and crow's-feet in the lower eyelids to provoke skin retraction, as well as a second fat injection of the facial folds. Two months after the second procedure I injected fat a third time into the facial folds (Figs. A2-24–A2-26).

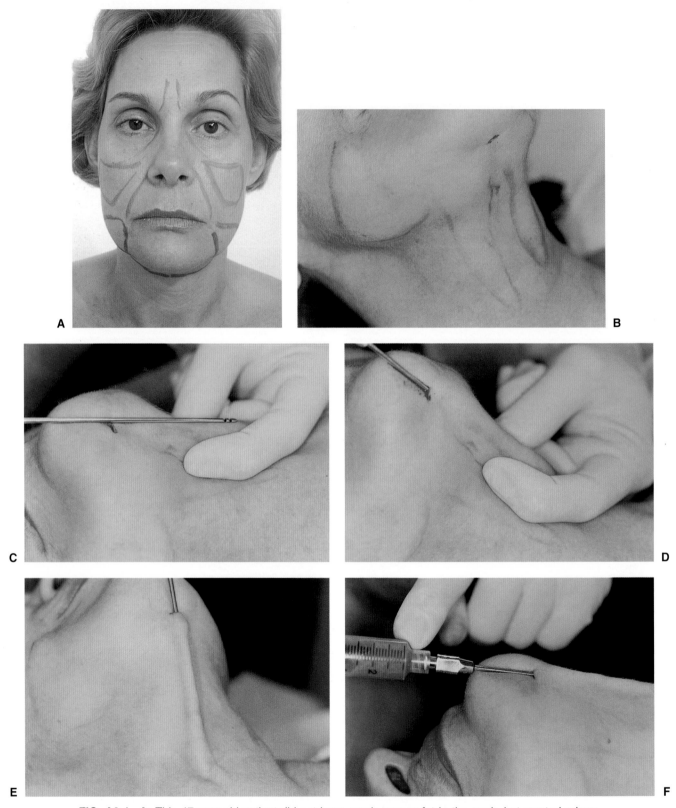

FIG. A2-1. A: This 47-year-old patient did not have much excess fat in the neck, but wanted rejuvenation without any visible signs or scars of plastic surgery. She needed fat injection in the malar, nasolabial and periorbital areas, and lips. She also wanted a light peel on the vertical wrinkles of her upper lip. **B:** The area of the so-called platysmal bands and jowls. **C:** After local anesthesia, superficial suction was performed using a 1.5-mm-gauge cannula. **D, E, F:** I directed the holes of the cannula first towards the platysma and then towards the dermis.

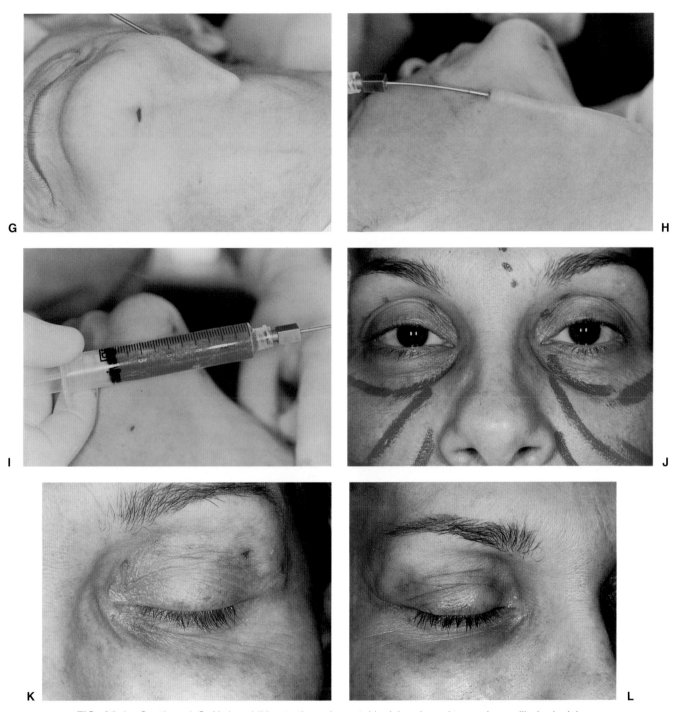

FIG. A2-1. *Continued.* **G, H:** In addition to the submental incision, I used two submandibular incisions, below the jaw line, for crisscrossing purposes. **I:** The total fat aspirated from this area was only 17 ml, but a good retraction of the skin was accomplished. **J:** The rejuvenation effect was completed with fat injection of the malar region, nasolabial and nasojugal folds, upper eyelids, and earlobes. **K, L:** Immediate postoperative pictures showing the injected fat placement within the orbital region. *Figure continues on next page.*

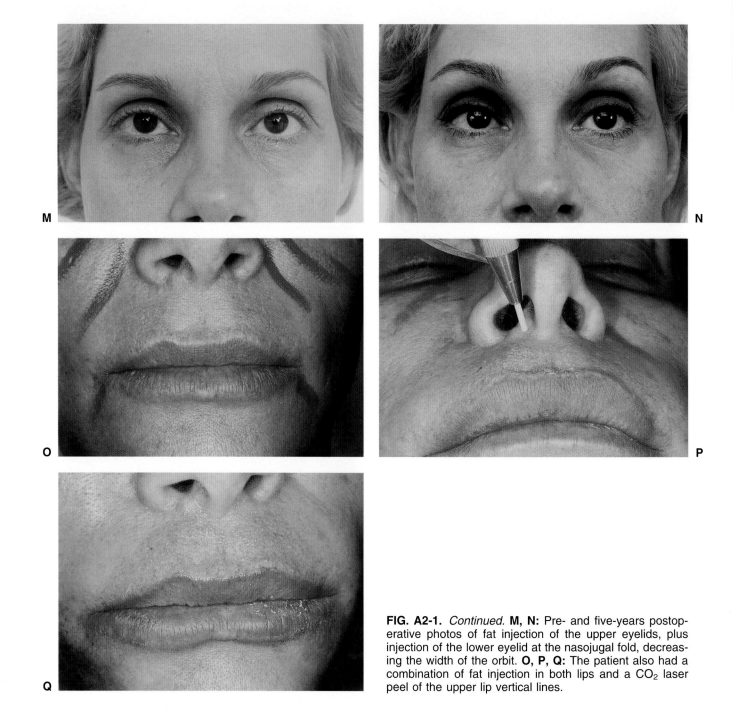

FIG. A2-1. *Continued.* **M, N:** Pre- and five-years postoperative photos of fat injection of the upper eyelids, plus injection of the lower eyelid at the nasojugal fold, decreasing the width of the orbit. **O, P, Q:** The patient also had a combination of fat injection in both lips and a CO_2 laser peel of the upper lip vertical lines.

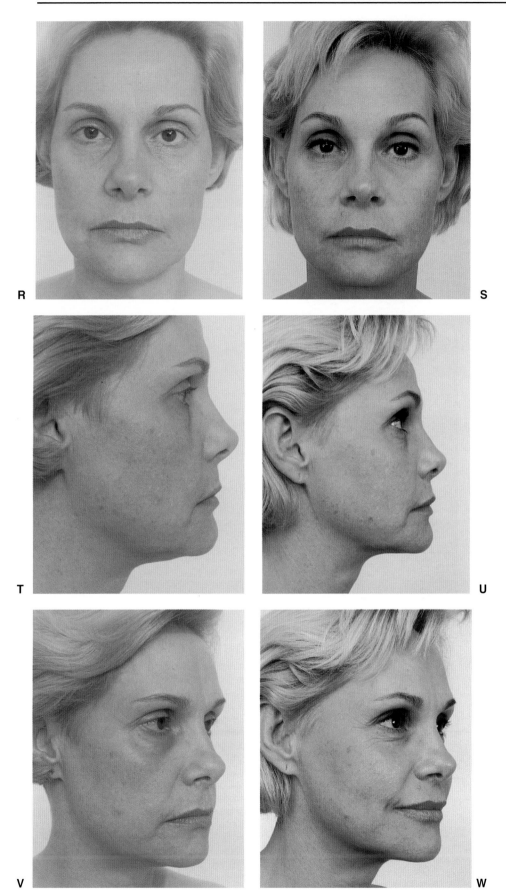

FIG. A2-1. *Continued.* **R, T, V:** Preoperative pictures. **S, U, W:** Five years postoperatively, 52 years old and without a face-lift scar.

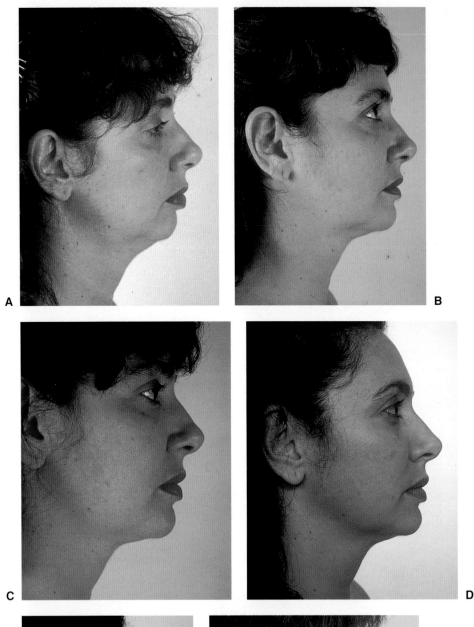

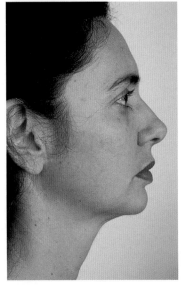

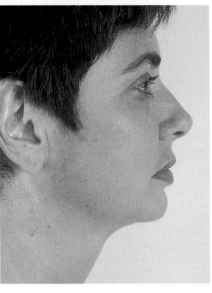

FIG. A2-2. A, B: Pre- and six-month post-operative photos after two injections of fat, two months apart, in the malars (3 cc each), nasolabial area (2 cc each), periorbital area (2 cc each), and lips (2 cc each). I aspirated 28 cc of fat from the submental area and inserted a silicone chin prosthesis. **C:** The patient had the third injection at six months and returned one year after the first procedure. I took pictures then but did not operate on her face. **D:** Two years after the first procedure she returned and I injected 3 cc of fat into each malar region. **E:** The patient returned three years after the initial procedure, wanting another fat aspiration of the neck. I aspirated 12 cc of fat and injected fat into her malar region (3 cc each) and nasolabial folds (2 cc each). **F:** Three years after the last procedure, six years after the first. The patient is now 45 years old.

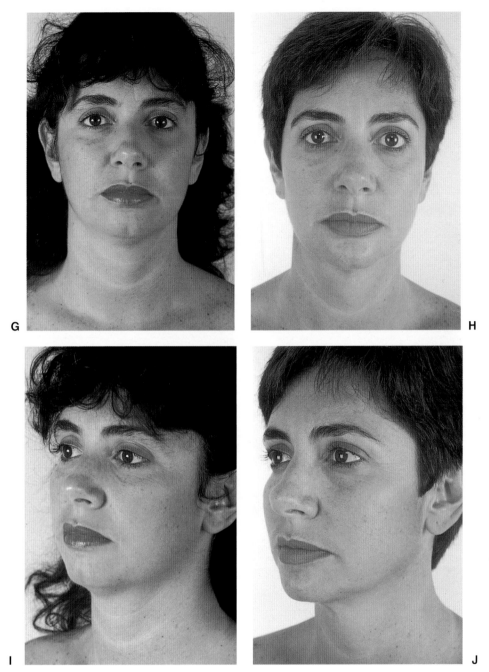

FIG. A2-2. *Continued.* Pre- **(G, I)** and six-year postoperative photos **(H, J)** of facial liposculpture. *Figure continues on next page.*

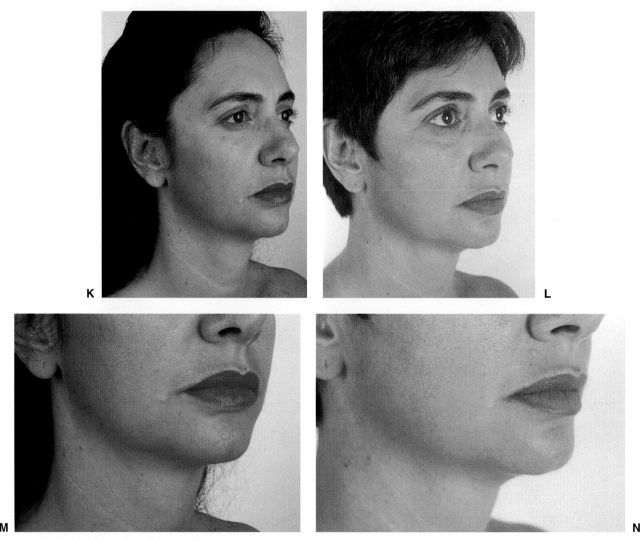

FIG. A2-2. *Continued.* Preoperatively **(K, M)** and three years after **(L, N)** the second fat aspiration of the neck. There is more definition of the jawline and no skin redundancy.

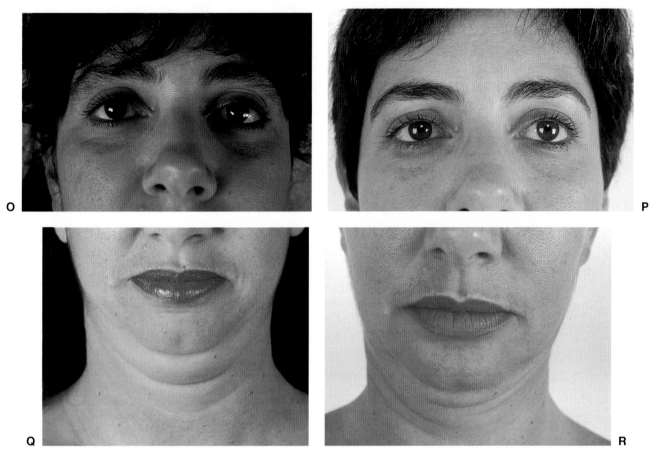

FIG. A2-2. *Continued.* **O, P:** Pre- and six-year postoperative photos of fat injection in the orbital area. There is a rejuvenating effect, reducing the size of the orbital cavity. The patient is now considering blepharoplasty. **Q, R:** Pre- and six-year postoperative photos of chin implant and fat aspiration of the submental area. She has had a second aspiration three years after the first. There was a good retraction of the area, even when the chin is down.

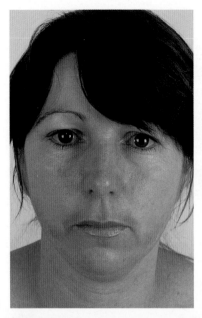
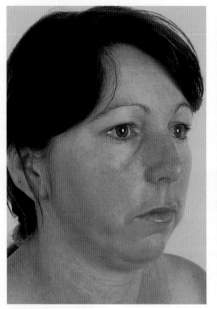
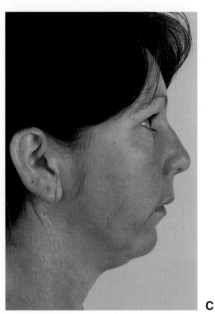

A,B

C

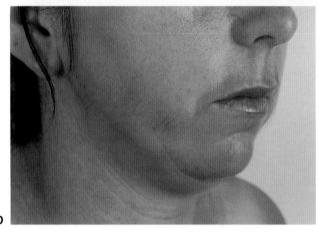

D

FIG. A2-3. A–D: Preoperative photos of a 33-year-old patient.

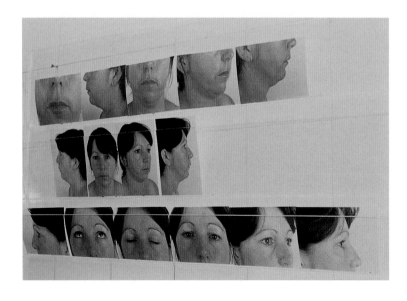

FIG. A2-4. I work with pictures of the patient in the operating room.

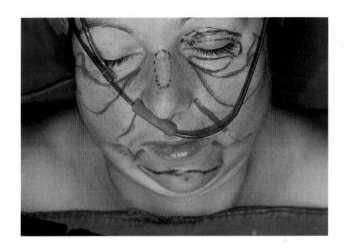

FIG. A2-5. Fat suction of the submental area and jowls. The areas to be suctioned are marked in blue, the areas for fat injection in red, and for blepharoplasty in purple.

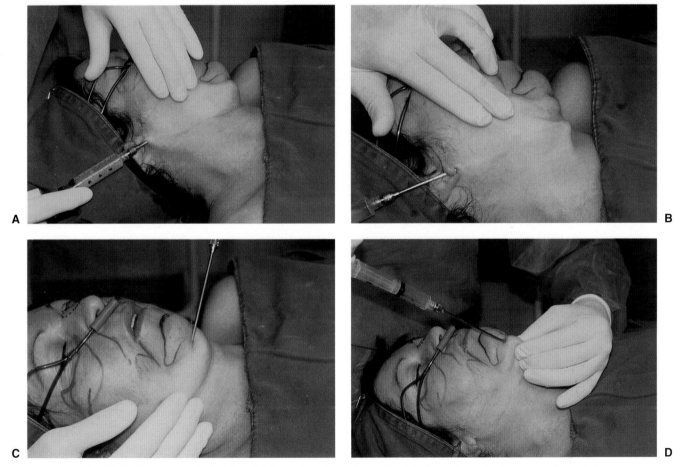

FIG. A2-6. A–D: I aspirated the fat from the deep layer though the retroauricular and submental incisions, close to the platysma, using a thicker, 3-mm-gauge cannula to improve the contour of the area.

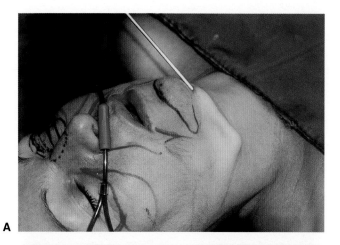

A

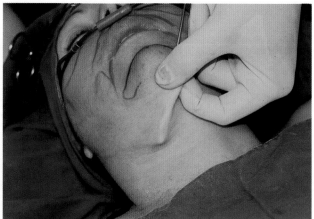

FIG. A2-7. A–C: A 1.5-mm-gauge 15-cm-long two-holed flat-tip cannula was used closer to the skin, in the subdermal area. The holes can be turned towards the dermis when more retraction is necessary.

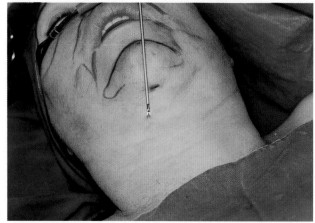

B

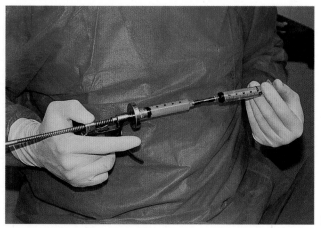

C

A

B

FIG. A2-8. A, B: Fat harvested from the flank area was anaerobically transferred to a syringe connected to a pistol.

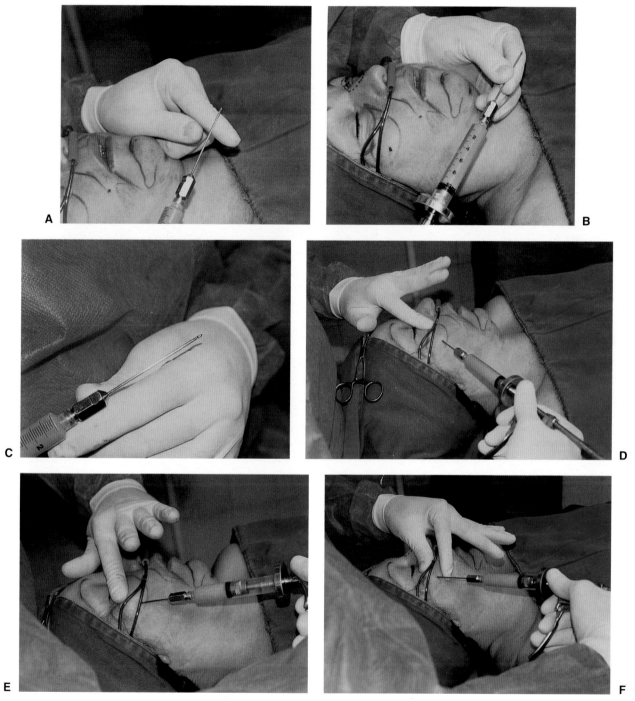

FIG. A2-9. A–F: This anesthesia formula injection anesthetizes the area, but also measures the amount of fat to be injected for a natural result. Injection of the anesthesia and fat with a blunt needle prevents unnecessary ecchymosis and edema provoked during injection.

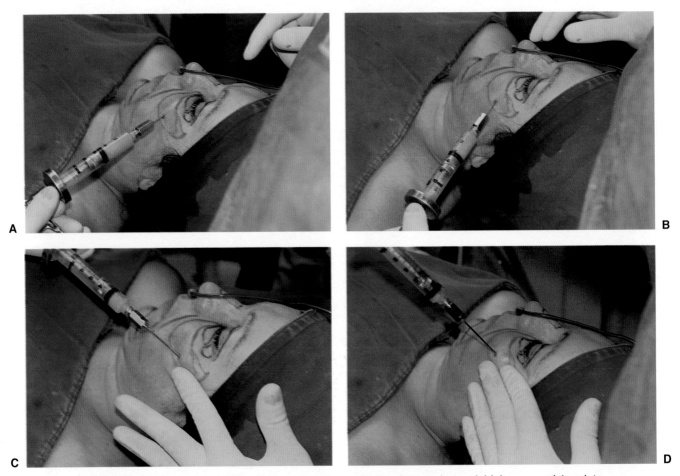

FIG. A2-10. A–D: Injection of 5 cc into each malar area, 4 cc into each nasolabial area, and 1 cc into each side of the marionette lines. Fat injected in the orbital rim area will improve the result of the blepharoplasty.

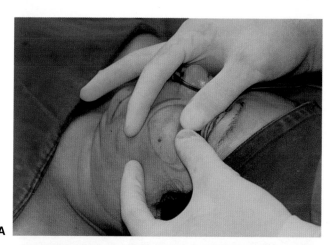

A

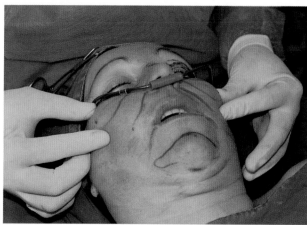

B

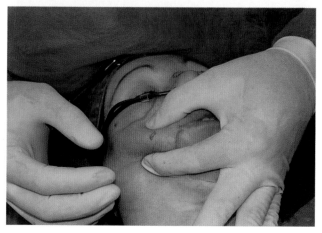

C

FIG. A2-11. A–C: Gentle molding and repositioning of the fat graft immediately after injection. If I feel there is excess fat, I can squeeze it through the incision point.

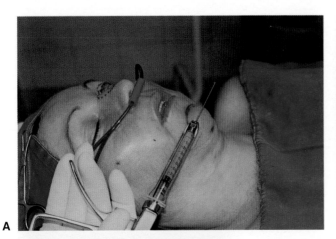

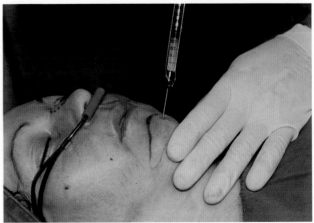

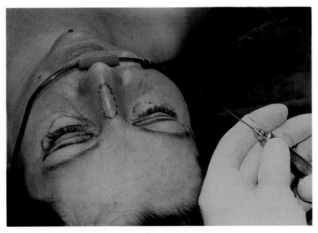

FIG. A2-12. A–C: The injection of Bioplastique is a very simple and direct method of improving the contour of the chin. Small quantities, such as the 0.8 cc injected here, will produce a dramatic change in the profile, without the patient having to undergo a more extensive, traditional chin prosthesis procedure.

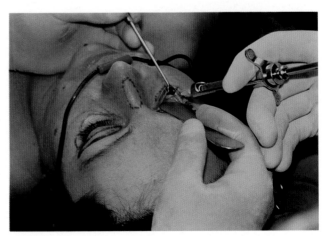

FIG. A2-13. A, B: Lower eyelid anesthesia. Local infiltration with 2% lidocaine with adrenaline 1: 100,000. The lower eyelid is pulled with a modified Desmarres retractor while an assistant covers the eyeball with a Jaeger plate.

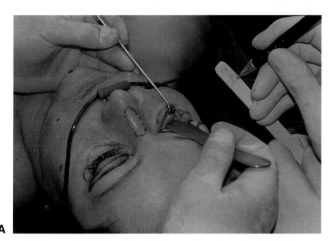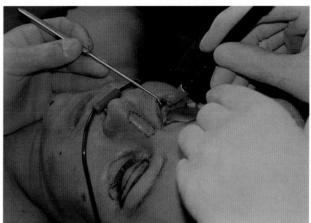

A   B

FIG. A2-14. A, B: First, the laser was tested on a wood spatula to check if the power was right. Then I performed a transconjunctival incision. The assistant, with the Jaeger plate and the modified Desmarres retractor, exposed the eyelid. The incision was 5 mm parallel to the tarsal border; it can be of variable length, according to the fat compartments.

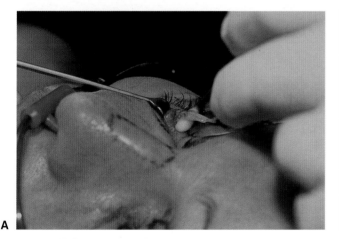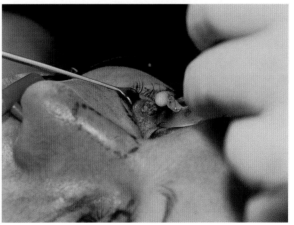

A   B

FIG. A2-15. A, B: With delicate one-toothed forceps, I pulled out the excess fat and placed it against a wet cotton tip. The laser beam easily cuts the excess fat. I did not suture the conjunctiva.

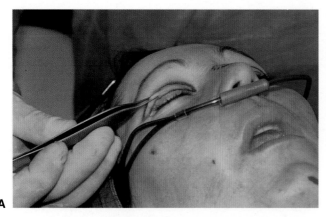

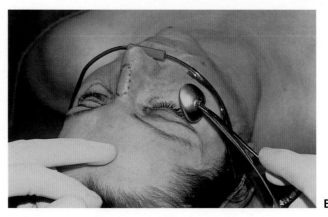

A   B

FIG. A2-16. A, B: The forceps measured the excess skin to be removed. A stainless steel eye protector was placed on the eyeball beneath the upper eyelid.

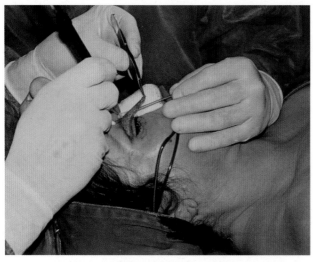

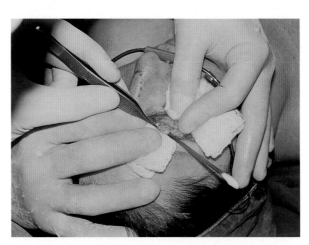

FIG. A2-17. Skin incision was performed with the laser in pulse mode.

FIG. A2-19. The septum was incised and the fat pockets were exposed by gently pressing the eyeball. The fat pocket was cut with the laser beam against a wet cotton tip.

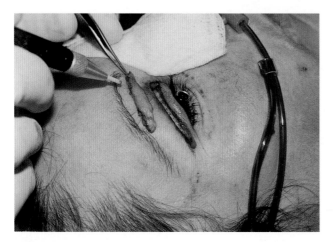

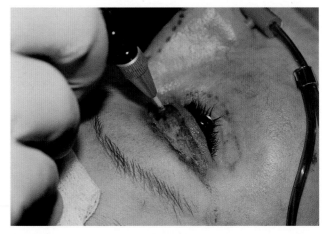

FIG. A2-18. The nose was protected with wet gauze.

FIG. A2-20. Hemostasis was checked. Hemostasis for the entire surgery is commonly performed with one or two cotton tips.

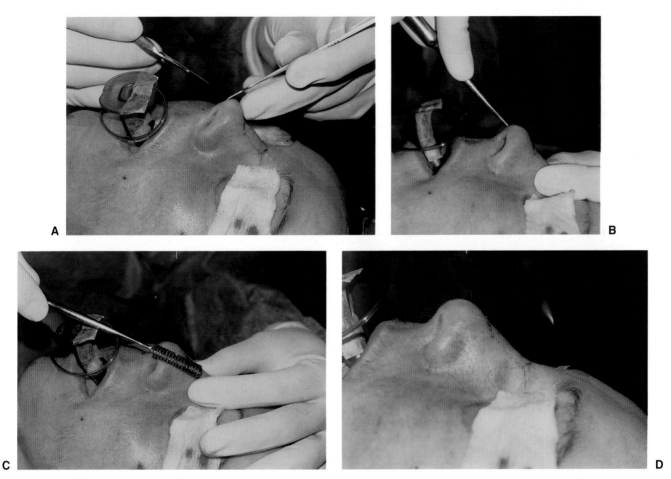

FIG. A2-21. A–D: Rhinoplasty. An intracartilaginous incision was performed in the left nostril. The dorsum periosteum was dissected and 2 mm of the dorsal hump was removed with the rasp. No suture was needed.

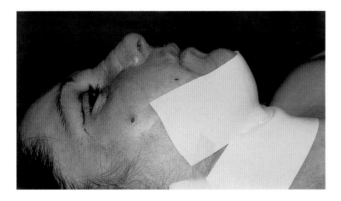

FIG. A2-22. The nose was taped with Micropore for five days. The neck was taped with Microfoam for 24 hours.

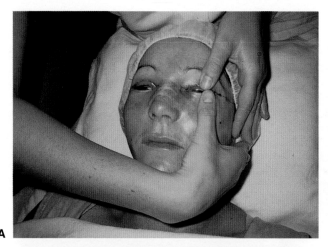

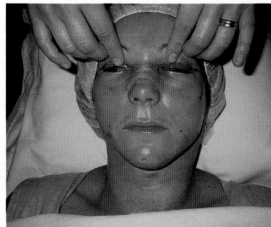

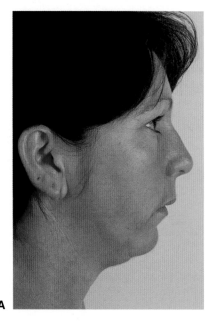

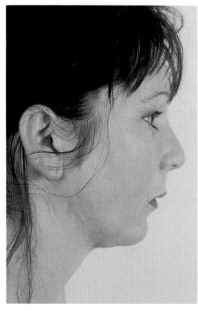

FIG. A2-23. A–C: Manual lymphatic drainage by the esthetician. This type of French light massage is usually well-accepted by patients in the early postoperative days. It helps to reduce swelling and bruising, and improves comfort. The patient should wear an elastic bandage to sleep for seven nights.

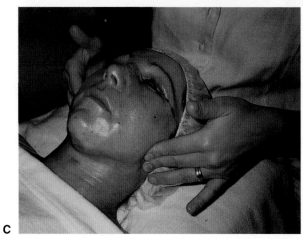

FIG. A2-24. Preoperative **(A, C)** and four-month postoperative **(B, D)** photos.

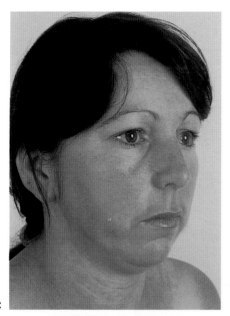

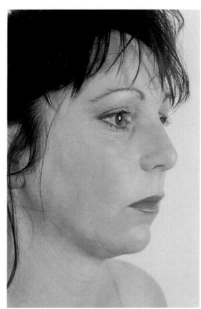

D   **FIG. A2-24.** *Continued.*

C

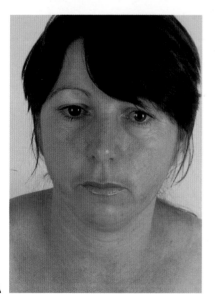

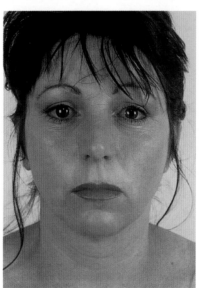

A   B

FIG. A2-25. Preoperative **(A)** and four-month postoperative **(B)** photos.

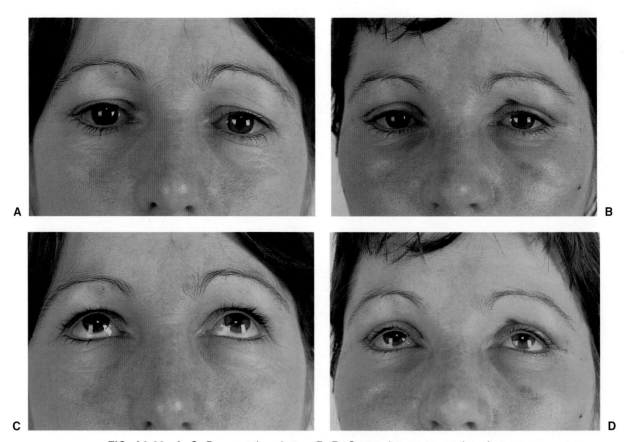

FIG. A2-26. A, C: Preoperative photos. **B, D:** Seven-day postoperative photos.

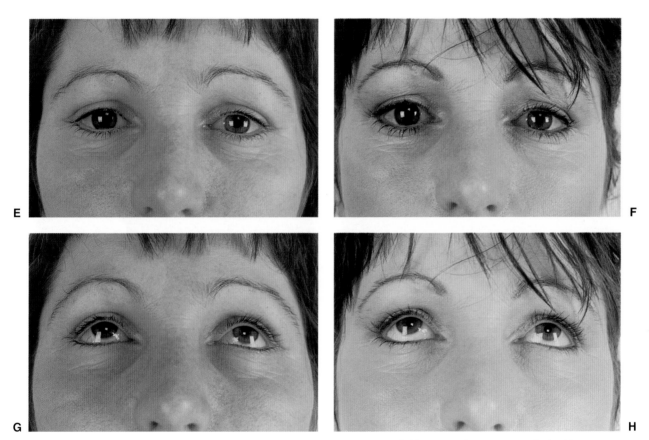

FIG. A2-26. *Continued.* **E, G:** 30-day postoperative photos. **F, H:** Four months postoperatively. Two months after lower eyelid laser resurfacing.

Subject Index

Note: Page numbers in *italics* refer to illustrations. Page numbers followed by a t refer to tables.